RESTORING MENTALIZING
in Attachment Relationships

Treating Trauma
With Plain Old Therapy

RESTORING MENTALIZING
in Attachment Relationships

Treating Trauma
With Plain Old Therapy

Jon G. Allen, Ph.D.

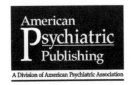

American
Psychiatric
Publishing
A Division of American Psychiatric Association

Washington, DC
London, England

Purchasers of 25–99 copies of this or any other American Psychiatric Publishing title are eligible for a 20% discount; please contact Customer Service at appi@psych.org or 800–368–5777. If you wish to buy 100 or more copies of the same title, please e-mail us at bulksales@psych.org for a price quote.

Disclosure of Interests: The author affirms that he has no commercial or financial involvements that could represent competing interests or an appearance of conflict of interest with the publication of this book.

Manufactured in the United States of America on acid-free paper
19   5 4 3 2
First Edition

Typeset in Berling Roman and Frutiger.

American Psychiatric Publishing, Inc.
A Division of American Psychiatric Association
1000 Wilson Boulevard
Arlington, VA 22209-3901
www.appi.org

Library of Congress Cataloging-in-Publication Data
Allen, Jon G.
  Restoring mentalizing in attachment relationships : treating trauma with plain old therapy / Jon G. Allen. -- 1st ed.
    p. ; cm.
  Includes bibliographical references and index.
  ISBN 978-1-58562-418-8 (pbk. : alk. paper)
  I. American Psychiatric Association. II. Title.
  [DNLM: 1. Stress Disorders, Traumatic--therapy. 2. Object Attachment. 3. Psychoanalytic Therapy--methods. 4. Theory of Mind. WM 172.5]
  616.85'21--dc23
                              2012021293

British Library Cataloguing in Publication Data
A CIP record is available from the British Library.

To Susan, Clifford,
and Yvonne

CONTENTS

PART I
Attachment Trauma and Psychiatric Disorders

PART II
Treatment and Healing

About the Author

Jon G. Allen is a senior staff psychologist and holds the Helen Malsin Palley Chair in Mental Health Research at The Menninger Clinic. He is professor of psychiatry in the Menninger Department of Psychiatry and Behavioral Sciences at the Baylor College of Medicine and an adjunct faculty member of the Houston-Galveston Psychoanalytic Institute and the Institute for Spirituality and Health in the Texas Medical Center. Dr. Allen received his B.A. degree in psychology at the University of Connecticut and his Ph.D. degree in clinical psychology at the University of Rochester. He completed postdoctoral training in clinical psychology at The Menninger Clinic. He conducts psychotherapy, diagnostic consultations, psychoeducational programs, and research, specializing in trauma-related disorders and treatment outcomes. He has taught extensively at the undergraduate, graduate, and postdoctoral levels. He is past editor of the *Bulletin of The Menninger Clinic*, associate editor of the *Journal of Trauma and Dissociation*, and a member of the editorial boards of *Psychological Trauma: Theory, Research, Practice, and Policy* and *Psychiatry: Interpersonal and Biological Processes*. His books include *Coping With Trauma: Hope Through Understanding; Coping With Depression: From Catch-22 to Hope;* and, with coauthors Peter Fonagy and Anthony Bateman, *Mentalizing in Clinical Practice*, all published by American Psychiatric Publishing. He is also author of *Traumatic Relationships and Serious Mental Disorders* and coeditor, with Peter Fonagy, of *Handbook of Mentalization-Based Treatment*, both published by John Wiley & Sons. He has authored and coauthored numerous professional articles and book chapters on trauma-related problems, psychotherapy, the therapeutic alliance, hospital treatment, and psychological assessment.

Foreword

Anyone considering reading this book should be prepared for a major surprise. There was a children's science fiction television series many decades ago on British TV, when I was an adolescent growing up in London. The hero's spaceship looked like a telephone booth from the outside, but as soon as Dr Who (the hero, who was a Time Lord) stepped inside, you magically found yourself in the Tardis, a spacious hi-tech vehicle capable of time travel. *Restoring Mentalizing in Attachment Relationships: Treating Trauma With Plain Old Therapy* reminds me of this kind of illusion. Under the guise of something ordinary, "plain old therapy," Jon Allen opens our eyes and creates an extraordinary clinical and scientific vista. The deceptively simple idea that trauma may be understood as a consequence of mental pain experienced in psychological isolation is unfolded with extraordinary mastery to provide a new vision of development, of trauma genesis, and of therapeutic interaction, creating a new multidimensional integration for the scientific foundations of psychosocial treatments.

Finding a single underlying theory for most forms of psychotherapy has been a major challenge during the century that marked the birth and subsequent rapid burgeoning of modalities of psychotherapy. Although we always had the suspicion that the many hundreds of "brands" of therapy could not all draw on unique psychological processes (Kazdin 2009), identifying the so-called common mechanisms has eluded all those who searched to find them (e.g., Frank 1988; Frank and Frank 1991). Plain old therapy is, in my view, that distillation of components of psychological therapies which comes closest to what we have been looking for to reduce the bewildering array of approaches to a few basic clinical and psychological processes: a reduction that may be compelling, evidence based, and also helpful in terms of generating understanding, facilitating learning, and assisting implementation for both clients and psychotherapists. Allen in several previous excellent monographs (Allen 1995, 2001, 2005, 2006; Allen et al. 2008) has built a body of theoretical and clinical contributions that should be appropriately considered alongside the work of John

Bowlby (1969), Aaron Beck (1976), Marsha Linehan (1993), and Sidney Blatt (2008). In this book, the threads from previous monographs are brought together to initiate a step-change in our understanding of trauma-related mental disorders and their treatment.

Like all significant contributors, Allen simplifies while at the same time adding a substantial new level of sophistication. His model is rooted in attachment theory and in the belief (which I of course share) that the relationship of caregiver and helpless infant is paradigmatic of the functioning of all intimate relationships. All such relationships are organizers of emotional responses and catalysts of the emerging capacity to understand behavior in terms of subjective experience in self and other. Indeed, it may be of great importance to psychotherapists that increased sophistication in social cognition evolved hand in hand with apparently unrelated species characteristics such as helplessness in infancy, the prolongation of childhood, and the emergence of intensive parenting.

Attachment relationships ensure the full development of the social brain. This constraint, of course, makes the infant-parent relationship into a training ground for teaching the infants about minds. The selective advantage to human infants conferred by intensive multi-adult parenting is the opportunity it affords for the full development of neurocognitive social capacities. The child discovers minds in attachment figures as she tries to find herself in their actions. The infant learns about the nature of mental states and learns to represent specific mind states symbolically.

But Allen takes this story further. Linking self-compassion to attachment, he is able to advance a fully integrated theory linking brilliantly the mentalizing, mindfulness, and attachment literatures. He writes: "In sum, mindfulness, mentalizing, and acceptance exemplify sensitive responsiveness; all three are essential to security in parent-child relationships, friendships, love relationships, and plain old therapy" (p. 31). This is a brilliant insight because it gives a "value" (of acceptance) to the psychotherapeutic approach focused on increasing the individual's capacity to mentalize. The "plain old therapist," through humble curiosity and a dogged determination to see the world through the patient's eyes, will implicitly and explicitly engender an attitude of tolerance, compassion, and acceptance toward subjective experience that gradually eases out the tendency we have to berate ourselves for our feelings.

Allen's brilliant clinical insight, building on nearly two decades of theoretical and clinical work finally fully expressed in this extraordinary book, is that while the felicitous co-occurrence of emotion regulation and social understanding ensure normal development, the disjunction of these two processes creates the background to trauma. If negative emotions normally come to be regulated through the sensitive responding of the other, what happens with states of mind when a sense of terror or grief in response to loss is not met by reasonably attuned comforting? When unbearable emotional states are repeatedly not reflected on, they become traumatic owing to the absence of another mind capable of resonating, reflecting on, and appropriately responding to the individual's anguish. Posttraumatic stress disorder and dissociation are shown by Allen to be partial failures of mentalizing, as in posttraumatic flashbacks where memories lose their connection with the continuity of subjectivity and are experienced with the full force of the experience of physical reality. In dissociative detachment, the failure to mentalize affect generates a feeling of unreality. Therapy re-creates a situation in which an appropriately sensitive individual is able to respond with compassion (mindful acceptance) to the subjective distress felt by the patient and enables the individual to fully experience, express, understand, and reflect upon (in a word, *accept*) the subjective state from which he or she sought constant refuge.

This book, using trauma as its springboard, actually tackles most of the psychiatric states that developmental psychopathology has linked with severe adversity (Cicchetti and Valentino 2006). There is something close to magical about the facility with which Allen can incorporate anxiety, depression, self-harm, eating disorder, suicide, and suicidal ideation into a single, person-centered frame that may at times leave the reader breathless. Yet his elegant writing hammers home his key point that all these states exemplify the need for plain old therapy—by which he means a mentalizing relationship in which the therapist's empathy allows the patient no longer to feel alone in emotional pain.

The exploring of the challenges inherent in this type of dyadic relationship is perhaps the most immediately practical implication of the book. Through vivid clinical examples, Allen shows how patients' destructive behavior can elicit unbearable emotional states in the person they find themselves with, which in turn effectively destroys the potential for secure attachment and, with it, the rekindling of mentalizing. Allen's important lesson for us is contained in the description of the traumatized patient who is further traumatized (in the sense of being alone with his emotional pain) through the isolation that is generated by his traumatic impact on others. The therapist, who is no less likely to feel frightened and overwhelmed than the patient's family, will be profoundly restricted in her capacity for compassionate understanding and will undermine, as opposed to helping, her patient.

This book opens a new chapter on psychological approaches to treatment. Allen's phenomenal powers of integration, his capacity for leaping across epistemological, clinical, and empirical boundaries, brings a new kind of creature into the twenty-first century consulting room. This "plain old" practitioner is neither plain nor set in his ways; far from it. He is familiar with evidence-based practice, with the biology of mental disorders, with diagnostic traditions emanating from the phenomenological tradition, with many of the complex psychological models of developmental and personality research, with brain imaging and epidemiology but also with psychodynamic thinking reaching well back to the last century. Remarkably, the therapeutic approach he advocates is respectful of knowledge gained from all these traditions.

But Allen also makes us aware of the limitations of this knowledge. He helps us recognize, for example, that psychiatric diagnoses have made a monumental contribution to research on the impact of attachment trauma, but he also evidences that the diagnosis of multiple disorders potentially undermines a coherent understanding of the individual. Similarly, he eschews the wholesale adaptation of the social psychiatry tradition and is uncomfortable with the generic conceptualization of trauma in the context of a broad domain of complex traumatic stress. He alights on a rigorously person-centered, developmental approach to understanding psychological disorder. Adroitly steering us through the minefield of evidence-based therapies, Allen arrives at "plain old therapy," a fresh combination of mindfulness, mentalizing, and attachment-based therapy that provides the diagnostic understanding which therapists and patient—implicitly or explicitly—both seek.

This book initiates a new form of treatment. The approach is marked by an oxymoronic characteristic that may be termed *rigorous flexibility*. It is an extraordinary feat of intellectual agility. Through his previous work, Allen has created a special form for communicating clinically relevant ideas simultaneously and with equal effectiveness to nonprofessional and professional readers. He does so through judicious use of science to guide and inform, to shine a helpful light on obscure phenomena, to reinforce common sense where necessary, and, above all, to admit ignorance where systematic understanding still fails us. This makes Allen's work miraculously accessible and true to the pedagogy that is at the core of his identity as a therapist and as a scientist. But this book (as indeed did the ones that preceded it) goes leagues beyond the simple summary and elucidation of clinical and scientific observations. The theory of plain old therapy is the first adequate "uni-theory" of psychotherapy, and as such its description in this book represents a gigantic achievement. Congratulations, Dr. Allen! It seems like we have almost arrived!

Peter Fonagy, Ph.D., F.B.A.
Freud Memorial Professor of Psychoanalysis, University College London
Chief Executive, The Anna Freud Centre, London

References

Allen JG: Coping With Trauma: A Guide to Self-Understanding. Washington, DC, American Psychiatric Press, 1995

Allen JG: Traumatic Relationships and Serious Mental Disorders. Chichester, UK, Wiley, 2001

Allen JG: Coping With Trauma: Hope Through Understanding, 2nd Edition. Washington, DC, American Psychiatric Publishing, 2005

Allen JG: Coping With Depression: From Catch-22 to Hope. Washington, DC, American Psychiatric Publishing, 2006

Allen JG, Fonagy P, Bateman A: Mentalizing in Clinical Practice. Washington, DC, American Psychiatric Publishing, 2008

Beck AT: Cognitive Therapy and the Emotional Disorders. New York, International Universities Press, 1976

Blatt SJ: Polarities of Experience: Relatedness and Self-Definition in Personality Development, Psychopathology, and the Therapeutic Process. Washington, DC, American Psychological Association, 2008

Bowlby J: Attachment and Loss, Vol 1: Attachment. London, Hogarth Press and the Institute of Psycho-Analysis, 1969

Cicchetti D, Valentino K: An ecological-transactional perspective on child maltreatment: failure of the average expectable environment and its influence on child development, in Developmental Psychopathology, 2nd Edition, Vol 3. Edited by Cicchetti D, Cohen DJ. New York, Wiley, 2006, pp 129–201

Frank JD: Specific and non-specific factors in psychotherapy. Curr Opin Psychiatry 1:289–292, 1988

Frank JD, Frank JB: Persuasion and Healing: A Comparative Study of Psychotherapy. Baltimore, MD, The Johns Hopkins University Press, 1991

Kazdin AE: Understanding how and why psychotherapy leads to change. Psychother Res 19:418–428, 2009

Linehan MM: Cognitive-Behavioral Treatment of Borderline Personality Disorder. New York, Guilford, 1993

Preface

This book addresses a major health problem: trauma in attachment relationships—at the extreme, childhood abuse and neglect. Traumatized patients and the therapists who endeavor to help them must contend with a large group of psychiatric disorders to which trauma makes a contribution, posttraumatic stress disorder (PTSD) being only one among many. In the face of this complexity, therapists also have too much of a good thing: an even larger array of treatment approaches for different psychiatric disorders and many different interventions for PTSD alone. Because of this professional fragmentation, we therapists and our patients can lose sight of the essence of trauma and its treatment. Aiming to be provocative, I contend that we must give due weight to the value of "plain old" therapy.

I don't mean to be frivolous; rather, I intend to make a research-based case for the venerable features of healing relationships that long antedated the creation of professional psychotherapy. But I also think we can refine our ability to offer healing relationships on the basis of new knowledge gained from research on attachment relationships. This research informs us about the nature of trauma in attachment relationships as well as the ways in which trauma can be ameliorated in relationships.

More specifically, growing appreciation for the cardinal importance of *mentalizing*—attentiveness to mental states such as thoughts and feelings in self and others—enables us to home in on what I believe to be the key to trauma and the pathway to recovery: mentalizing in the context of attachment relationships. With the inclusion of mentalizing, attachment theory and research provide a solid foundation for trauma treatment that offers us therapists and our patients a clearer idea of what we're doing.

This book addresses a wide audience. Having written the first edition of *Coping With Trauma* for patients, I was delighted to learn that therapists liked it, too, because it was written in plain language and reflected patients' experiences. Thus, I wrote the second edition with therapists as well as patients in mind. Similarly, I wrote this book for professionals and laypersons as an expression of my conviction that we all need to speak a common language. Although the book is thoroughly grounded in theory and research, its style is conversational, no technical background is required to understand it, and, as I explain in the Introduction, it all boils down to common sense.

Working at The Menninger Clinic for over three decades has provided me with a unique opportunity to learn about trauma and to articulate what I have learned to a broad readership. I've conducted long-term psychotherapy with inpatients and outpatients; in recent years, my practice has consisted of providing therapy in the context of intensive inpatient treatment spanning several weeks—a rare luxury in contemporary hospital psychiatry. In addition, my work at the clinic has provided an unusual opportunity to develop and conduct psychoeducational groups on trauma, depression, attachment, and mentalizing. I've discovered that teaching patients is one of the best ways to learn from them; they are the true experts, and they have been gracious in sharing their knowledge. In this book, I have used many clinical examples from this recent practice. Factual details have been altered and elements from various patients have been combined to protect confidentiality.

Acknowledgments

I thank many colleagues who have reviewed various portions of the manuscript along the way: Chris Frueh, Chris Fowler, Daniel Garcia, Len Horwitz, Jim Lomax, Mario Mikulincer, Elizabeth Newlin, Ken Pargament, Debbie Quackenbush, Shweta Sharma, and Rebecca Wagner. I continue to enrich my understanding of applied mentalizing by working with Flynn O'Malley, Michael Groat, and Harrell Woodson, who have enthusiastically embraced our efforts to educate patients. I also thank Tom Ellis and John Hart for lending me their expertise in cognitive-behavioral approaches. I am grateful to my colleague Roger Verdon, senior editor in marketing at The Menninger Clinic, who reviewed the entire lengthy first draft during its creation and whose expert counsel sustained my effort. My profound debt to Peter Fonagy will be obvious throughout the pages of this book. Peter's genius is matched only by his generosity, and I have been privileged to benefit from both for the better part of two decades. I've also been fortunate to confer, teach, and write with Anthony Bateman, whose down-to-earth clinical approach has affirmed my affinity for plain old therapy. And I am most grateful to my wife Susan, whose discriminating blend of enthusiasm and criticism contributed immeasurably to the readability of the book. I could not have written this book without the support of the administration of The Menninger Clinic, which afforded me the time I needed to do the work. In this regard, I thank especially Ian Aitken, president; John Oldham, chief of staff; and Sue Hardesty, medical director. Finally, I express my continuing gratitude to Robert Hales, editor-in-chief, and John McDuffie, editorial director, of the Books Department at American Psychiatric Publishing, whose guidance and support were crucial throughout this book's evolution and contributed substantially to its focus and coherence. I also thank Roxanne Rhodes, Senior Project Editor, for her skillful editorial oversight in the final production.

Introduction

This book challenges a well-established practice: therapists diagnose a psychiatric disorder and then prescribe an evidence-based treatment—that is, a structured approach that has been demonstrated through controlled research to be effective in ameliorating the disorder. What could be more sensible? Yet, over the past few decades, psychiatric diagnoses and evidence-based therapies have proliferated like rabbits. The scourge of what I have dubbed "acronymania" has accompanied this proliferation. We have acronyms for disorders: PTSD, GAD, OCD, MDD, SAD, DID, and BPD. We also have acronyms for empirically supported treatments: PE, EMDR, ERP, CBT, EFT, SIT, DBT, DIT, TPP, PCT, and IPT, to pick a few. Putting them together, we have EMDR for PTSD, DBT for BPD, ERP for OCD, and so on. Who can remember them all—much less learn to practice all these acronymed therapies? But a therapist without an acronym is a professional without an identity. In this book, I don't conceal my aversion to excessive specialization—a multitude of therapies for each of a multitude of psychiatric disorders. Yet, being unable to resist the need for a therapeutic identity, tendentiously, I now declare myself a practitioner of "plain old therapy"—though I'll refrain from using the acronym lest the reader confuse it with marijuana.

I remember vividly a moment at the end of a talk on trauma that I gave in a workshop for patients' family members at The Menninger Clinic. When I invited questions and comments, a father in the back of the room stood up and challenged, "Isn't all you've said just common sense?" I responded with pleasure, "You've understood me perfectly!" I remarked that common sense, however, is a high aspiration in the field. Unknowingly, I was on a path to plain old therapy. As the length and complexity of this book attest, the path is neither short nor straight. To illuminate the path while reassuring readers that I am far from dismissing the entire field of psychiatry, I begin by laying bare the commonsensical story of trauma and treatment.

Security in attachment relationships is our best means of regulating emotional distress. We all have a prototype in mind: a mother comforting her frightened child. The mother comforts her child through her psychological attunement to her child's distress. Anticipating her empathy, her child becomes securely attached—that is, confident in turning to his mother for comfort in times of distress. In my view, trauma stems from repeatedly being left *psychologically alone in unbearable emotional pain.* Early attachment trauma—maltreatment—is most pernicious in this regard, because the attachment figure's natural function in the mind of the child is to provide comfort and safety. Instead, the traumatic attachment relationship engenders emotional distress while failing to relieve it. This confluence places the child in the ultimate bind of needing yet fearing attachment. The traumatic outcome of this experience is the bane of the psychotherapist: psychotherapy is beneficial by virtue of a trusting relationship, yet the patient is unable to trust.

Jargon though the term may seem, I've found the concept of "mentalizing" to be indispensable in understanding and treating attachment trauma. In brief, mentalizing entails attunement to mental states in self and others—in Peter Fonagy's felicitous phrase, *holding mind in mind.* To continue the commonsensical story: mentalizing begets mentalizing. The parent who mentalizes—holds the child's mind in mind—not only thereby comforts the child but also helps the child understand his or her feelings. Held psychologically, the child becomes attuned to feelings and, ultimately, able to regulate emotions with and without direct help from attachment relationships. The child also develops greater empathy for others and, ultimately, might become an empathic parent who provides his or her child with a secure attachment relationship. In a straightforward process of social learning, from one generation to the next, mentalizing begets mentalizing and, concomitantly, secure attachment begets secure attachment. Conversely, attachment trauma undermines the development of mentalizing and secure attachment, thereby impairing the capacity to manage emotional distress—with or without the help of attachment figures. Like secure attachment and mentalizing, attachment trauma and impaired mentalizing can be passed on from generation to generation.

To conclude the commonsensical story, the antidote to trauma—and the means of interrupting the transmission of trauma from one generation to the next—is strengthening the capacity for secure attachment through mentalizing emotional pain. In plain language, the traumatized person needs caring, empathic relationships to render the emotional pain bearable and understandable. Thankfully, attachment security can be strengthened by a wide variety of caring relationships, including extended family members, close friends, members of the clergy, and romantic partners. Sadly, attachment trauma commonly is alienating, and alienation can block these natural avenues to healing. In the past century, psychotherapy has evolved to fill this gap, but in my view, the means by which psychotherapy promotes healing from trauma is not fundamentally different from all these other attachment relationships, with mentalizing at their core. Plain old therapy is a modern professional variant of plain old caring relationships, which sustained the human species for millennia.

Armed with common sense, one could stop reading here. But common sense is no substitute for science, and my conviction of the soundness of this commonsensical story and its implications for the practice of psychotherapy has been greatly strengthened by burgeoning attachment research. I aim to persuade readers to adopt this way of thinking about trauma and psychotherapy by reviewing this line of compelling research in considerable detail. Though my enthusiasm for attachment and mentalizing may come across as missionary zeal, I have no wish to convert anyone. I don't aim to challenge or contradict other ways of thinking and practicing but rather to enrich them. I'd rather build bridges than inhabit islands. Thus, I review the literature on psychiatric disorders and traditional psychotherapies from the perspective of attachment trauma—in effect, offering a new conceptual lens.

The plan is simple. In the first chapter, I lay the foundation in attachment trauma, but I need to work up to it. I start at the beginning, with the wellspring of attachment in infancy and childhood. This research on childhood has established stark prototypes of secure and insecure attachment, which are dramatic for their parallels in adult attachment. Accordingly, for better or for worse, attachment patterns can be transmitted from one generation to another, as attachment research demonstrates. The development and intergenerational transmission of attachment is intertwined with mentalizing, as I'll discuss at length. Building a bridge, I include mindfulness in the review of mentalizing, because these two overlapping concepts are mutually enhancing. This foundation in attachment and mentalizing will put readers in a position to understand attachment trauma as it develops in childhood and influences the course of adulthood.

Using the lens of attachment trauma, we need stereoscopic vision, because we therapists and patients are working in the well-established field of psychiatry wherein treatments have evolved in relation to psychiatric disorders. Too often, trauma is equated with PTSD. Like PTSD, dissociative disorders commonly stem from trauma, and dissociation is thoroughly intertwined with PTSD. Accordingly, I devote a chapter to these disorders. Attachment trauma, however, puts persons at greater risk for the development of many different psychiatric disorders and problems beyond PTSD and dissociation, leading to the concept of complex traumatic stress disorders, the subject of an additional chapter.

Walking a tightrope while relying on stereoscopic vision, I devote two chapters to trauma treatment. Although trauma cannot be reduced to PTSD, the official recognition of PTSD as a psychiatric diagnosis has been a boon in stimulating the development of different treatment approaches and research on their effectiveness. Patients and therapists alike need to know about these evidence-based treatments, and I devote a chapter to them. Yet attachment trauma goes far beyond the bounds of PTSD and calls for an integrative approach to treatment that transcends specific psychiatric disorders, treatment methods, and theoretical schools. Reaching the end of the long path, I make my case for plain old therapy, now grounded in contemporary research on attachment and mentalizing as well as venerable research on the contribution of the therapeutic relationship to treatment outcomes. Plain old therapy, as I envision it, is neither entirely plain nor old, and we must continue to refine it through ongoing research. Although in this book I advocate the practice of plain old therapy in the context of treating attachment trauma, I intend the book to have general applicability on two grounds: first, I take a broad view of trauma; second, I've found that understanding the roles of attachment and mentalizing in psychotherapy sharpens my work with the full range of patients I see.

Now I can state the overall aim of this book with utmost simplicity. As is true in general medicine, the field of psychotherapy needs generalists and specialists. Ostensibly, in our field of psychotherapy, the specialists have a corner on science with their evidence-based treatments. On the contrary, I aim to show that we generalists—practitioners of plain old therapy by whatever name—also have a firm basis in scientific evidence for our practice.

Moreover, I view the practice of plain old therapy, though informed by science, as an ethical endeavor, as pertains to all caring relationships. Hence, we have much to learn from philosophy as well as science. In this vein, having reached the end of the path, the final chapter exposes a wide open field. Not leaving science behind altogether, this last chapter goes beyond the bounds of psychiatry to address existential-spiritual aspects of trauma, which I consider even more challenging than all the psychiatric disorders.

Attachment Trauma and Psychiatric Disorders

Attachment, Mentalizing, and Trauma

This chapter lays the foundation for the rest of the book. To cement the book's developmental perspective, I start at the beginning: reviewing attachment in childhood. Through a wealth of research, we can see starkly the basic prototypes of secure and insecure attachment that establish a foundation for ways of relying on others—or not—to manage distress. In the chapter's second section, I recapitulate these secure and insecure attachment patterns as they play out in adulthood; the parallels to early childhood are dramatic and instructive. Of course, attachments change dramatically over a person's lifetime, but the basic functions of attachment pertinent to infancy do not change, and this makes the comparison of adulthood and childhood worthwhile.

The third section of this chapter elucidates what I consider to be the psychological glue that bonds attachment relationships: Mary Ainsworth (Ainsworth et al. 1978) called it sensitive responsiveness, Peter Fonagy (Fonagy et al. 2002) refined it as mentalizing, and I will mix it with mindfulness. With attachment and mentalizing in mind, the reader is prepared for the section on attachment trauma. I propose simply that traumatic attachments stem from mentalizing failure, wherein relationships become unglued. Plain old therapy restores connections.

Childhood

We should start with some basic concepts in attachment theory, all of which revolve around the main function of attachment: *emotion regulation*. These concepts set the stage for discussing three prototypical attachment patterns. In short, sensitive responsiveness promotes secure attachment. Correspondingly, in the face of limited responsiveness, the child has two basic options: to try harder (ambivalent attachment) or to go it alone (avoidant attachment). In this section, I elaborate these patterns and describe some ways that caregivers might contribute to them. I also consider the role of the child's temperament and the environmental context of care, which contributes to stability and change in attachment. The section concludes with a summary of the developmental advantages of attachment security.

Key Concepts

Attachment relationships are like other close relationships that involve *affectional bonds* (Ainsworth 1989), which are evident in a desire for closeness, distress upon separation, joy upon reunion, and grief upon loss. Yet attachment relationships are distinct in providing *security and comfort in the face of distress*—hence their fundamental role in trauma. Beginning in infancy, attachment develops in the context of a *goal-corrected partnership* (Bowlby 1982) in which two behavioral systems become coordinated: infant attachment and parental caregiving. The infant attaches to the parent, and the parent bonds with the infant. Infants' attachment security and strategies to cope with insecurity are tied closely to the quality of parental caregiving. Notably, although parents must establish affectional bonds with their children, parental *attachment* to children is anomalous inasmuch as parental reliance on children for security and comfort is problematic.

Attachment relationships are patterned on the basis of *internal working models* (Bowlby 1982)—that is, relatively stable *mental representations* built up from repeated child-caregiver interactions. These mental models include not only representations of the caregiver (e.g., as loving and dependable) but also self-representations (e.g., as lovable and worthy of care). Like any other representations—maps, for example—these internal working models can be more or less accurate or distorted. Yet John Bowlby (1973) asserted that working models are predominantly realistic: "the varied expectations of the accessibility and responsiveness of attachment figures that different individuals develop during the years of immaturity are *tolerably accurate* reflections of the experiences those individuals have actually had" (p. 202, emphasis added).

Internal working models are implicit as well as explicit. *Explicit* models are conscious and thus can be thought about and talked about: "My mother could be cruel and sometimes glared at me with such contempt that I felt as low as a cockroach." *Implicit* models are nonconscious; they become automatic procedures for interacting that guide behavior without awareness. These models are based on procedural learning and memory, akin to learning to ride a bicycle. Thus, the child might learn, without thinking about it, to avoid the mother's contempt by means of ingratiating behavior, always striving to please. Bowlby's (1982) concept of *working* models is crucial: such models are potentially employed flexibly and are subject to modification. Explicating implicit models in psychotherapy is one route to change, for example as ingratiating behavior in the patient-therapist relationship is identified, discussed, and surmounted. Yet, more pervasively, working models also are modified implicitly, without awareness, in the course of relationship changes (e.g., mother becoming less irascible and more consistently affectionate) or new relationships (e.g., with an even-tempered partner).

The universal prototype of attachment is a mother lovingly cradling a frightened or distressed infant in her arms. This prototype exemplifies the fundamental function of attachment: providing the infant a *safe haven* that offers protection from harm. Bowlby (1958) proposed that attachment evolved in a wide range of species—mammals prototypically—to provide protection from predation: mothers are naturally motivated to remain close to their infants, as infants are motivated to stay close to their mothers; when separated, for example, a mother and infant are reunited by the infant's cries of distress. Although physical protection remains a crucial function of caregiving, attachment research has come to give greater weight to the value of restoring a *feeling of security* (Sroufe and Waters 1977), which relates to the previously mentioned cardinal function of attachment: emotion regulation. As I discuss further in the context of mentalizing (see section Mentalizing in Attachment Relationships), the prolonged period of dependency in humans is now more fully appreciated not only as providing needed protection and felt security but also as constituting the foundation for social learning—nothing less than learning to be a person in relation to other persons (Fonagy et al. 2002).

Although the safe-haven function of attachment is intuitively evident, those who are unfamiliar with attachment theory are less likely to appreciate its complementary function: attachment provides a *secure base for exploration*. Bowlby (1988) asserted, "No concept within the attachment framework is more central to developmental psychiatry than that of the secure base" (p. 202). One needs merely to picture the toddler and his mother at the playground: Checking back periodically to make sure his mother is available, the toddler explores the playground confidently. Losing sight of his mother, the toddler stops playing, perhaps crying and searching for her. Or the toddler may play enthusiastically until a barking dog approaches. In either case, the toddler will seek the safe haven of maternal comfort to restore a feeling of security and relief from distress. Conjointly, the safe haven and secure base afford *psychological security*— that is, security in attachment and security in exploration, confidence in others, and self-confidence (Grossman et al. 2008).

Ingeniously, based on her extensive in-home observations of mother-infant interactions from Uganda to Baltimore, Mary Ainsworth (Ainsworth et al. 1978) developed a 20-minute laboratory procedure to assess attachment security in infancy. This procedure is the experimental analogue to the playground. Ainsworth designed the Strange Situation to be moderately stressful to the infant by scripting two brief separations in a playroom environment that includes a stranger and a set of toys (see Table 1–1). The infant's responses to the mother's departure play some role in the evaluation of attachment security, but the most crucial question relates to the reunions: how do these interactions affect the infant's distress? The assessment involves the partnership—that is, the infant's behavior in relation to the mother's behavior. In the Strange Situation, trained investigators can discern the three fundamental attachment patterns. I present these patterns in idealized forms; readers should keep in mind that reality is messier than the following neat categorizations.

Secure Attachment

Introduced to the playroom with his mother present, the securely attached infant explores the toys and engages in play, sometimes with assistance from his mother and perhaps in interaction with the stranger. Left alone with the stranger, the secure infant will show varying degrees of distress, likely in conjunction with diminished interest in play. The infant might seek comfort from the stranger to some extent but will strongly prefer his mother's comfort when she returns. Left completely alone in the second separation, the infant is liable to become more intensely distressed and to be in even greater need of comfort. Upon reunion in relation to either separation, the secure infant seeks proximity to his mother, typically desiring close bodily contact. His mother effectively provides comforting and reassurance, such that the infant settles down and returns to exploration and play.

Extensive research confirms Ainsworth's original observation that sensitive responsiveness on the part of the caregiver is conducive to secure attachment in the infant (Weinfield et al. 2008). Sensitive responsiveness

TABLE 1–1. Strange Situation episodes

1. The infant and the mother are brought into an unfamiliar but comfortable room filled with toys.
2. The infant is given the opportunity to play with the toys, potentially with the mother's assistance.
3. A stranger enters the room and plays with the infant.
4. The mother departs, leaving the infant with the stranger and the toys.
5. The mother returns, pausing to give the infant a chance to respond to her return, and the stranger leaves the room.
6. The mother leaves the infant alone in the room.
7. The stranger comes back into the room and interacts with the infant.
8. Then the mother returns, and the stranger leaves the room.

is the basis of the safe haven insofar as the mother is warm and affectionate as well as attuned to the infant's signals of distress, interpreting them accurately and responding to them promptly and appropriately. In addition, sensitive responsiveness provides a secure base for exploration insofar as the mother is engaged in the infant's activities in a way that is cooperative and helpful without interfering with her infant's intentions.

Ambivalent-Resistant Attachment

The ambivalently attached infant clings to the (insufficiently) safe haven, with attachment predominating over exploration. The ambivalent infant finds separations extremely distressing; upon reunion, he demands care yet angrily resists comforting. As he rejects the care he desperately needs, his ambivalence may be blatant: he may demand to be picked up and then push his mother away, squirm out of her grasp, yet continue to cling to her. Hence, he is distressed but his frustration renders him inconsolable.

Ainsworth and colleagues (1978) observed ambivalent infant attachment in conjunction with chronically unresponsive or inconsistent care. Thus, the infant's intensification of distress and angry protests (e.g., tantrums) are implicit strategies learned to command attention and to force more responsiveness from caregivers who are lacking in psychological attunement. Ambivalent infants thus *hyperactivate* their attachment needs—in effect, turning up the dial to elicit care. To the extent that it is (intermittently) effective in evoking responsiveness, this hyperactivating strategy is rewarded. Yet the attachment remains ambivalent: the desire for care is intermingled with feelings of deprivation and frustration, and the coercive behavior infuses the relationship with resentment.

Avoidant Attachment

Whereas ambivalent infants cling ineffectively to the safe haven, avoidant infants are stuck in exploration—in effect, on their own in the playground. Thus, in the Strange Situation, the avoidant infant may appear precociously independent as he plays and ostensibly ignores his mother. In contrast to the securely attached infant, who involves his mother in play, the avoidant infant is more likely to engage in solitary play. In contrast to the ambivalent infant, he shows no overt distress in response to his mother's departure; when she returns, he shows little desire for contact. If she picks him up, he is unresponsive, preferring to be put down so he can return to play.

Ainsworth observed mothers of avoidant infants to be subtly rejecting, averse to bodily contact, perhaps irritated by their infant but suppressing their anger. She also found the mothers to be rigid and compulsive, not wanting the infant to interrupt their activities and becoming frustrated quickly when the infant didn't comply immediately with their wishes. Avoidance appears to be a reasonable strategy for managing distress in relation to a consistently emotionally unavailable and subtly irritable caregiver who is communicating, "Don't bother me with your needs or distress." The infant strives to avoid bothering the mother, *deactivating* his attachment needs, turning down the dial, and attempting to manage his emotional distress as best he can on his own.

Child Temperament

The early attachment research elicited intense debate about the likely influence of infant temperament on the research findings (Karen 1998). Intuitively, for example, one would expect the infant or child who is temperamentally anxious, distress prone, or "difficult" to be a likely candidate for developing ambivalent attachment. This controversy about the relative contribution of temperament and caregiving to attachment patterns has inspired extensive research with surprising results: the patterns of caregiving just described exert a far stronger influence on attachment classification than do a child's genetic or temperamental factors.

Yet this broad conclusion obscures complexity (Vaughn et al. 2008). Temperament, although rooted in genetic and physiological characteristics, is not immutable. On the contrary, temperament is subject to environmental influence, prominently including caregiving. Moreover, the infant's temperament may influence the parent's caregiving behavior. For example, a more distress-prone infant could evoke a stressed-out parent's irritability or inconsistency. To add a further layer of complexity, owing to genetic differences, some children are more responsive than others to patterns of caregiving (Belsky and Fearon 2008). For those children who are genetically predisposed to be more responsive to caregiving, the relations I just summarized will be more evident than for those children who are less responsive to variations in caregiving.

Environmental Influences on Caregiving

Attachment researchers have been criticized for blaming parents—mothers in particular—who would be better served by compassionate understanding that takes into account the environmental context of caregiving. Sensitive responsiveness—or lack of responsiveness—doesn't occur in a vacuum. Many factors have been found to influence caregiving and attachment: parental age, education, and socioeconomic status; parental psychiatric disorders; and stressful life circumstances. Moreover, underscoring the importance of attachment, the mother's attachment security influences her caregiving: the child is likely to be more insecure with a mother who is a single parent, struggling with marital conflict, or relatively lacking in other sources of social support (Belsky and Fearon 2008). Plainly, an accumulation of vulnerabilities is most likely to be detrimental to attachment security (Belsky 2005), as would be true, for example, of a mother without any confidants who is living in poverty and raising a temperamentally difficult infant along with a number of siblings while embroiled in a turbulent marriage.

Thus, as I elaborate in this chapter, we therapists must remain mindful of the context of care. The capacity of humans for attachment (and for mentalizing) evolved in the context of communal caregiving (Hrdy 2009), in which multiple caregivers were available to assist the mother. Thus, in our culture, the mother (or other caregiver) who raises a child single-handedly will be challenged to provide consistent sensitive responsiveness. For better or for worse, marriage plays a critical role: parents might support each other and compensate for each other's limitations, or they might undermine each other and exacerbate each other's limitations (George and Solomon 2008).

Stability and Change

Stability warrants our interest in attachment patterns, and potential for change justifies our interventions. Longitudinal research on stability of attachment from infancy into early adulthood (Grossman et al. 2005) shows substantial continuity as well as lawful patterns of change (Thompson 2008). One key factor is that stability and change in attachment patterns will occur in tandem with stability and change in environmental influences.

I consider it nothing short of astounding that *any* correspondence—no matter how modest—can be found between infant attachment behavior in a 20-minute laboratory observation and security of attachment measured by an interview many years later. Yet Strange Situation attachment classifications at 12 months have been found to correspond to interview-based attachment assessments at ages 19 (Main et al. 2005), 21–22 (Crowell and Waters 2005), and 26 (Sroufe et al. 2005). On the flip side of this coin, less than perfect correspondence between infant and later attachment classifications in these studies attests to evidence for change. For example, detrimental changes in attachment security are associated with trauma, stressful life events, divorce, parental death, and serious illness in the child or parent. Fortunately, parent-infant interventions (Belsky and Fearon 2008) as well as psychotherapy (Sroufe et al. 2005) have the potential to enhance attachment security, sooner or later.

Developmental Benefits of Attachment Security

On the basis of their longitudinal research on the developmental impact of infant attachment, Alan Sroufe and colleagues (2005) made the strong claim that "nothing is more important in children's development than how they are treated by their parents, beginning in the early years of life" (p. 288). The subsequent benefits of infant attachment security have been studied in toddlers, in preschoolers, and in middle childhood.

Secure attachment is associated with multiple forms of adaptation (Berlin et al. 2008). In comparison with those who are insecurely attached, securely attached children are more capable of regulating emotional distress with the help of caregivers and on their own; are relatively easygoing; and are more socially competent, empathic, and caring. Therefore, they form more positive relationships with siblings, peers, friends, and teachers. Given their security in exploration, they are relatively curious and persistent in problem solving, while also able to seek help when they need it. Accordingly, their security promotes cognitive and academic development.

We naturally associate security with independence, but this association is misleading. Secure attachment is associated with *effective dependence*, which also promotes effective independence. In comparison with their secure counterparts, ambivalent children are more anxious and easily frustrated; more passively helpless and excessively dependent; and less able to perform well in novel and cognitively challenging situations that call for active mastery. Notwithstanding their relative immaturity and passivity, they are less socially isolated than avoidant children, who tend to be more hostile and aggressive as well as emotionally insulated. Avoidant children are likely to bully and victimize ambivalent children, and classmates and teachers single out avoidant children as being disliked. Hence, just as secure attachment broadly enhances development, insecurity compromises it.

Adulthood

While delineating substantial developmental changes, Bowlby (1988) maintained that "attachment behaviour…is characteristic of human nature throughout our lives—*from the cradle to the grave*" (p. 82, emphasis added). Although attachment phenomena can be observed in a range of relationships, parent-child relationships are paradigmatic of attachment in childhood, and romantic relationships are their prototypical adulthood counterparts. I start there. But we adults maintain internal working models of our childhood attachments to our parents, and these working models influence our romantic relationships as well as our patterns of caregiving with our children. Accordingly, there are two main domains of adult attachment research: attachment to romantic partners and attachment to parents. Both domains are central to treating attachment trauma, and I distinguish research methods in each. With this foundation, I explicate the three basic patterns of attachment (secure, ambivalent, and avoidant) in each of the two domains (romantic partners and parents).

At this point, readers should be alerted to two complications. First, we have three main domains paired with different methods for assessing attachment security: infant attachment using the Strange Situation, adult attachment to romantic partners using questionnaires, and adult attachment to parents using the Adult Attachment Interview. The terminology for the different attachment patterns varies from one domain and method to another. Second, as I discuss later in conjunction with attachment trauma, a fourth pattern of profoundly insecure (disorganized) attachment was discovered belatedly in conjunction with maltreatment. Table 1–2 summarizes the variations in methods and terminology.

After reviewing the three basic patterns of attachment, I consider the extent to which adult attachment is relationship specific, the import of matches and mismatches in attachment patterns between romantic partners, and evidence for stability and change in attachment patterns in adulthood.

Attachment in Romantic Relationships

Debra Zeifman and Cindy Hazan (2008) developed an interview to assess the four defining characteristics of attachment relationships: seeking proximity at times of distress, feeling distressed upon separation, using the relationship as a safe haven for comfort, and relying on the relationship as a secure base for exploration. They found that children showed clear-cut attachment (i.e., all four features) only in relation to parents, whereas adolescents showed clear-cut attachment in relation to peers, almost invariably a boyfriend or girlfriend. Interviews of adults ranging in age from 18 to 82 years showed that full-blown attachment was most characteristic of romantic relationships lasting 2 or more years. We can become enamored quickly, but we become attached far more slowly.

As just implied, attachment is only one facet of adult romantic relationships, which also involve sex and caregiving along with much else. We humans are a relatively monogamous species, and thus sex, attachment, and caregiving often are combined in a partnership; however, romantic relationships also are characterized by great diversity, as these three facets also are somewhat independent (e.g., a person could be attached to a spouse yet engage in casual sex with others). This diversity also encompasses same-sex romantic relationships, which are similar to heterosexual relationships with respect to attachment (Mohr 2008).

Measuring Adult Attachments to Romantic Partners

In collaboration with Phil Shaver, Hazan developed what I consider a do-it-yourself approach to attachment classification. They wrote the following brief descriptions of the romantic counterparts of Ainsworth's categories (Hazan and Shaver 1987, p. 515):

- *Secure:* I find it relatively easy to get close to others and am comfortable depending on them and having them depend on me. I don't often worry about being abandoned or about someone getting too close to me.
- *Ambivalent:* I find that others are reluctant to get as close as I would like. I often worry that my partner doesn't really love me or won't want to stay with me. I want to merge completely with another person, and this desire sometimes scares people away.
- *Avoidant:* I am somewhat uncomfortable being close to others; I find it difficult to trust them completely, difficult to allow myself to depend on them. I am nervous when anyone gets too close, and often, love partners want me to be more intimate than I feel comfortable being.

Hazan and Shaver published these descriptions as a "love quiz" in a local newspaper and invited readers to indicate which description best fit their

TABLE 1–2.   Variations in terminology for attachment classifications

Method; domain	Terminology			
Strange Situation; infant with parent	Secure	Ambivalent-resistant	Avoidant	Disorganized-disoriented
Questionnaire; adult with romantic partner	Secure	Ambivalent-anxious	Avoidant	Fearful
Adult Attachment Interview; adult with parents	Secure-autono-mous	Preoccupied	Dismissing	Unresolved-disorganized

most important relationship and to mail in their answers. In so doing, they launched what has become a prolific and informative self-report tradition of adult attachment research (Mikulincer and Shaver 2007a).

Subsequent self-report assessments of adult romantic attachment have become more refined (Crowell et al. 2008), consisting of many questions that permit the assessment of attachment security in degrees. Such questionnaires can be scored on two dimensions: anxiety and avoidance (Brennan et al. 1998). I use Figure 1–1 to depict such a scheme in educating patients about attachment. Secure attachment is evident in low scores on anxiety and avoidance (i.e., comfort with closeness); ambivalent attachment is associated with high scores on anxiety and low scores on avoidance (i.e., anxiety with closeness); and avoidant attachment is associated with low scores on anxiety and high scores on avoidance (i.e., comfort with distance). This depiction also yields a fourth category called *fearful* attachment, characterized by high anxiety and avoidance. This plight of feeling afraid and alone epitomizes attachment trauma, as I elaborate later in this chapter in the Attachment Trauma section.

The diagram shown in Figure 1–1 helps patients to understand the differences among the various attachment categories and to appreciate the differences in degrees of security and insecurity. The diagram also illustrates the potential for differences in security between relationships as well as the possibility for shifts over time within relationships. To take one example, in our psychoeducational group on attachment and mentalizing in the Professionals in Crisis program at The Menninger Clinic, we frequently discuss how patients who have functioned at high levels of success in the upper-right quadrant (avoidant) collapse into the lower-right quadrant (fearful) in the face of extreme stress. In part, such collapses result from the lack of support that secure attachment would provide. We also use the diagram to highlight pathways to security (e.g., as illustrated by the dotted line). We propose in the group that movement from avoidant or fearful to secure attachment entails a pathway through ambivalence, given that avoidance stems from painful prior attachment experiences and that moving closer inevitably evokes anxiety.

Measuring Adult Attachments to Parents

In contrast to the questionnaire assessment of attachment in romantic relationships, which initiated a line of research in social and personality psychology, Mary Main and colleagues developed a clinical interview to assess adults' experiences of attachment with their parents (Hesse 2008). This hour-long Adult Attachment Interview is intended to be emotionally evocative, potentially stimulating painful memories and strong feelings. The interview begins with an orientation toward the participant's family constellation and asks for five adjectives characterizing mother and father (e.g., *affectionate, distant, controlling*). For each adjective and each parent, the participant is asked for concrete examples—that is, detailed early memories of events exemplifying the adjective (e.g., an incident in which the parent was "controlling"). In addition, participants are asked about feelings of closeness to their parents; the ways their parents responded to distress or illness; experiences of separation; and feelings of being rejected or threatened by their parents. The interview asks about childhood attachments with other adults as well as experiences of significant loss throughout the lifetime. As would be the case in psychotherapy, all experiences are explored in detail, drawing on specific memories.

The Adult Attachment Interview also asks participants to reflect on the meaning of early experiences and their long-term influences. For example, they are asked for their understanding of the reasons for their parents' behavior; the influence of their early attachment experiences on their personality; and changes in their relationships over the course of development. The interview also inquires about relationships with children, actual or anticipated. In addition, the interview inquires about traumatic experiences—not only regarding losses but also related to neglect and abuse. Although the interview includes an estimation of the quality of actual relationships (e.g., the extent to which each parent was loving), assessments are made not on the basis of these estimates but rather on the basis of the participant's *current overall state of mind with respect to attachment*. Hence, some participants with a history of abuse and neglect are able to demonstrate secure attachment in their valuing of attachment and the capacity to give an emotionally rich and coherent account of their at-

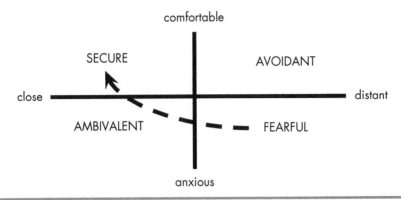

FIGURE 1–1. Dimensional view of attachment categories for patient education.

Dotted line indicates movement from fearful attachment through anxious ambivalence to secure attachment.

tachment relationships despite their history of trauma—a state of mind we therapists aim to achieve through psychotherapy. In parallel with the infant attachment research, attachment classifications are assigned, albeit with the slightly different terminology indicated in Table 1–2: secure-autonomous, preoccupied with attachment (corresponding to *ambivalent*), and dismissing of attachment (corresponding to *avoidant*).

As I hope to have made clear, these two traditions—questionnaires regarding romantic attachments and clinical interviews for state of mind regarding attachments to parents—were developed to measure adult counterparts to Ainsworth's three attachment categories. Despite their overlapping aim to arrive at attachment classifications, these two research traditions involve different methods (questionnaires versus interviews) and different relationships (romantic partners versus parents). Moreover, they were developed for fundamentally different purposes: the questionnaires were developed to relate attachment security to other facets of adult romantic relationships and general adjustment, whereas the Adult Attachment Interview was developed specifically to establish correspondence between parents' discussions of their childhood attachments and their infants' security of attachment with them in the Strange Situation. Thus, albeit to varying degrees, children's attachment classifications match their parents' attachment classifications in the Adult Attachment Interview.

Given the different methods, targets, and purposes of the questionnaire assessments and the Adult Attachment Interview, it's not surprising that researchers have found limited agreement among the attachment classifications (Mikulincer and Shaver 2007a). Notwithstanding this limited agreement between these two parallel traditions, I find it instructive to juxtapose research findings for each of them with respect to the major attachment classifications. Again, in the following section, I present idealizations—pure types; reality is rarely so neat. I begin each attachment category with a review of romantic relationships, followed by a discussion of interview findings regarding adults' attachment to their parents. We therapists need to have a clear image of secure attachment relationships in adulthood inasmuch as a cardinal goal of trauma treatment is increasing the capacity for secure attachment, often in all domains—with parents, partners, and children—and predicated partly on establishing security in the patient-therapist relationship.

Secure Attachment in Adults

Case Example

Aaron sought hospitalization in his mid-40s after he became severely depressed for the first time in his life. He felt blindsided by his depression, characterizing himself as generally outgoing and upbeat. But he had experienced a series of losses, and his wife's sudden illness was the proverbial last straw that culminated in a depression so severe that he withdrew from all his social activities and ultimately was unable to continue working in his highly successful real estate business.

Aaron had grown up in a close and loving family, but he moved far away from his parents and two sisters when he went to college, met his wife, and established his career. His parents both died young—his father when Aaron was in his late 20s and his mother when he was in his 30s. In hindsight, he traced the beginning of his depression to the death of his business partner, who had a fatal heart attack 2 years prior to Aaron's hospitalization. His partner, several years his senior, had been like an older brother to him, a mentor and confidant on whom he had come to rely after his father died.

Aaron was active in his community and had a substantial social network, but he began to lose his "verve" after his partner died; then he began spending more time at home. He had a close and loving relationship with his wife, and their active family life with their two adolescent children kept him from being too withdrawn and inactive. Three months prior to his hospitalization, however, his wife had a stroke, which he said "pulled the rug out" from under him. With the loss of his parents in the background and his partner's death from a heart condition in the foreground, Aaron became "petrified" that he would lose his wife, even though she was recovering from the stroke.

Aaron faced a dilemma, because he had always confided in his wife and drawn comfort from her, particularly with the deaths of his parents and then his partner. But he felt unable to confide in her regarding his fear about her death, believing that he needed to "be strong" for her. His hospitalization provided a refuge for Aaron because he was accustomed to relying on others for support, and there were no barriers to his talking openly about his losses and his fears. He relied on individual and group psychotherapy as well as informal contacts with his fellow patients to overcome his isolation and to regain an appreciation for the value of social activities in his life.

With the help of marital counseling, Aaron discovered that his wife had been distressed by his withdrawal from her, which resulted from his deepening depression and reluctance to talk with her about his fears about death. He came to realize that his wife also could "be strong" and that she was able to accept his fears as well as to talk with him openly about her own fears. At the same time, he reached out to two close friends, letting them know about his depression and hospitalization, and he found them to be understanding and eager to help him become reconnected to his social network. Thus, his lifelong capacity to form emotionally supportive connections enabled him to rebound from his severe depression over the course of several weeks, at which point he said he could "reclaim" his life.

With images of secure attachment in childhood in mind, the adulthood counterparts are unsurprising. Moreover, as Aaron's experience attests, the adaptive benefits of secure attachment are as evident in adulthood as they are throughout childhood.

Secure romantic relationships are characterized by trust, commitment, and stability; emotionally open communication; empathy and emotional availability conducive to providing comfort for the partner's distress; sexual intimacy and monogamy; reciprocity and interdependence; and high levels of satisfaction with the relationship. Secure relationships are not free of conflict but rather entail a level of trust that fosters communication, negotiation, and a propensity to forgive; accordingly, attachment security fosters confidence that relationship problems can be addressed and resolved, thus promoting stability in the relationship. Although attachment theory distinguishes sex, love, exploration, and caregiving from attachment, attachment security tends to glue all these facets together in romantic relationships. Of course, security doesn't provide immunity to breakups, but it does foster resilience, in part by enabling a person to make use of emotional support in other relationships.

Jim Coan and colleagues (2006) conducted a remarkable experiment that I use to impress upon patients and colleagues the centrality of attachment in distress regulation. These researchers recruited couples who were satisfied with their marriages, and they exposed the wife in each couple to the threat of shock, reinforced by administering shock in a minority of trials. The wives experienced the threat under three conditions while their brain activity was monitored: 1) holding their husband's hand, 2) holding a stranger's hand, and 3) not holding anyone's hand. Broadly speaking, threat activates two processes in the brain: stress responses and corresponding efforts to dampen distress. The researchers found that both patterns of brain activity were lowest while wives were holding their husband's hand and highest while they were not holding anyone's hand. Moreover, the greater the satisfaction in the marital relationship, the lower the level of brain activity while holding the husband's hand. Coan (2008) thus makes a compelling case that secure attachment is the most efficient way to regulate stress; as I view it simplistically, attachment gives the brain a break from the strain of experiencing and managing stress.

Implicitly and explicitly, secure attachment is associated with working models of others as benevolent and trustworthy. For securely attached persons, such models not only apply to romantic relationships but also extend to a more generalized positive view of human nature. Expectations that partners are well-intentioned, dependable, and forgiving are conducive to problem solving in the relationship. As in childhood, secure attachment in adulthood is associated with a model of self as being worthy and lovable. Secure attachment doesn't entail viewing relationships through rose-colored glasses; on the contrary, security allows room for criticism and self-criticism, making for a balanced view of others and oneself, a capacity to tolerate the negative as well as the positive, and thus openness to influence and change.

Those who report security in their romantic attachments also are likely to characterize their relationships with parents as being warm and supportive in questionnaire studies. As I noted earlier, however, the Adult Attachment Interview focuses not on the actual history but rather on the participant's manner of recounting that history in the interview. More specifically, the hallmark of secure-autonomous attachment is *narrative coherence*, a concept that applies directly to psychotherapy. Main and colleagues (2008) examine interviews for several core characteristics: truthfulness backed by specific evidence, succinctness, completeness, relevance, clarity, and organization. Accordingly, secure interviews are marked by emotionally authentic and convincing accounts of childhood experience, and they have a quality of freshness: participants are actively reflecting, thinking on their feet, sometimes coming up with new perspectives and realizations—a process we strive to achieve in psychotherapy. The antithesis of freshness is a stale account, full of generalizations or clichés, likely to be boring to hear—a sign in therapy of distance and insecurity.

More generally, persons demonstrating attachment security convey a positive attitude toward attachment; that is, regardless of the nature of their early history, they value attachment relationships. As it was intended to do, secure-autonomous attachment as evidenced in the Adult

Attachment Interview predicts infant attachment security in the Strange Situation, exemplifying the intergenerational transmission of attachment patterns (see Table 1–3). I discuss the reasons for the relation between parental and infant attachment security later in this chapter in the context of mentalizing (see section Mentalizing in Attachment Relationships).

Ambivalent-Preoccupied Attachment in Adults

Case Example

Bruce had become "crippled" with anxiety and depression in the context of escalating conflict in his second marriage. He traced his emotional instability back to high school when his parents' tumultuous marriage ended in divorce. Bruce said he'd been shy and socially "insecure" as long as he could remember, and he said he was just like his mother, who'd "fly off the handle at the drop of a hat."

In his senior year of high school, Bruce developed his first serious romantic relationship with Clarissa, a girl who was struggling with a similarly tumultuous household in which her parents' marriage was disrupted by her father's alcoholism. Bruce said they clung to each other "like Velcro." Bruce and Clarissa went away to the same college and married before graduation. Their marriage deteriorated when Clarissa gave birth to their son, and Bruce complained that he'd been "replaced." Two years later, they divorced, and Clarissa took custody of their son.

TABLE 1–3. Prototypical developmental pathway: secure attachment

Parent's discussion of childhood attachment experience	Coherent, at ease, open, free to explore, comfortable discussing painful emotions and experiences, balanced in views of self and others
Parent's behavior with infant	Sensitively responsive, consistently emotionally available
Infant's behavior with parent	Explores environment and checks back with parent; focuses on parent around separation; misses parent; initiates contact on reunion; gives flexible attention to parent and environment
Developmental outcomes	Is accepting of dependency; is effectively dependent *and* independent; has feelings of self-worth and self-confidence; is empathic and caring toward others; has capacity for trust and intimacy; is open to positive and negative emotions; is skillful in emotion regulation; has comforting memories of attachment relationships

Bruce started drinking more heavily after the divorce and, within a few months, he met Donna at a bar. She was a "soul mate" who easily matched all his resentments with resentments of her own. He said it was "us against the world." Bruce and Donna married "on the rebound" after a few months. But their marriage went downhill after Bruce was terminated from his job and despaired of finding alternative work. Whereas Bruce felt increasingly help-less, he characterized Donna as a "fighter," and she took a second job to make ends meet. While she worked, Bruce would just "veg" around the house, watching TV and half-heartedly applying for jobs. Although they needed the money, Bruce increasingly resented Donna's being out at work so much, es-pecially on evenings and weekends. He pleaded with her to take time off from work, recognizing that he tried to cling to her "like Velcro," as he'd done with Clarissa. But Donna's absences just kept "ripping" them apart.

At one point when he grabbed her arm as she was going out to work, Donna blurted out that she wished she had three jobs so she'd never have to see Bruce's "sorry ass." At that point, Bruce's anxiety and despair be-came so unbearable that he started thinking about suicide and ultimately started downing a bottle of pills in Donna's presence. Thus, he was pro-pelled into treatment in desperation.

As Bruce's experience attests, ambivalent attachment in romantic re-lationships is associated with a fast pace: falling in love quickly, passion-ately, and perhaps indiscriminately. This fast pace includes a high level of emotional openness and self-disclosure—too much too fast, potentially including rapid sexual intimacy. Minimizing differences and idealizing the partner—having found the perfect love—is a setup for disillusion-ment. As it is in childhood, the need for closeness is driven by the fear of abandonment. Yet, coupled with possessive and controlling behavior, the demand for closeness is liable to push the partner away. Vicious circles en-sue as the partner's distancing fuels intensified anxious clinging.

As it is in childhood, ambivalent attachment in adulthood is associated with anxiety, feelings of deprivation, and frustration. My colleague Helen Stein calls it the *kick-and-cling* pattern. The ambivalent partner is liable to suppress the direct expression of anger, thereby building up resentment, which may be expressed indirectly (e.g., in sullen withdrawal) and in pe-riodic angry outbursts. Such outbursts serve the same function in adult-hood as they do in childhood: protesting unresponsiveness to force attentiveness. Of course, such strategies might be effective in the short run but are likely to alienate the partner in the long run, leading to increasing mutual resentment. Furthermore, the dependent-helpless stance that characterizes ambivalent attachment undermines the development of au-tonomy and competence, thereby cementing dependency and adding fuel to fears of abandonment and inability to manage on one's own.

Ambivalent attachment is predicated on working models of attach-ment figures as being capable of providing care yet undependable. Thus, ambivalence intermingles hope with expectations of disappointment. Also inherent in the concept of ambivalence is conflict and contradiction, expecting the partner to be both loving and rejecting. The anxiety inherent in ambivalence leads to wariness and hypervigilance; the ambivalent partner is continually on the lookout for hints of rejection and potential abandonment. Such hypersensitivity leads to misperceptions or overreactions to ordinary failures in attunement or responsiveness that are ubiquitous in relationships (e.g., interpreting preoccupation as disinterest). Self-fulfilling prophecies ensue as minor problems escalate into major conflicts, reinforcing the ambivalent working models. These models entail a high level of self-criticism, including feelings of being inadequate, unworthy, weak, and unlovable. Such feelings fuel sensitivity to rejection and criticism, thereby contributing to conflict and further self-fulfilling prophecies. Feelings of inadequacy fuel dependency and failure to develop competence and self-reliance; these failures block successes that would be needed to develop more positive working models of self.

Although I've painted a rather unattractive picture of ambivalent attachment, there is a positive side to it: a high level of persistence in seeking and maintaining attachment relationships. Thus, ambivalence entails a level of engagement that keeps the door open to developing secure attachments. As I noted earlier, in the subsection Measuring Adult Attachments to Romantic Partners, ambivalence is likely to be on the pathway from avoidance to security.

As the label implies, preoccupied attachment as demonstrated in the Adult Attachment Interview entails an inability to move beyond conflict and frustration with early attachments, as shown in ongoing entanglement in attachment-related distress. Preoccupied interviews lack coherence and are rambling, vague, overly detailed, tangential, and thus hard to follow. These interviews are infused with continuing resentment, as evident in complaints about parental failures as well as blame—not only blaming parents but also self-blame. As these interview findings attest, merely thinking about childhood attachment relationships is emotionally distressing, thus activating attachment needs as well as the frustration associated with unmet needs.

As is the case with security, the child's insecure attachment classification is likely to match the parent's. Thus, parental attachment preoccupation in the Adult Attachment Interview is associated with infant ambivalence in the Strange Situation in the prototypical intergenerational pattern summarized in Table 1–4. The infant's distress and attachment needs are liable to evoke the preoccupied parent's ongoing problems with attachment and emotion regulation, thereby interfering with the parent's capacity to respond sensitively and consistently to the infant's distress.

TABLE 1–4.   Prototypical developmental pathway: preoccupied-
              ambivalent attachment

Parent's discussion of childhood attachment experience	Poor capacity to focus, long-winded, vague, tangential, preoccupied with anger toward parents, blaming and self-blaming
Parent's behavior with infant	Inconsistent, unavailable, unresponsive, under-involved
Infant's behavior with parent	Wary and distressed; focuses attention on parent to the exclusion of play; is difficult to soothe or comfort on reunion; shows anger mixed with effort to maintain contact
Developmental outcomes	Anxious, hypervigilant, worried about attachment figure's availability and responsiveness; exaggerates threat and fear to elicit care; seeks reassurance; has negative beliefs about self and world; punishes attachment figure to discourage unresponsiveness

The positive side of ambivalence, however, also is evident in parenting as it is in romantic relationships: albeit inconsistently, the parent is likely to remain emotionally engaged with the infant.

Avoidant-Dismissing Attachment in Adults

Case Example

Elaine, a bright and attractive woman in her early 30s, sought treatment when her alcohol abuse escalated to the point that she was arrested at 2:00 A.M. and jailed overnight for driving under the influence after a night of barhopping. This incident was humiliating, especially because she was a "rising star" in a law firm.

Recognizing that her life was "out of control," Elaine sought psychotherapy. But she started every session presenting herself as bubbly and cheerful, routinely saying with a smile that everything was "rosy." Without a hint of distress, she talked about what seemed to be a painful history of emotional isolation—inside and outside her family. She said she admired her father from afar. Although she "walked in his footsteps," she hardly knew him. He was a "high-powered" attorney who was rarely at home, and he was emotionally disengaged from the family when he was there. Thus, she was left at the mercy of her mother, whom she flatly characterized as a "cold bitch" who was demanding and perfectionistic.

Elaine was socially isolated throughout her school years, with the exception of having one friendship with a girl her age who was a "kindred spirit." She said the two were alike in being equally "mean and cruel," taking pleasure in the "pranks" they played on their peers. But they were both ostracized socially. Elaine was able to get by on her intelligence, however, and she graduated high school near the top of her class. She said she'd learned to "suck up" to her teachers to "stay out of trouble."

Relying on "wits and charm," Elaine excelled in college and law school. She said that, regarding romantic relationships, she was content with a series of exciting "flings" that didn't involve any commitment. She surprised herself in one therapy session, however, when she was blind-sided by tearfulness as she talked about one romance that "got out of hand." Contrary to her usual "flings," she dated Fred for 3 years, although the relationship was "on again, off again." When they were together, she started to "open up" to him, but then she would distance herself. She acknowledged that she'd even started to fantasize about having children, but then she said with disdain that she considered this a "house-with-a-white-picket-fence pipe dream." She became tearful when she talked about spending a weekend away with Fred at the end of which he brought out an engagement ring and proposed marriage. She "panicked" and cut off the relationship, at which point her drinking escalated.

As Elaine's experience illustrates, low levels of intimacy, closeness, affection, commitment, and emotional dependence characterize avoidant attachment; the prototype is the self-sufficient loner. This is not to say that avoidant persons are asocial; on the contrary, they may be extroverted—downright charming and witty. Yet their relationships are superficial, devoid of emotional confiding and comforting. Avoidant attachment is conducive to sex without love—that is, associated with positive attitudes toward casual sex concomitant with promiscuity, sex with strangers, and one-night stands. Sex may serve the purpose of bolstering the self-image, as evident in bragging about sexual exploits and conquests. Moreover, avoidance is antithetical to providing care and nurturance; avoidant persons are likely to be emotionally unavailable in the face of their partner's distress or even to respond to distress with hostility.

In adulthood, as in infancy, avoidance is an *attachment strategy*—that is, a way of maintaining *attachment at a distance*, or a strategy to maintain connection while minimizing rejection. As stated earlier, avoidant children acquiesce to the implicit command, "Don't bother me with your unhappiness." In adulthood, this strategy goes both ways: "I won't bother you, and I don't want you to bother me." Moreover, given repeated experience of unmet attachment needs, the avoidant person suppresses not only the *expression* of distress but also the *experience* of distress. Distress is associated with a feeling of weakness, vulnerability, and inferiority; hence, the avoidant person blocks awareness of the full range of distressing emotions, including anxiety, fear, shame, guilt, loneliness, and sadness. Irritation and anger may be the exception to this general rule.

Plainly, avoidant attachment is associated with negative working models of others—that is, expecting others consistently to be rejecting or unavailable. More generally, avoidance is likely to be associated with suspiciousness and distrust, which is conducive to hostility. Such negative attributions of others' intentions can reflect sheer projection of one's negativity onto others. Of course, such attributions contribute to self-fulfilling prophecies: hostility and suspiciousness beget rejection. Avoidant attachment is patently defensive in being self-protective, and defensiveness also may be evident in the avoidant person's sense of self. That is, avoidance is associated with defensive self-inflation, coupled with a penchant for externalization—namely, casting blame for problems onto others. In contrast to ambivalence, which is likely to be associated with feeling one-down in relationships, avoidance is associated with an effort to remain in control, one-up in relationships.

In the Adult Attachment Interview, dismissing attachment makes for a short story—literally, because interviews tend to be brief (i.e., the opposite of preoccupied interviews). Attachment is devalued, memories are sparse, and descriptions of relationships are abstract; thus, descriptive adjectives are not backed up with convincing evidence. Some dismissing interviews are marked by idealizing parents as being "wonderful" or "the best," without evidence. Sometimes idealizations are blatantly contradicted by the ostensibly supportive evidence: "Yeah, he used to hit me with a board when I got out of hand, but that was just his way of showing love, doing it for my own good."

Parents who are dismissing in the Adult Attachment Interview are likely to have infants who are avoidant in the Strange Situation, the prototypical intergenerational pattern summarized in Table 1–5. Children are likely to adapt to their parents' attachment pattern. Dismissing parents aspire to downplay, suppress, and reject emotional distress; to reiterate, the dismissing parent conveys "Don't bother me," and the avoidant infant acquiesces, for example, by directing attention to the toys.

Relationship Specificity of Adult Attachments

The Adult Attachment Interview yields a single classification intended to capture the individual's overall state of mind in relation to attachment. Similarly, questionnaires about adult attachment generally yield an overall classification. We have reason to rely on generality: these assessments of overall attachment patterns have shown enormous predictive power in research (e.g., most impressively, predicting an infant's attachment behavior from a parent's attachment classification). As the evidence reviewed here implies, working models stemming from earlier relationships influence the development of later relationships, generalizing from one relationship to

TABLE 1–5. Prototypical developmental pathway: dismissing-avoidant attachment

Parent's discussion of childhood attachment experience	Poor memory for childhood; downplays negative experiences; idealizes or devalues attachments; presents self as strong and independent
Parent's behavior with infant	Rejects infant's bids for comfort when distressed; unemotional with infant; intrusive, controlling, overstimulating
Infant's behavior with parent	Directs attention toward environment and away from parent, whether parent is present, departing, or returning; unemotional with parent
Developmental outcomes	Downplays threat, worry, vulnerability, need for comfort; rejects help; shows lack of emotional awareness, sometimes coupled with physiological reactivity; shows defensive self-inflation; is unwilling to provide comfort and support; shows outward emotional health but collapse of defenses with extreme stress

another. As also implied, these models are likely to be self-perpetuating, for better or for worse: securely attached persons anticipate benevolence and demonstrate caring and empathy, and thus others are likely to respond positively to them; ambivalently attached persons bring anxiety and resentment into relationships in a way that evokes conflict; and avoidant persons tend to maintain distance, which blocks engagement altogether.

Yet, being relational, attachment also is relationship specific to a considerable degree, based on the history of interactions between individuals. The most compelling evidence for relationship specificity is the finding that an infant may be securely attached to one parent and insecurely attached to the other (Steele et al. 1996). These differences within a family make sense in light of the fact that attachment strategies are responses to patterns of caregiving: if one parent is sensitively responsive and the other is inconsistently responsive or consistently rejecting, the infant will demonstrate security in one of these relationships and insecurity in the other. Such relationship specificity is conducive to flexibility in attachments, and we must count on it in conducting psychotherapy: to use Ainsworth's language, plain old therapy requires a level of sensitive responsiveness that promotes patients' security in the relationship. Also counting on generality, we hope that such enhanced security will generalize to other relationships, and we aspire to help this process along by examining and potentially modifying insecure working models in these other relationships. Yet, as I'll emphasize repeatedly throughout the book, individual psychotherapy has its

limits, and we therapists also rely on couples and family therapy to promote relationship-specific changes in attachment security.

Matches and Mismatches

Given that attachment is relational and to some degree relationship specific, attachment researchers have investigated the occurrence and impact
of matches and mismatches of attachment patterns in romantic partners
(Feeney 2008). The complexity in these findings is considerable in light of
the number of possible combinations. Unsurprisingly, securely attached
persons are likely to pair up with one another, and their relationships are associated with better adjustment and higher levels of satisfaction. There is
also some evidence for greater than chance levels of partner matching between insecure individuals (i.e., ambivalent-ambivalent and avoidant-
avoidant). Mismatches can be advantageous if one partner is secure: the security of one may buffer the insecurity of the other, and this particular mis-
match offers a crucial pathway to positive change (e.g., as might occur in a
good romantic relationship or in an effective psychotherapy relationship).
Ideally, each partner relies on the level of security the other partner shows,
and this allows them to ratchet up their conjoint security.

Of course, insecurity also can beget insecurity: ambivalence begets
ambivalence, and avoidance begets avoidance. As hinted earlier, the pair-
ing of ambivalence with avoidance is liable to lead to escalating conflict in
vicious circles. The avoidant partner's distancing stokes the ambivalent
partner's anxiety and resentment; anxious clinging and angry protests on
the part of the ambivalent partner promote further withdrawal and stonewalling on the part of the avoidant partner. Not uncommonly, ambivalent
wives are dissatisfied with avoidant husbands. In contrast, two avoidant
spouses are liable to have an emotionally distant marriage—at worst characterized by an emotional divorce.

Stability and Change

As in childhood, attachment patterns show a mixture of stability and
change over the course of adulthood, and the stability of a relationship
will depend on the stability of many other factors. Perhaps supporting the
idea of self-perpetuation, studies of stability in adult attachment over periods ranging from 1 week to 25 years show consistency in 70% of participants on average (Feeney 2008). As in childhood, instability is associated
with lawful discontinuity (Mikulincer and Shaver 2007a). Secure attachment can be destabilized by experiences of rejection or betrayal, as well as
by separations and losses. Conversely, insecure attachment can be ameliorated by the formation of positive and stable relationships—entering

into a good marriage, becoming a loving parent, or engaging in psychotherapy. For better or worse, experiences that disconfirm working models are associated with change in attachment security. We cannot avoid one brute fact: disconfirming insecure models requires a trustworthy partner.

Mentalizing in Attachment Relationships

Thus far, I have adopted Ainsworth's concept of sensitive responsiveness as the linchpin for secure attachment. We easily appreciate how a mother's sensitive responsiveness to her child's distress will give the child confidence in turning to her for solace. And we need only make a short leap to imagining that we adults will turn to sensitively responsive persons when we need comfort and understanding. Fonagy and Target (2005) have refined Ainsworth's insights in relating parental mentalizing capacity to children's attachment security as well as relating impaired mentalizing to attachment trauma. *Mentalizing* is not an easy word to adopt, as Jeremy Holmes (2010) contends: "When I first encountered the term 'mentalising' I found it off-putting, with its abstract pseudo-technical ring." Yet he adds, "I have come round to the view that mentalising captures a crucial aspect of psychological health, and psychotherapists' efforts to promote it" (p. 9).

I agree with Holmes on both counts and, sensitive to the potentially jarring sound of *mentalizing*, I like to introduce the concept to patients and colleagues alongside *mindfulness*, which is intuitively meaningful and user friendly. Yet I'm more interested in substance than semantics in this regard; mentalizing and mindfulness are overlapping concepts, and we can learn something about mentalizing from mindfulness research. Thus, I start this section with a discussion of mindfulness, then move on to review mentalizing, and conclude by summarizing the overlap and differences between mindfulness and mentalizing.

Mindfulness

In brief, mindfulness refers to *attentiveness to present experience* coupled with an *accepting attitude* toward experience—including emotionally painful and traumatic experience. Acceptance of emotionally painful experience, as contrasted with strategies to diminish emotional pain, has led to a significant shift in contemporary cognitive-behavioral therapies. Steven Hayes and colleagues (1999) contrast *experiential acceptance* with two forms of avoidance, each of which is pertinent to trauma. *Situational avoidance* encompasses avoiding situations that evoke painful emotions (e.g., a person who was assaulted in a parking garage might avoid parking garages). *Experiential avoidance* entails avoiding distressing thoughts and feelings, in effect, trying to avoid one's own mind—a futile endeavor. Mindfulness practice (e.g., through meditation) can promote experiential acceptance by demonstrating that mental states, including painful thoughts and feelings, are transient phenomena and not inherently toxic if one can adopt a nonjudgmental attitude of curiosity toward them. This attitude requires a complex amalgam of engagement (attentiveness) and detachment (i.e., observing one's thoughts and feelings, not taking them too seriously, and allowing them to pass through one's mind).

I find the mindfulness literature appealing, in part because of its explicit ethical foundation. Although many therapists approach mindfulness from a secular perspective, mindfulness has roots in Buddhism and hence in spirituality. The mindfulness tradition advocates compassion toward all beings, including the self. The practice of self-compassion has garnered increasing attention (Neff 2011), and compassion toward oneself is conducive to experiential acceptance. For example, you can bear emotional pain more easily if you empathize with yourself rather than berating yourself for your feelings.

Mindfulness took hold in the clinical research literature with Jon Kabat-Zinn's (1990) development of an 8-week group intervention, Mindfulness-Based Stress Reduction. Kabat-Zinn designed this program to help patients with general medical conditions (e.g., heart disease and chronic pain) who did not respond fully to standard medical care. Mindfulness practice has since become a mainstream intervention incorporated into contemporary cognitive-behavioral therapies for a wide range of symptoms and disorders (Roemer and Orsillo 2009). A review of nearly 40 studies with over 1,000 patients showed significant decreases of anxiety and depression with mindfulness interventions, and a substantial subset of these studies showed enduring benefit in follow-up assessments (Hoffmann et al. 2010). This research suggests that, paradoxically, accepting emotional distress rather than aspiring to suppress it is a helpful strategy for emotion regulation. This suggestion appears less paradoxical, however, in light of research on attachment security: sensitive responsiveness implicitly entails mindfulness—attentiveness and acceptance—and sensitive responsiveness ameliorates distress by enhancing feelings of security.

Mentalizing

Mentalizing entails mindfulness in the context of *attentiveness to mental states* in oneself and others—in short, holding mind in mind. The technical sound of the word *mentalizing* is misleading in implying something esoteric. On the contrary, mentalizing is a natural human capacity that we typically take for granted. Barring autism, we all become natural psychologists, inclined to make sense of ourselves and others.

Yet, as summarized in Table 1–6, mentalizing is complex in that the term encompasses many facets (Fonagy et al. 2012). Most fundamentally, we distinguish between self and others; knowing one's own mind is not the same as knowing the mind of another person. In addition, we distinguish explicit (controlled) from implicit (automatic) mentalizing. Explicit mentalizing is conscious and deliberate, typically involving language (e.g., putting feelings into words) and narrative (e.g., constructing a story to explain a problematic action). Implicit mentalizing is intuitive and nonconscious (e.g., as in turn-taking in conversations and automatically adjusting one's posture and voice quality in the process of empathizing with a friend's discouragement). We also distinguish an external focus (e.g., on a coworker's scowling face) from an internal focus (e.g., on the reasons for her scowl). In addition, we distinguish between mentalizing cognitive processes and affective processes (i.e., mentalizing thoughts versus emotions). Moreover, the time frame of mentalizing can vary: one can mentalize in relation to the present (e.g., a current desire), the future (e.g., anticipating the impact of a planned confrontation), or the past (e.g., reconstructing the basis of a misunderstanding). Finally, the scope of mentalizing may be narrow (e.g., a current thought) or broad (e.g., as in constructing an autobiographical narrative).

Understanding the development of our mentalizing capacity is tantamount to fathoming how we come to have a full-fledged human mind—no small feat (Fonagy et al. 2002). My colleagues and I have reviewed pertinent developmental research elsewhere (Allen et al. 2008); here, I focus merely on the contribution of secure attachment to the development of mentalizing. As a prelude, however, you must understand a fundamental and counterintuitive principle: the mind develops from the outside in. That is, you develop a sense of a self and come to know your own mind by virtue of others—caregivers most prominently—relating to you as a person with a mind.

TABLE 1–6. Different facets of mentalizing

- Focus on self versus others
- Explicit (deliberate, verbal) versus implicit (automatic, intuitive, nonverbal)
- External focus (observable behavior) versus internal focus (mental states)
- Thoughts versus feelings
- Present versus past and future
- Narrow (present state) versus broad (autobiographical)

Consider the process of coming to learn what you feel, beginning in the first year of life. Fonagy and colleagues (2002) explained how infants come to recognize their feelings by virtue of caregivers mirroring their emotional states in a complex fashion. The caregiver is not a simple mirror: it won't help the crying infant for his mother to cry just as hard; the infant will not be soothed! Rather, the mother shows the infant that she appreciates how he feels and empathizes: she integrates compassion and caring into her expression of sadness, using a soothing voice. Thus, she represents the infant's emotion to him. Similarly, if the infant is frustrated, the mother doesn't express her frustration with the infant but rather imitates his frustration in conjunction with an attitude of sympathy; she shows what *he* feels, not what *she* feels. Through this process, he comes to learn what he feels. This emotional learning process is the crucible for the development of subsequently more refined mentalizing, which, ultimately, enables a person to label feelings, understand the reasons for them, and put them into an autobiographical narrative.

As I noted in the section on adulthood, Main and colleagues (1985) demonstrated correspondence between parents' Adult Attachment Interview classifications and their infants' Strange Situation classifications. Extending this research, Fonagy and colleagues (1991a) conducted a remarkable study. They administered the Adult Attachment Interview to 100 mothers who were pregnant with their first child, and then they observed the mother-infant interactions in the laboratory when their infants were 12 months old. They found significant concordances between mothers' attachment classifications and infants' classifications. They subsequently replicated these results for fathers (Steele et al. 1996). The way the parent talked about attachment before the child was born predicted the way the child would interact with the parent in the lab 1 year after being born. This finding calls for explanation.

How does parental security of attachment lead to infant attachment security? Although the research is complex and arduous to conduct, the developmental principle is simple: mentalizing begets mentalizing. Fonagy and colleagues (1991b) demonstrated, for example, that parental mentalizing in the adult interview was the strongest predictor of infant attachment security. This finding makes sense if we suppose that parents who are able to mentalize in relation to their own attachment history (i.e., to reflect in a coherent and emotionally engaged manner) are likely to be more capable of mentalizing in relation to their infant's attachment needs and emotions. Subsequent research bears out this supposition. Securely attached parents mentalize their infants. They engage in what Elizabeth Meins (Meins et al. 2006) called *mind-minded commentary* on their infants' behavior, spontaneously commenting on what the infants might be thinking, feeling, and intending to do. Secure parents also talk about their infants in a psychologically attuned way, attentive to their feelings, desires, and needs (Slade et al. 2005). Naturally, intuitively anticipating a mentalizing response, infants turn to them for help when distressed; they're securely attached. Moreover, securely attached infants develop better mentalizing capacities in childhood; for example, they're able to appreciate what other children are thinking and feeling.

These research findings relating mentalizing to secure attachment constitute substantial refinements to Ainsworth's pioneering discovery of the importance of sensitive responsiveness (Fonagy and Target 2005). To reiterate the commonsensical story foretold in the book's Introduction, we would expect that infants would seek and find comfort from parents who are attuned to their emotional states, and we shouldn't be surprised that children learn to mentalize by virtue of engaging in mentalizing interactions, just as children learn to speak by virtue of being spoken to.

Integrating Mindfulness and Mentalizing

I find the overlap between the concepts of mindfulness and mentalizing remarkable inasmuch as they come from such diverse traditions: mindfulness has roots in Buddhism, philosophy, and ethics, whereas mentalizing derives from psychoanalysis and developmental psychopathology. Research on both has been motivated by the desire to relieve suffering (see Figure 1–2). Hence, each has a place in psychotherapy. I cannot imagine a psychotherapy that does not entail mindful attention to mental states. Moreover, mindfulness and mentalizing entail a stance of curiosity toward mental states as well as an accepting attitude toward experience. In sum, mindfulness, mentalizing, and acceptance exemplify sensitive responsiveness; all three are essential to security in parent-child relationships, friendships, love relationships, and plain old therapy.

Yet mentalizing is not equivalent to mindfulness. Five differences stand out. First, mindfulness is not restricted to mental states (e.g., you can be mindful of a flower or your breath); hence, I construe mentalizing as *mindfulness of mind*. Second, mentalizing is more social than mindfulness in two senses: mentalizing includes attention to mental states in others as well as in oneself; more fundamentally, mentalizing is intrinsically social insofar at it comes into being in the context of social interactions. Third, our understanding of mentalizing, related to its social nature, comes from developmental research. Thanks to this research, we now understand how mindfulness of mind comes into being and how we might enhance its development. Fourth, whereas mindfulness entails *bare attention*, mentalizing also involves *reflection* and narrative—that is, elaboration

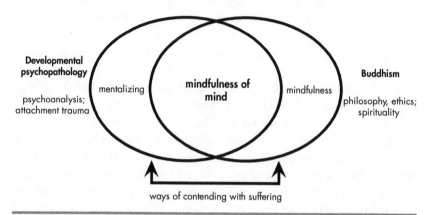

FIGURE 1–2. Overlap between mentalizing and mindfulness.

and interpretation of mental states. Fifth, short of being stripped down to its bare bones in secular applications, an ethical perspective is explicit in mindfulness while remaining implicit in mentalizing.

Finally, there is a seeming contradiction between the mindfulness and mentalizing literatures: the Buddhist tradition advocates nonattachment, whereas the mentalizing literature emphasizes attachment. In the Buddhist literature, attachment connotes grasping, clinging, and possessiveness; yet these inclinations are characteristic of insecure attachment. Accordingly, research by Shaver and colleagues (2007) has shown that mindfulness is associated with secure attachment—that is, lower levels of anxiety and avoidance. This finding makes sense, because secure attachment is conducive to acceptance of emotional experience—neither being anxious about it nor pushing it aside. Accordingly, if somewhat ironically, secure attachment also relates positively to measures of nonattachment as construed in the Buddhist literature (Sahdra et al. 2010). For example, securely attached persons are nonattached in the sense that they are able to accept the flow of events and experiences (without obsessing about them or avoiding them) and are less encumbered by possessiveness. Hence, these two views of attachment are complementary rather than contradictory.

Attachment Trauma

I use the term *attachment trauma* in two senses: first, to refer to trauma that takes place in attachment relationships; second, to refer to the adverse impact of such trauma on the capacity to develop secure attachment relationships. Attachment trauma creates a *dual liability* (Fonagy and Target 1997): it simultaneously evokes emotional distress and undermines the development of the capacity to regulate distress. I've been building the case in this chapter that mentalizing in secure attachment relationships is the foundation of emotion regulation. Hence, my main thesis about attachment trauma that provides the fundamental rationale for plain old therapy is as follows:

> The experience of being left psychologically alone in unbearable emotional states repeatedly for prolonged periods is potentially traumatic owing in part to the absence of mentalizing. Treatment entails creating a secure attachment context conducive to mentalizing in which previously unbearable emotional states can be experienced, expressed, understood, and reflected upon—and thereby rendered meaningful and bearable.

To confirm this proposition, we therapists merely need to be attentive to all the ways in which traumatized patients express their core experience of feeling *invisible*—ignored, overlooked, dismissed, misunderstood, unheard, unseen—in the present as well as the past.

Thus, consistent with its profound and pervasive adverse developmental impact (Strathearn 2011), I place neglect—lack of psychological attunement—at the center of attachment trauma. From this perspective, neglect is inherent in abuse. Mentalizing failure—psychological unavailability—lies at the core of emotional neglect. But mentalizing failure, and neglect in this sense, also lies at the core of every form of abuse—physical, sexual, and psychological. Abusing a child, or an adult, for that matter, is incompatible with mentalizing—that is, mindful attentiveness to the child's (or adult's) experience. Accordingly, mentalizing puts the brakes on violence, and being violent requires releasing the mentalizing brakes (Fonagy 2004).

Our understanding of attachment trauma comes from Main and colleagues' (Main and Solomon 1990) recognition of a fourth attachment category in conjunction with seemingly anomalous infant behavior in the Strange Situation. Main classified this anomalous pattern as *disorganized* attachment, and this atypical pattern was discovered to originate in maltreatment. After reviewing the research on the organized patterns of attachment (secure, ambivalent, and avoidant), I have established a conceptual template for understanding attachment trauma. Here, too, an intergenerational pattern emerged: parents' unresolved-disorganized attachment in the Adult Attachment Interview predicts infants' disorganized attachment in the Strange Situation (Main and Hesse 1990). Trauma begets trauma. This groundbreaking discovery spawned two decades of research that has refined our understanding of attachment trauma and its development, including its roots in mentalizing failures.

Infant Disorganization in the Strange Situation

Classifying infants as being disorganized in the Strange Situation requires careful observation and clinical sensitivity, because disorganized behavior often is short-lived—potentially occurring in bouts as brief as 10–30 seconds (Main et al. 2005). Hence, the disorganized classification is superimposed on the predominant pattern (i.e., secure, ambivalent, or avoidant) rather than substituting for it. Notwithstanding their brevity and subtlety, indications of disorganization portend significant developmental problems, potentially extending into psychiatric disturbance in adulthood.

Disorganized behavior is seemingly inexplicable in lacking an obvious intention or goal. Main and colleagues realized that the reason for this confusing behavioral pattern was the infant's irresolvable conflict: in the most glaring instances, the abusive attachment figure is frightening, and the infant's primary strategy for reducing fear—seeking proximity—only exacerbates the fear. Hence, Main construed disorganized attachment as stemming from *fright without solution*. Here is a painful example: When the mother leaves the room in the Strange Situation, the infant runs after her, screaming and pounding on the door through which she has exited. When the mother returns, the infant becomes frightened and runs to the opposite side of the room. Thus, despite the infant's extreme distress, there is no reunion and no solace. Other examples of disorganized behavior include a cheerful greeting followed by a frozen, dazed expression; clinging to the parent while turning away and averting gaze; extended rocking or automaton-like movements; direct expressions of fear of the parent, such as jerking back with a frightened expression; aimless wandering; sudden eruptions of fear or anger into otherwise contented play; and prolonged, trancelike states.

Notably, some of these observations suggest that *dissociative states*, a common trauma-related symptom, have origins in infancy. Thus, I touch on dissociation in this chapter before considering it at more length in the next. In brief, dissociation entails either *alterations* in consciousness (e.g., detached, dazed, trancelike states) or *alternations* in consciousness (e.g., contradictory and seemingly compartmentalized behavioral states, such as the sudden intrusion of fear). In either form, painful experience is dissociated in the sense of being disconnected or kept separate from ordinary consciousness.

Disabled Caregiving and Infant Disorganization

Infant disorganization is relationship specific; rarely does an infant show disorganized behavior with more than one parent (Lyons-Ruth and Jacobvitz 2008). Extensive research links disorganization to maltreatment (van IJzendoorn et al. 1999). For example, in Sroufe and colleagues' meticulous longitudinal study (Carlson 1998), disorganization was associated with physical abuse (e.g., intense and frequent spanking, angry parental outbursts resulting in serious injuries), psychological unavailability (e.g., parental unresponsiveness or detachment), and neglect (e.g., failure to provide physical care or protection).

Plainly, maltreatment exemplifies the infant's plight of fright without solution. Yet Main and colleagues' (2005) research also has shown more subtle contributors to disorganized attachment. Indeed, it is now clear that a wide range of parental behavior beyond blatant maltreatment is conducive to infant disorganization. That is, the parent may be directly *frightening* (e.g., abusive) or *frightened* (e.g., in a traumatized state). In either case, the parent is psychologically unavailable. In a related vein, Karlen Lyons-Ruth and colleagues (2005) have identified two patterns of misattunement conducive to infant disorganization: hostile intrusiveness and helpless withdrawal. More generally, Lyons-Ruth (Lyons-Ruth and Jacobvitz 2008) linked disorganization with *disrupted emotional communication*, which takes many forms: negative-intrusive behavior (e.g., mocking the infant), withdrawal (e.g., silence), communication errors (e.g., giving contradictory cues such as encouraging closeness while physically withdrawing), and disorientation (e.g., unusual and perplexing voice changes). The crucial discovery was that even in the absence of directly abusive or frightening behavior, signs of disrupted emotional communication predict infant disorganization. This is what I had in mind when I commented earlier that relationships have become unglued in attachment trauma.

More than any other study I have seen, Beatrice Beebe and colleagues' (2010) study of mother-infant interactions highlights the role of psychological disconnection in attachment trauma. In contemplating her research, one should keep in mind my basic proposition that being left psychologically alone in distressed states lies at the heart of attachment trauma. Beebe studied 150 seconds of mother-infant interactions in a free play situation, coding second-by-second segments. These interactions occurred when the infants were 4 months old, and the codings subsequently were found to be related to infants' Strange Situation classifications at age 12 months. Lack of maternal emotional attunement characterized interactions predictive of attachment disorganization: in the face of their infant's distress, a misattuned mother would look away, show a lack of facial responsiveness, or display discordant emotion (e.g., smiling while the infant cried). In addition to stonewalling, these mothers might show intrusiveness or loom unpredictably into the infant's space. When we consider the adverse implications of disorganized attachment, to be described later, it is no exaggeration to construe such misattunement to infant distress as potentially traumatic. In considering the import of these findings, one should keep in mind that the misattunement was evident in a brief laboratory interaction when mothers were instructed to attend to their infants (i.e., to play with them), and they were being observed. Presumably, such instances in the lab are indicative of more pervasive misattunement or psychological unavailability in the child's natural environment.

In work consistent with recent research findings, Judith Solomon and Carol George (2011) have construed infant disorganization as resulting from a disabled caregiving system, including helplessness in the caregiver, which results in an abdication of care. They describe mothers of disorganized infants as being emotionally flooded and overwhelmed by feelings of inadequacy that impair their capacity to engage emotionally with their infant's distress and thereby to provide comfort. In addition, caregiving can be disabled by pervasive emotional constriction (e.g., as might occur with severe depression or emotional detachment), with the same result. I discussed the importance of the environmental context of caregiving earlier in this chapter (see section Environmental Influences on Caregiving), and it shouldn't be overlooked here. As Solomon and George contend, abdication of care is associated with assaults to the caregiving system, which can include perinatal loss of a previous child; parental psychiatric disorders and substance abuse; divorce; and living in a violent environment, including in the midst of terrorism or a war zone.

Notably, disorganized attachment appears to be the exception to the rule that infant genetic factors play a limited role in attachment behavior (Spangler 2011). Yet genetic factors exert their influence on disorganization in interaction with the caregiving environment. That is, some genetic anomalies appear to be risk factors in combination with unresponsive care; conversely, different genetic factors appear to be protective (i.e., lowering the risk of disorganization in the face of unresponsive care). In addition, the wider developmental context of care needs to be considered: as discussed next, the parent's history of trauma and loss can contribute to infant disorganization in an intergenerational process.

Disorganization in Adulthood

Analogous to their infants' disorganized behavior demonstrated in the Strange Situation, parents' disorganized thinking can be evident in the Adult Attachment Interview (Hesse 2008). Just as secure attachment is marked by narrative coherence in the interview, disorganized attachment is evident in narrative incoherence. Such disorganization is liable to occur when parents are invited to think and talk about their history of attachment trauma and loss. Such lapses in coherence may take the form of brief dissociative states, as the parent seems momentarily detached or disoriented, perhaps lost in the past. These interviews are coded as unresolved-disorganized (i.e., unresolved with respect to past trauma or loss). As little as a few sentences of disrupted coherence can lead the researcher to code the interview as unresolved-disorganized. Hence, as in infant classifications, the disorganized coding is assigned alongside the best-fitting organized classification (i.e., secure, preoccupied, or dismissing). Alternatively, some parental interviews are coded as "cannot classify" on the basis of intermingling of contradictory patterns (e.g., dismissing and preoccupied) or pervasive incoherence that renders interviews relatively incomprehensible. Like the unresolved-disorganized classification, these unclassifiable interviews are predictive of infant disorganization.

Many studies have confirmed the relation between parents' unresolved trauma and loss as evident in the Adult Attachment Interview and infant disorganization in the Strange Situation (van IJzendoorn et al. 1999). As just noted, these parental interviews are coded on the basis of momentary disruptions in narrative coherence. However, Lyons-Ruth and colleagues (Melnick et al. 2008) also found more pervasive signs of disturbance in the interviews to be predictive of infant disorganization— that is, disturbance evident beyond discussions of trauma and loss. Recall that hostile-helpless parental behavior in the Strange Situation is associated with infant disorganization in that situation. These researchers found that hostile-helpless states of mind with respect to attachment in the adult interview also are associated with infant disorganization in the Strange Situation. These hostile-helpless states of mind reflect identifications with hostile or helpless childhood attachment figures, based on a history of traumatic attachment relationships. For example, persons in the hostile subtype might describe themselves as acting just like a terrorizing parent; those in the helpless subtype are likely to be more passive and fearful, identifying with a parent who was disengaged from the caregiving role.

All these findings are connected: the parents' hostile-helpless stance in the Adult Attachment Interview is related to their hostile-helpless interactions with their infants in the Strange Situation; in turn, these hostile-helpless interactions are related to infant disorganized behavior. This prototypical intergenerational pattern of unresolved-disorganized attachment is summarized in Table 1–7. Presumably, if these hostile-helpless states are evident in clinical interviews and laboratory observations, they also occur routinely in the natural environment, potentially pervasively disrupting the kind of attunement and communication needed for emotional support and secure attachment.

TABLE 1–7. Prototypical developmental pathway: unresolved-disorganized attachment

Parent's discussion of childhood attachment experience	Unresolved with respect to trauma or loss; shows momentary lapses in attention and dissociative states or alteration in consciousness; incoherent; unclassifiable
Parent's behavior with infant	Frightened/frightening behavior; dissociative states; hostile intrusiveness or fearful withdrawal; emotionally overwhelmed in response to infant's distress; disrupted communication; role confusion; disabled caregiving or abdication of care
Infant's behavior with parent	Fright without solution: fear; trancelike and dissociative states; disorientation; dramatically contradictory behavior
Developmental outcomes	In childhood, is controlling (punitive or caregiving) with parents; in adulthood, shows continuing disorganization or is vulnerable to dissociation and other psychiatric disorders

Impaired Mentalizing in Disorganized Attachment

With your thinking about mentalizing now well primed, I hope that you've been connecting the dots while reading about this research on disorganized attachment in parents and infants. To make the connections explicit, the disruption in narrative coherence in the Adult Attachment Interviews of parents whose infants become disorganized can be construed as evidence of impaired mentalizing (Fonagy et al. 1991b). For parents classified as unresolved-disorganized, mentalizing is compromised when the interview evokes a history of attachment trauma or loss. For those in the "cannot classify" category, mentalizing is more pervasively compromised during the interview inasmuch as they are unable to present a coherent picture of their attachment history. Similarly, hostile or helpless states of mind that pervade the interview exemplify impaired mentalizing. In all these instances, evoking memories and feelings associated with attachment derails mentalizing.

Paralleling what happens in the parent's interview, the infant's attachment needs expressed in Strange Situation reunions are liable to evoke distress in the parent (e.g., at the extreme, evoking memories of attachment trauma, such as neglect or abuse); hence, by evoking memories and feelings associated with past trauma, such interactions may undermine parental mentalizing, resulting in misattunement to the child's distress.

Such misattunement is evident in parents' frightening or frightened behavior, their hostile or helpless behavior, or their more pervasively disrupted emotional communication. In stark form, as Beebe and colleagues (2010) demonstrated, the parent may simply turn her attention away from her infant's distress. All such behavior is the antithesis of mindfully holding the infant's mind in mind.

Research supports the chain of reasoning I've just outlined. For example, Arietta Slade and colleagues (2005) directly assessed parents' capacities to mentalize their infant in the 90-minute Parent Development Interview. The interview covers the mother's perception of her infant; her experience of separations from her infant; her view of herself as a parent; and her understanding of the influence of her parents on her way of parenting. As anticipated, the researchers found that parental unresolved-disorganized attachment was associated with relatively poor mentalizing of the infant in the Parent Development Interview and, in turn, with infant disorganization in the Strange Situation. Moreover, poor maternal mentalizing in the interview also was associated with disrupted parent-infant communication in the Strange Situation, and disrupted communication was associated with infant disorganization (Grienenberger et al. 2005).

Disorganized attachment has two prominent adverse consequences. First, the infant is unable to find solace when distressed and thus experiences repeated emotional dysregulation—distress without respite. Second, because a person learns to mentalize by virtue of being mentalized, the disorganized infant's development of mentalizing capacity is compromised. Just as mentalizing begets mentalizing, nonmentalizing begets nonmentalizing. Accordingly, Fonagy and colleagues (2007) reviewed research showing multiple impairments in children's mentalizing in conjunction with a traumatic attachment history: difficulty appreciating what others are thinking and feeling, limited capacity to talk about mental states, difficulty understanding emotions, failure to empathize with other children's distress, and difficulty managing emotional distress. These mentalizing impairments can contribute to problems in a wide range of relationships—not only with parents, but also with siblings, peers, and teachers.

This research shows the sheer extent of the dual liability associated with early attachment trauma that I mentioned at the beginning of this section. The trauma evokes distress and undermines the development of capacities to regulate distress. Children learn to regulate distress through mentalizing interactions; moreover, they learn to identify what they feel through these interactions, setting the stage for them to manage feelings on their own as well as with the help of others. Without the capacity to mentalize, they can be relatively helpless in regulating their distress. We easily imagine vicious circles in which impaired mentalizing contributes to interpersonal conflicts, interpersonal conflicts evoke distress, impaired emotion regulation escalates distress and conflicts, and so on.

Nonmentalizing Modes of Experience

Fonagy and colleagues (2002) delineated three prominent nonmentalizing modes of experience stemming from attachment trauma that lay the foundation for further developmental adversity. I will be referring back to these modes in later discussions of psychiatric disorders.

Psychic equivalence is the most fundamental failure of mentalizing: mental states are equated with reality. Dreaming is the prototype: the dreamer believes the dreamed events are really happening. Posttraumatic flashbacks are another example: a memory is experienced as a current reality—a "daymare" as one patient described it. Paranoid delusions also reflect psychic equivalence: the deluded individual is convinced of the truth of his beliefs, not considering that they could be false. He has no doubts that people really are conspiring against him. Understanding psychic equivalence helps one to understand mentalizing: the crux of mentalizing (and mindfulness) is awareness of the distinction between mental states and reality. Beliefs can be false, and feelings can be unwarranted. Mentalizing is fundamental in coping with traumatic flashbacks; people with posttraumatic stress disorder (PTSD) must learn to recognize that they are remembering trauma, not reliving it.

The *pretend* mode represents the opposite of psychic equivalence: rather than mental states being too real (i.e., equated with reality), they're too disconnected from reality. Dissociatively detached states have a pretend quality—and are commonly associated with trauma. At the extreme, these states are evident in feelings of unreality (e.g., feeling as if one were an actor in a play). Most commonly, the pretend mode is evident in the disconnection between thoughts and feelings; conversation in the pretend mode carries no emotional weight or conviction. Thus, functioning in the pretend mode is a significant threat to psychotherapy in that the illusion of collaboration is maintained without any serious work being done. For example, the pretend mode is evident in speech riddled with clichés or psychobabble.

In the *teleological* mode, action replaces thought and emotion; that is, goal-directed behavior takes the place of experiencing and expressing mental states. Accordingly, impulses and emotions quickly lead to action, in effect bypassing deliberation, reflection, or even emotional awareness. In this mode, intense emotional distress is not mentalized but rather is directly expressed in such behavior as substance abuse, nonsuicidal self-injury, bingeing or purging, sexual promiscuity, suicide attempts, and so forth. Such problematic behavior led Maria Holden, a postdoctoral fellow working with me, to propose the need for a *pause button* (Allen 2001), shorthand for the need to mentalize.

Developmental Impact of Disorganized Attachment

Like the organized patterns of attachment, disorganized attachment shows a mixture of stability and change in longitudinal studies. On the whole, with assessments in infancy and reassessments ranging from 1 month to 5 years later, researchers find substantial stability (van IJzendoorn et al. 1999). Moreover, long-term longitudinal studies reveal some continuity from disorganization in infancy to unresolved trauma in the Adult Attachment Interview administered in late adolescence (Main et al. 2005) and early adulthood (Sroufe et al. 2005).

Yet disorganization frequently changes in form by early childhood. Main and colleagues (2005) discovered that many children who showed disorganization in infancy develop an organized *controlling* pattern of interacting with their parents by early childhood. Moreover, their controlling behavior takes one of two forms. Some children become *punitive* in their interactions, perhaps ordering the parent around (e.g., "Sit down and shut up, and keep your eyes closed!"), whereas others adopt a *caregiving* stance, becoming solicitous (e.g., "Are you tired, Mommy? Would you like to sit down and I'll bring you some [pretend] tea?") (p. 283). These controlling strategies in child-parent interactions belie the fact that these formerly disorganized children remain extremely anxious and insecure. For example, children who show this pattern give fearful responses to projective storytelling tests about separation experiences, which include catastrophic fantasies about injuries to the parents or the child.

Ellen Moss and colleagues (2011) found that controlling-punitive children are more disruptive and aggressive than their controlling-caregiving counterparts. They are more difficult to raise, and they perform more poorly in school. The controlling-caregiving children were more likely to have mothers who had suffered loss of an attachment figure during the child's early years, consistent with the child's developing a caregiving stance. Notably, although many disorganized infants develop a controlling strategy by early childhood, a substantial minority remains disorganized. Moss and colleagues' description of one such 4-year-old boy is noteworthy in suggesting dissociation. When reunited with his mother after a brief separation, the child made "bizarre, frightened, and selfdepreciative comments" and then "seemed to completely forget about this part of the conversation when his mother answered him back." Also, the child "seemed to experience abrupt changes of state evidenced by a sudden shift of affect and disruption in his discourse" (p. 64). These children showing ongoing disorganization tended to come from families with a high level of marital tension and, like the punitive group, showed especially high levels of behavioral and academic problems.

As these findings suggest, infant disorganization portends diverse developmental problems from childhood to adulthood (Lyons-Ruth and Jacobvitz 2008), especially when it occurs in combination with maltreatment (Melnick et al. 2008) and other developmental risk factors such as broader family adversity (Deklyen and Greenberg 2008). Worryingly, disorganization in infancy increases the likelihood of developing PTSD symptoms in response to trauma later in childhood (MacDonald et al. 2008). More generally, infant disorganization was the strongest predictor of global psychopathology at age 17½ in the Minnesota longitudinal study of attachment and adaptation across development (Sroufe et al. 2005). That study exemplifies a broad principle of crucial importance: maltreatment and infant disorganized attachment are *nonspecific risk factors* for a wide range of subsequent disturbances.

Further attesting to the presence of nonspecific risk associated with attachment trauma, continuing unresolved-disorganized attachment in adulthood, as measured by the Adult Attachment Interview, is associated with a wide range of concurrent disorders in adulthood. Combining findings from studies that included more than 4,200 participants, researchers found a strong relationship between adult disorganization and the likelihood of psychiatric disorder (van IJzendoorn and Bakermans-Kranenburg 2008). Disorganization was relatively uncommon in the nonclinical adolescent and adult participants (16.5% and 15%, respectively) and relatively high in the adult clinical sample (41%). These combined studies showed disorganization to be most strongly related to borderline personality disorder, suicidality, and PTSD in relation to a history of abuse.

One intriguing exception to the principle of nonspecific risk is that some instances of disorganized behavior in the Strange Situation have a dissociative quality, such as dazed, trancelike states or sudden eruptions of contradictory behavior. Notably, such infant behavior may mirror parents' dissociative states in the Adult Attachment Interview (e.g., bouts of confusion and disorientation, such as talking about deceased parents as if they were still living). With data from the Minnesota longitudinal study, Elizabeth Carlson (1998) found infant disorganization to be associated with dissociative and self-injurious behaviors in grade school and high school; moreover, disorganization in infancy related significantly to dissociative disturbance assessed by interviews and self-report questionnaires in late adolescence. This is truly remarkable developmental continuity.

Consistent with Carlson's findings, extensive evidence now shows that infant disorganization is associated with dissociative disturbance (Dozier et al. 2008). Most crucial to my view of attachment trauma, Lyons-Ruth and colleagues (Melnick et al. 2008) proposed specifically that chronically disrupted communication and lack of caregiver responsiveness might be *more* predictive of later dissociative disturbance than is outright abuse. If one thinks of dissociation as disconnection—disconnection from the self and disconnection from others—and thinks of mentalizing as psychological glue for attachment with others and with oneself, then the research findings make sense: disconnection begets disconnection. To reiterate, the feeling of disconnection—at the extreme, invisibility—lies at the heart of attachment trauma. Dissociative disturbance is a dramatic instance of this pervasive experience.

Synthesis

In his wonderfully integrative book *Polarities of Experience*, Sidney Blatt articulated a developmental framework that puts the attachment research I've reviewed in this chapter into broader perspective. As Blatt (2008) explained,

> Every person throughout life confronts two fundamental psychological developmental challenges: (a) to establish and maintain reciprocal, meaningful, and personally satisfying interpersonal relationships and (b) to establish and maintain a coherent, realistic, differentiated, integrated, essentially positive sense of self. ... The articulation of these two most fundamental of psychological dimensions—the development of interpersonal *relatedness* and of *self-definition*—provides a comprehensive theoretical matrix that facilitates the integration of concepts of personality development, personality organization, psychopathology, and mechanisms of therapeutic change into a unified model. (p. 3, emphasis added)

I find downright elegant the correspondence between Blatt's (2008) contrast of relatedness and self-definition, on the one hand, and Bowlby and Ainsworth's concepts of the safe haven and secure base, on the other hand. Thus, as the safe haven provides a secure base for exploration, Bowlby and Ainsworth ingeniously showed how relatedness fosters self-definition. Similarly, in their work on the complex mirroring process through which children learn what they feel, Fonagy and colleagues (2002) showed how relatedness promotes self-definition. Conversely, as Blatt argues, self-definition promotes relatedness; relationships are predicated on two individualities coming together. Beginning in infancy, relationships and self-definition are forged from oscillating patterns of engagement and disengagement—being together and being on one's own.

In my mind, secure attachment relationships have an accordion-like quality; we oscillate between closeness and distance while remaining connected. Our capacity to mentalize—encompassing self-awareness and awareness of others—maintains our sense of separateness while keeping us related (i.e., as we hold mind in mind). Mindful that we must view attachment through the dual lenses of science and ethics, I was captivated by the book *Virtue Ethics* by New Zealand philosopher Christine Swanton (2003). Swanton referred to nineteenth-century German philosopher Immanuel Kant's differentiation of two grand moral forces: love and respect. Kant viewed love as coming close—no surprise there. Less intuitively, Kant viewed respect as maintaining distance. Thus, respect entails keeping one's distance in the sense of giving the other person space and supporting autonomy. Failures of respect are evident in being controlling, possessive, intrusive, and demeaning. Kant contended that in any good relationship, these two moral forces must be kept in balance. Love and respect maintain each other: the secure base of relatedness supports autonomy, and granting autonomy is crucial to maintaining healthy relatedness. As attachment theory shows, possessiveness (as in ambivalent attachment) undermines relationships, as does excessive distance (as in avoidant attachment). Plainly, from this perspective, attachment trauma in the most extreme form of neglect and abuse exemplifies our most glaring—and all too common—moral failure: neglect is a failure of love, and abuse is a failure of respect.

Just as secure attachment maps onto an optimal balance between relatedness and self-definition (love and respect), insecure attachment patterns map onto imbalance. As diagrammed in Figure 1–3, ambivalent attachment reflects preoccupation with relatedness to the exclusion of self-definition and autonomy; conversely, avoidant attachment entails dismissing of relatedness with an overemphasis on self-definition and autonomy. Lastly, disorganized or fearful attachment entails a failure to establish relatedness coupled with a failure to sustain self-definition and autonomy, leaving the person alone in distress and unable to manage.

With Patrick Luyten and others, Blatt made a strong case that we therapists should view psychiatric disturbance from a developmental perspective and that we should approach treatment from a person-centered rather than a disorder-centered perspective (Luyten et al. 2008). But reformulating our understanding of psychiatric disturbance remains a work in progress, and meanwhile we cannot discard the lens of psychiatric diagnoses, nor can we afford to ignore everything we have learned from dis-

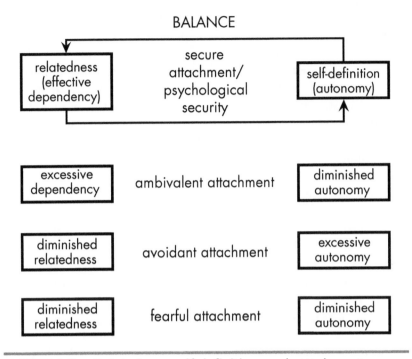

FIGURE 1–3. Relatedness, self-definition, and attachment categories.

order-centered treatments. Accordingly, I review these trauma-related disorders and treatments in the next few chapters, while keeping in mind what we've learned about relatedness and self-definition, secure and insecure attachment, and mentalizing and mindfulness. To reassert the ethical perspective, we must strive to overcome attachment trauma by creating relationships that embody a balance of love and respect. These two great moral forces, exemplified in relatedness and autonomy, form the ethical foundation for plain old therapy.

Key Points

◆ Attachment evolved not only to ensure physical protection but also to provide a feeling of security. Secure attachment is the foundation of emotion regulation. In providing a safe haven (for comfort) and a secure base (for exploration), secure attachment optimally balances the fundamental developmental dialectic of relatedness and autonomy; the securely attached child or adult is effectively dependent *and* independent.

◆ Attachment security and insecurity are maintained by internal working models of the self, the attachment figure, and the relationship. These internal models are based on patterns of infant-caregiver interactions and show a balance of stability and change over the lifetime. Secure attachment stems from the caregiver's consistent emotional responsiveness, and the typical patterns of insecure attachment are adaptive strategies to maintain attachment in the face of suboptimal care. For example, the avoidant pattern might entail deactivating attachment needs in the face of consistent rejection; the ambivalent pattern might entail hyperactivating attachment needs to elicit care in the face of inconsistent or unresponsive care.

◆ Parents' attachment proclivities are passed on to their children: extensive research demonstrates that a parent's state of mind in relation to his or her childhood attachments influences the parent's pattern of caregiving, which in turn influences the child's attachment pattern. This intergenerational pattern is influenced by the parent's mentalizing capacity; ideally, mentalizing begets mentalizing and attachment security.

◆ Attachment trauma stems from mentalizing failures: the child is left psychologically alone in unbearably painful emotional states. Abuse and neglect represent the extreme of attachment trauma, but less conspicuous disruptions of parenting, evident in hostility, helplessness, or disrupted emotional communication, also can lead to profoundly insecure (disorganized) attachment that carries a high risk of subsequent psychopathology. Such disabled caregiving stems from a failure of parental mentalizing, which also compromises the child's development of mentalizing. Hence, as mentalizing begets mentalizing (and attachment security), nonmentalizing begets nonmentalizing (and, potentially, profound insecurity).

CHAPTER 2

Posttraumatic Stress and Dissociative Disorders

This and the next two chapters cover psychiatric diagnoses related to trauma and specialized treatment approaches. In these three chapters, I'm juggling two perspectives. On the one hand, I intend to maintain the developmental, person-centered approach to understanding trauma-related disturbance established in the first chapter ("Attachment, Mentalizing, and Trauma"). This approach is consistent with my argument for the enduring value of plain old therapy. On the other hand, I want to make full use of the knowledge gained from research on trauma-related psychiatric disorders and the associated evidence-based treatments. As an advocate of plain old therapy, I am a generalist, but I'm keen to make use of whatever we generalists can learn from our specialist colleagues. As I hope to have exemplified in the first chapter, I believe that we generalists, like specialists, must ground our work in ongoing research evidence.

Yet I take a critical stance toward diagnoses, owing to the limitations associated with our efforts to categorize trauma-related disturbance. I want to dissuade people from taking diagnoses too seriously. And I want to dissuade them from the idea that we need to match a neatly tied box of symptoms to a tidy package of treatment interventions. As all clinicians who make diagnoses and patients who receive them know, symptoms are not neatly packaged. In my mind, the boxes are not well sealed; their contents spill out and intermingle; and it's often hard to figure out into which box to put the particular contents (symptoms). Symptoms don't come with labels. Also, psychiatry is continually reorganizing what symptoms go into what boxes as well as changing the boxes. Besides, many people resent being put into a box in the first place. As will become obvious in this chapter and the next, this image of difficulty finding the right boxes for widespread symptoms is particularly apt for problems in diagnosing disorders related to attachment trauma. I ask you to keep in mind a basic principle I proposed in the previous chapter: attachment trauma and disorganized attachment are *nonspecific risk factors* for psychiatric disorders; they increase the risk of a large number of psychiatric disorders rather than of any specific disorder.

I include dissociative disorders together with posttraumatic stress disorder (PTSD) in this chapter not only because attachment trauma plays such a central role in their development but also because of their overlapping symptoms. Unfortunately, attachment trauma can contribute to a wide range of psychiatric problems and disorders beyond PTSD and dissociation, and I consider these other problems in the next chapter. After reading these chapters, you should have no illusion of neatly tied boxes but rather an appreciation for the sheer diversity of trauma-related problems and the challenges in conceptualizing them. In the face of all this complexity, we need to see the forest for the trees. I use attachment theory to remain oriented.

Posttraumatic Stress Disorder

The diagnosis of PTSD came into being in the context of social controversy, and controversy persists. The significant clinical and scientific problems with the diagnosis of PTSD have implications for how treatment is viewed. Throughout this section, I discuss research on a wide range of traumatic experiences beyond those in attachment relationships because these wider experiences have greatly informed the understanding of PTSD. For example, much has been learned about PTSD from research on combat trauma. Of course, attachment trauma can set the stage for vulnerability to later trauma. Notably, this adverse developmental impact includes vulnerability to combat trauma (Bremner et al. 1993).

In this section, I summarize current research evidence to dissuade readers from equating trauma with PTSD and from viewing PTSD as a distinct illness resulting solely from exposure to traumatic stress. I take a long road, starting with long-standing controversies. I review problems in defining trauma and PTSD; discuss the unusual nature of traumatic memories and the impact of trauma on identity; and summarize evidence attesting to the complex developmental pathways to PTSD, highlighting the role of traumatic attachments and mentalizing failures. I conclude by circling back to my main agenda, the need for a person-centered approach to diagnosis. Table 2–1 provides a summary of the many areas of controversy and disagreement about PTSD that I take up in this section.

TABLE 2–1.   Controversies in diagnosing posttraumatic stress disorder (PTSD)

Social context

The creation of the PTSD diagnosis was based on social-political pressure.

Diagnosing PTSD pathologizes normal responses to stress.

Clinicians erroneously attribute symptoms to trauma.

Zealous trauma treatment generates false memories of abuse.

Diagnosing PTSD contributes to a culture of victimization and invalidism.

Diagnosing PTSD fosters malingering for purposes of compensation.

Compensation for PTSD provides an incentive to remain ill.

Defining traumatic stress

There is no bright line indicating what level of stress qualifies as traumatic.

The objective definition of traumatic stress has been criticized as too broad and too narrow.

Most persons exposed to traumatic stress do not develop PTSD.

Subjective distress goes far beyond fear to encompass a wide range of emotions.

Some persons develop the full PTSD syndrome without exposure to traumatic stress.

Some experts argue that traumatic stress exposure should be dropped from the PTSD criteria.

Diagnostic criteria

Research does not consistently support grouping symptoms into three clusters.

PTSD symptoms overlap extensively with those of other disorders.

PTSD is heterogeneous; patients with the diagnosis differ markedly from one another.

PTSD, specific symptoms, and functional impairment occur in degrees.

Experts disagree on the occurrence of delayed-onset PTSD.

Researchers debate the accuracy of traumatic memories, especially for childhood trauma.

Researchers disagree about whether traumatic memories are fragmented or exceptionally well organized.

Controversy

The history of PTSD is beset with contentiousness. Over the past 150 years, trauma—notably, childhood abuse and neglect—has come and gone from professional and public consciousness. In DSM-III in 1980 (American Psychiatric Association 1980), psychiatry officially acknowledged trauma by establishing PTSD in the diagnostic lexicon. Yet this diagnosis has brought its own controversy. Crystallizing the contention, Chris Brewin (2003) distinguished between Saviors and Skeptics. Saviors take the position that "after years of neglect, the special suffering brought about by psychological trauma has at last been recognized." Moreover, this diagnosis lessens the risk of blaming the victim, as research shows that a wide range of traumatic events "have in common a mental and physical response that is caused by the traumatic incident and *has nothing to do with any personal weakness* or vulnerability" (p. 1, emphasis added).

Powerful social and political forces antedating DSM-III pushed trauma to the forefront. War recurrently brings trauma to public attention, and antiwar sentiment associated with the Vietnam War was a political force in the recognition of trauma in DSM. Indeed, the extent of PTSD associated with the Vietnam War continues to be researched (Dohrenwend et al. 2006), and now the wars in Iraq and Afghanistan have resulted in more cases of extensive trauma—not only PTSD but also traumatic brain injury and much else. But war was hardly the only social impetus for codifying PTSD into the diagnostic system; a wide range of trauma also was being documented: battering of children (Kempe et al. 1962), childhood sexual abuse (Herman 1981), rape (Burgess and Holmstrom 1974), and battering of women (Walker 1979). For the Saviors, creating a well-defined illness was a major social achievement: an official diagnosis helps justify allocating resources needed for treatment, prevention, and research.

Amidst the controversy, no one denies the extent of suffering associated with trauma or the need to help those who suffer. Yet, as Brewin (2003) pointed out, Saviors can go overboard: "An unquestioning acceptance of the literal reality of any experience claimed to be traumatic was matched by the assumption that any symptoms should be if possible prevented, certainly treated, and at any rate compensated" (p. 222). Moreover, symptoms to which trauma *might* make a contribution, such as depression and eating disorders, could be erroneously attributed by therapists to trauma such as childhood sexual abuse—simply on the basis of symptoms that could stem from a multiplicity of causes. Not surprisingly, as Brewin put it, a moral backlash arose in response to "the new 'victim culture' in which traditional virtues of fortitude were being eroded, lawyers were encouraging people to obtain compensation they did not deserve, and therapists were conjuring up trauma that never existed" (p. 222). Hence, with the Saviors come the Skeptics.

Skeptics argued, for example, that diagnosing PTSD could pathologize or medicalize normal responses to extreme stress from which gradual recovery is to be expected. At worst, zealous clinical interventions that convey expectations of severe and chronic disorder can become a self-fulfilling prophecy and promote invalidism. Perhaps the most striking form of skepticism was the furor that erupted over false memories of childhood sexual abuse (Loftus 1993). Of course, ostensibly false memories must be distinguished from false reports and false accusations, which also occur in relation to childhood trauma. Although painful for patients, affected family members, and therapists, the uproar about the validity of memories of childhood trauma had the salutary effect of bringing research-informed balance to the field. Now, a great deal more is known about conditions that impair or distort memory for trauma, especially in the earliest years. Yet there is also robust evidence for the alarming prevalence of trauma as well as evidence for the global accuracy of memories of trauma. Hence, in the midst of the controversy, I concluded that the extent of patently false memories remains uncertain, but the extent of trauma is glaringly evident (Allen 1995). The attachment research reviewed in the first chapter attests to that fact.

Saviors and Skeptics alike can be zealots. But Brewin (2003) also made the compelling point that to advance, the field requires both Saviors and Skeptics (in moderation). Science is founded on a combination of passion and skepticism, and both are important to the understanding and treatment of trauma: "The field of traumatic stress therefore provides an almost unrivaled opportunity for assessing the extent to which scientific research is able to settle enduring controversies between the Saviors and Skeptics and produce original insights into the processes responsible for human suffering" (p. 3). As reviewed next, the diagnosis of PTSD has provided much impetus for research.

Definition of Trauma

The word *trauma* is used ambiguously to refer to exposure to potentially traumatic (i.e., extremely stressful) *events* and to the traumatic *effects* of such exposure (i.e., in the sense of having been *traumatized*). We treat effects, not events. PTSD is well named, referring to a disorder that develops in the aftermath of traumatic stress; indeed, PTSD is evidence that the stress was *traumatic*. Yet, while effects are the primary concern of therapists, exposure to events is included in the current diagnostic criteria, and stress exposure is the one diagnostic criterion that most clearly sets PTSD apart from other diagnoses. I believe we therapists must take seriously the challenges in deciding what constitutes "trauma," because our patients often have a narrow view (e.g., sexual abuse, rape, combat trauma). This narrow view obscures their vision of their development. From the perspective of attachment trauma, the DSM criteria perpetuate this narrow vision. Thus, the full extent of the definitional problems warrants the attention of therapists and patients alike.

There is ample room for disagreement about what level of stress counts as being potentially "traumatic." In DSM-IV-TR, the potentially traumatic stressors are defined objectively and subjectively. Objectively, in Criterion A1, traumatic stress is defined as

> involving direct personal experience of an event that involves actual or threatened *death* or serious *injury*, or other threat to one's *physical* integrity; or witnessing an event that involves death, injury, or a threat to the physical integrity of another person; or learning about unexpected or violent death, serious harm, or threat of death or injury experienced by a family member or other close associate. (American Psychiatric Association 2000, p. 463, emphasis added)

Subjectively, Criterion A2 specifies, "the person's response involved intense fear, helplessness, or horror" (American Psychiatric Association 2000, p. 467). Both objective and subjective stressor criteria have come in for substantial criticism from the scientific community.

As my focus on attachment trauma implies, I think the DSM focus on physical threat is too narrow: psychological abuse (e.g., being sadistically tormented, terrorized, humiliated) can be profoundly damaging (Bifulco et al. 2002), as can psychological neglect (Erickson and Egeland 1996). Underscoring the significance of psychological threat, Emily Holmes and colleagues (Grey and Holmes 2008; Holmes et al. 2005b) investigated the experience of threat associated with exposure to traumatic events by studying the content of intrusive memories and hotspots within these memories. *Hotspots* are "specific parts of the trauma memory that cause high levels of emotional distress, that may be difficult to recall to mind deliberately, and that are associated with intense reliving of the trauma" (Holmes et al. 2005b, p. 5). A hotspot might include the moment the door was locked for a child confined in a dark closet or the first sight of the knife for a woman who was raped.

As the researchers expected, the vast majority of intrusive memories are associated with hotspots (e.g., being pinned down and unable to move, feeling helpless and vulnerable). Of relevance to understanding the nature of threat, however, Holmes and colleagues systematically identified the core psychological themes in the traumatic experiences. Consistent with DSM criteria, fear of injury and death were prominent themes. Yet *the majority of themes related to psychological threat*—that is, to the victim's sense of self. Moreover, within the domain of psychological threat, prominent themes related to Sidney Blatt's (2008) polarities of relatedness and self-definition. That is, one theme related to abandonment (e.g., being let down and feeling outraged), and another theme related to self-esteem (e.g., self-blame and criticism). Although these two themes might be prominent in anyone's experience, feelings of abandonment might be especially characteristic in conjunction with ambivalent attachment, whereas self-criticism might be highlighted in the context of avoidant attachment.

Failing to arrive at satisfactory objective criteria for what constitutes traumatic stress, we therapists might see the extent of trauma as being in the eye of the beholder and focus on the individual's subjective experience. Yet the subjective criterion also has come in for criticism. The focus on fear is too narrow, excluding a host of emotions that also contribute to PTSD, including shame, guilt, anger, sadness, surprise, and disgust (Brewin 2003). In their research on the content of intrusive memories and hotspots, Holmes and colleagues (2005) tallied the frequencies of different emotions experienced in the midst of trauma. Consistent with DSM, fear was by far the most prominently experienced emotion. Yet collectively, fear, helplessness, and horror proportionately comprised only half the emotions; the other emotions just listed were included in the rest—along with positive emotions (e.g., relief when out of danger). Needless to say, for those who have experienced traumatic stress and those who aspire to help them, subjective experience means everything—DSM notwithstanding. I agree completely with Meaghan O'Donnell and colleagues (2010): *"the bottom line is that our patients do not really care how we define Criterion A in the DSM; they are concerned only with the distress they experience and the impact this distress is having on their social and occupational functioning"* (p. 67, emphasis added).

There are two additional glaring problems in trying to relate a certain level of traumatic stress to the syndrome of PTSD. First, despite the fact that the majority of men and women have been exposed to potentially traumatic events in their lifetime, only a small minority (5%–10%) have a history of PTSD (Kessler et al. 1995). Second, the symptom cluster of PTSD is sometimes evident in the absence of objectively defined traumatic events. The entire PTSD syndrome has been observed in relation to common stressors such as family or romantic relationship problems, occupational stress, parental divorce, and serious illness or death of a loved one (Gold et al. 2005). Mary Long and colleagues (2008) found that with some assessment methods, participants reported *higher* levels of PTSD symptoms in response to more ordinary stressors than to traumatic stressors. Notably, the most frequently chosen ordinary stressors related to attachment: the breakup of a romantic relationship or the sudden death of a loved one.

Notwithstanding the foregoing, we therapists have reason to be concerned about the severity of stress, however we define it; robust evidence exists for a dose-response relationship: the more severe the stressor, the greater the likelihood of the person's developing PTSD (Friedman et al. 2007). I view the efforts in DSM to draw a bright line between traumatic and nontraumatic stress with a combination of admiration and amusement. Ambiguity reigns. Accordingly, some authors have proposed dropping the stress-exposure criteria altogether (Brewin et al. 2009). Plainly, defined objectively (observable events) or subjectively (emotional distress), stress and trauma lie along a continuum. As my colleague Chris Frueh and coworkers contend, "the assumption that exposure to life-threatening stressors is the primary cause of a *unique* set of stress response symptoms is highly problematic and represents a disconnection from and failure to incorporate the larger body of general stress literature" (Frueh et al. 2010, p. 263, emphasis in original). In the long run, we may learn more from more nuanced assessments of stressful events that go beyond identifying some arbitrary cutoff point of severity and seek to determine what kinds and combinations of stressful events lead to what kinds of symptoms and disorders (Dohrenwend 2010). Meanwhile, we clinicians must aspire to clarify the history of stress and its impact on each individual's development. Next, I make a similar argument in relation to the syndrome of PTSD.

Definition of PTSD

The question "What is PTSD?" is remarkably difficult to answer and requires walking the reader through a series of complications. To start, I summarize the current diagnostic criteria for PTSD, then present alternative ways of arranging symptoms and mention new symptoms being considered for introduction in DSM-5. Next, I introduce the challenge of distinguishing PTSD from its close cousin, or perhaps its fraternal or identical twin, depression. Finally, I come back to the alternative of thinking in terms of degrees of problems rather than categories, which throws into question the idea of PTSD as a distinct illness.

DSM-IV-TR (American Psychiatric Association 2000) lists the first symptom of PTSD as persistent reexperiencing of the traumatic event, which may take several forms: intrusive images, thoughts, or perceptions;

recurrent dreams; a feeling of reliving the event as in flashbacks; intense distress at exposure to reminders; and physiological reactivity to exposure to reminders. For example, a woman who was terrorized in childhood by her mother's enraged tirades can panic when she hears a mother berating her child in a department store. In my view, there is a poignant cruelty to these reexperiencing symptoms: the person not only suffers through the stressful events in the first place but then continues to be exposed to the stress in her mind thereafter. These symptoms add insult to injury: the brain and body are assaulted by stress stemming from memories as well as the original events. Moreover, going to sleep may provide no respite but rather may be frightening when nightmares are in the offing.

Two remaining DSM-IV-TR criteria for PTSD are avoidance and hyperarousal. The *avoidance* criteria include not only avoiding activities, people, or places that arouse memories of trauma (situational avoidance) but also avoiding thoughts, feelings, or conversations about the trauma (experiential avoidance). Lumped in with these avoidance criteria are several others that involve *numbing* of emotional responsiveness: inability to recall aspects of the trauma, feelings of detachment, loss of interest in activities, restricted range of emotion or emotional numbing, and a sense of a foreshortened future. The *hyperarousal* criteria include two that are more specific to trauma—that is, hypervigilance (excessive alertness to threat) and exaggerated startle—and three that are characteristic of anxiety and high levels of arousal more generally—namely, problems falling or staying asleep, irritability, and difficulty concentrating.

We are now in a position to address the problem of putting the symptoms into boxes within boxes. Through statistical means, researchers have investigated the extent to which the 17 PTSD symptoms fall into the three clusters distinguished in DSM-IV (i.e., reexperiencing, avoidance, and hyperarousal). However, the symptoms don't readily group into these clusters. For example, avoidance, a relatively deliberate coping strategy to block the eruption of symptoms, is distinct from numbing, a more automatic blunting of emotional distress (Asmundson et al. 2004). Moreover, recent research with survivors of domestic violence suggests an additional symptom cluster intermingling anxiety and depression (Elhai et al. 2011a). As it currently stands, DSM-5 is headed toward incorporating a large cluster of symptoms beyond reexperiencing, avoidance, and hyperarousal; these include inability to remember aspects of the events; negative expectations about the self, others, and world; blame of self or others; negative emotions such as fear, horror, anger, guilt, or shame; diminished interest in activities; feelings of detachment; and inability to experience positive emotions, including psychic numbing. This expansion will keep the statisticians busy sorting out the sortings.

In addition to having problems defining the syndrome of PTSD, we have reason to question the extent to which PTSD is distinct from other disorders: not only do its symptoms overlap with those of other disorders, but also PTSD frequently is diagnosed alongside other disorders with which its symptoms are intertwined. Depression is a prime example of overlap, as evident in three ways: First, many patients who are diagnosed with PTSD also are diagnosed with depression. Second, painful intrusive memories and images are not only characteristic of PTSD but also common in depression (Brewin et al. 1999). Third, and perhaps most surprising, depression is *more common* as a trauma-related disorder than PTSD (Bryant 2010). To investigate this overlap, Jon Elhai and colleagues (2011b) studied co-occurring symptoms of PTSD and major depression in a large national sample of persons with a history of trauma exposure. These researchers found strong evidence for *one major factor,* combining symptoms of PTSD and depression, within which symptoms could be arrayed on a scale of severity. For example, intrusive thoughts and efforts to avoid them were at the lower end of severity (i.e., least frequently endorsed); flashbacks and impaired recall were in the middle range; and severe depression was at the high end, with thoughts of death and worthlessness toward the top. Notably, the inclusion of mood symptoms and negative cognitions in the DSM-5 draft criteria is likely to increase the overlap of PTSD and depression.

As this review attests, like the rest of medicine, DSM is based on categories—boxes, in my metaphor. A person either has or hasn't been exposed to "traumatic" stress. The person either has PTSD or doesn't. Yet general medical conditions also allow for degrees. Diseases like cancer and diabetes can be graded in severity, and symptoms like hypertension are measured in gradations. Akin to physicians measuring hypertension, we psychologists tend to measure everything in degrees—intelligence being a prime example. We construct scales to measure everything we can imagine, and we have a multitude of scales to measure common problems such as PTSD (Keane et al. 2007). Like stress, symptom severity is a matter of degree. Moreover, to qualify for a diagnosis of *disorder,* symptoms not only must be present but also must be associated with clinically significant levels of distress or impairment in functioning (e.g., preventing a person from maintaining a household or adequately performing a job). All these are matters of degree with no clear cutoff points. And degrees are important: for example, patients with significant symptoms of PTSD but too few to meet the diagnostic cutoff point show significant functional impairment yet may not be identified as needing treatment (Grubaugh et al. 2005).

Such considerations argue for a dimensional approach (Friedman et al. 2007) in which PTSD would be regarded not as a qualitatively different response to stress but rather as the upper end of a stress response spectrum (Broman-Fulks et al. 2006). This proposal applies to traumatic memories as well as other symptoms. This is a crucial point because, aside from exposure to traumatic events, the reexperiencing cluster of symptoms most distinguishes PTSD from related disorders (Brewin et al. 2009). Moreover, among traumatic memories, flashbacks are most distinctive of PTSD (Brewin 2011), particularly insofar as they entail the experience of reliving past trauma in the present. Flashbacks represent the most extreme form of nonmentalizing—namely, psychic equivalence (taking mental states as real). Treatment of PTSD helps patients move from psychic equivalence (reliving trauma as if it were happening in the present) to mentalizing (recognizing intrusive symptoms as memories while feeling safe in the present).

Given the extensive overlap of PTSD with other disorders, Brewin and colleagues (2009) have proposed that the criteria for PTSD be narrowed to make the syndrome relatively distinctive. They would eliminate the stress-exposure criteria, confine the intrusive symptoms (flashbacks and nightmares) to those that evoke fear, limit the avoidance criteria to active efforts to avoid reminders, and include only the hyperarousal criteria most related to trauma (hypervigilance and startle). This narrowing would better distinguish PTSD from depression. Nonetheless, the authors recognize that PTSD by no means captures the entire effects of exposure to traumatic stress, and that it will likely be diagnosed alongside a number of other conditions such as dissociation, depression, substance abuse, and other anxiety disorders.

Rather than proposing seemingly arbitrary cutoff points to put people in boxes, we might aspire to measure separately the nature and severity of stressful events to which they have been exposed, the severity of their various symptoms, and the extent of associated impairment. But don't hold your breath; all of us find it easier to deal with categories than to think of various points on a series of lines or to plot a point in multidimensional space—especially a space with four or more dimensions. As I discussed in the first chapter, attachment researchers have debated the same contrast between categories (secure versus different types of insecure) and dimensions (degrees of closeness and anxiety). We'll always use categories, but we shouldn't take them too literally.

Delayed-Onset PTSD

Nothing about PTSD is without controversy. Brewin (2011) distinguished four basic patterns in the course of PTSD after exposure to traumatic events: 1) *resilient*, with a low level of symptoms throughout; 2) *recovery*, with significant initial symptoms that diminish over time;

3) *chronic*, with symptoms starting at a high level and remaining so; and 4) *delayed onset*, with symptoms starting at a low level and then increasing later. The delayed-onset pattern is controversial, and some researchers propose that it is rare and may be a reflection of delayed help-seeking rather than delayed illness (Spitzer et al. 2007). Also contributing to the controversy is the concern that delayed-onset PTSD is an artifact of misguided memory-recovery therapy. Prototypically, in the misguided treatment scenario, a therapist erroneously attributes a common symptom (e.g., anxiety about sexual intimacy) to repressed childhood sexual abuse; potentially suggestive memory retrieval techniques (e.g., ill-informed use of hypnosis) lead the patient to begin constructing false memories and beliefs about being abused; and these memories evolve into PTSD. Patients and therapists must be mindful of such scenarios but should be careful not to overrate their frequency. Many factors bring traumatic memories to mind long after the traumatic events—inside or outside of therapy— and remembering trauma often is accompanied by a great deal of emotional upheaval along with a variety of symptoms (D. Brown et al. 1998).

A review of research (Andrews et al. 2007) revealed that delayed-onset PTSD isn't rare; it occurs in 15% of civilian and 38% of military cases of PTSD. But there's an important caveat here: going from no symptoms to meeting full PTSD criteria is rare indeed, whereas *gradual* escalation of symptoms into full-blown PTSD is not. Accordingly, a careful study of the development of delayed-onset PTSD (B. Andrews et al. 2009) in combat veterans suggests that there's nothing mysterious about it. Symptoms of anxiety (hyperarousal) begin developing gradually, even *before* exposure to the major traumatic event. Compared with those who develop PTSD immediately and are apparently overwhelmed at the time, those with delayed-onset PTSD are less likely to experience dissociation, anger, and shame around the time of the trauma. The delayed-onset group, however, reported higher levels of depression and alcohol abuse. Moreover, prior to the delayed onset of PTSD, they were likely to have experienced severe life stress unrelated to combat. The authors concluded, "the delayed-onset type is characteristic of individuals who develop general stress responses in a cumulative fashion rather than characteristic of those who are overwhelmed by a single traumatic experience" (p. 775). Notably, this cumulative stress ultimately leads to reexperiencing the combat trauma, memories of which had previously been held at bay. Analogously, I have worked with many patients whose stress pileup began with attachment trauma in childhood and culminated in severe depression in adulthood, opening the door to PTSD in the form of intrusive memories of childhood trauma—which the patients' stressful lifestyle had kept at bay.

Traumatic Memory

PTSD has a notoriously all-or-none quality. For example, overwhelming emotions with intrusive memories alternate with emotional numbing and life-constricting avoidance. A similar all-or-none quality relates to a paradoxical combination of too much memory and too little memory (van der Kolk 1994). This combination is included in the DSM criteria, which include intrusive memories along with amnesia for aspects of trauma. With the combination of too much and too little, it's no wonder that patients are confused about their traumatic memories—and lack of memory. The research literature on traumatic memory is mind-bogglingly complex. But patients and therapists need some rudimentary understanding to guide treatment.

I begin by using Edna Foa's work to make the simple point that intrusive traumatic memories are problematic owing to their poor fit with current reality. Then I use Brewin's proposal on different types of memory to sort out the too-much versus too-little paradox. Brewin's work also helps resolve the debate between those who believe traumatic memories are fragmented and those who regard them as excessively organized. This debate sets the stage for the impact of trauma on identity, which I take up in the next subsection (Identity).

Foa proposed a straightforward account of traumatic memory as it relates to PTSD (Foa et al. 2007). Plainly, we need to learn what has hurt us in the past so as to avoid it in the future. We're well equipped to do so but are liable to go overboard in this regard when we're utterly terrified. As Foa and colleagues (2007) wrote, on the basis of our experience and memory we develop *cognitive fear structures* that enable us to escape danger: "The fear structure includes representations of the feared stimuli (e.g., bear), the fear responses (e.g., heart rate acceleration), and the meaning associated with the stimuli (e.g., bears are dangerous) and responses (e.g., fast heartbeat means I am afraid)" (p. 12). Normal fear structures are based on realistic threats, and they serve as guides for action. PTSD is associated with maladaptive fear structures that do not accurately represent threat; harmless stimuli (e.g., the mother berating her child in the department store) are perceived as threatening, and they evoke excessive physiological and emotional arousal (e.g., panic) as well as maladaptive escape and avoidance responses (e.g., rushing out of the store).

Pointing out that a traumatized person is "overreacting," as frustrated caregivers may be inclined to do, only antagonizes the person, to whom this is all too obvious. My colleague Kay Kelly came up with a handy alternative, the "90-10 response." We use this phrase in educating patients

(Lewis et al. 2004): 10% of the emotion comes from the present (harm-less stimulus), and 90% comes from the past (traumatic events). Of course, these percentages are arbitrary and the proportions vary. We present this 90-10 response as a consequence of having become *sensitized* by virtue of traumatic levels of stress—that is, more reactive to lesser degrees of stress over time (Griffin 2008). Presented in the context of sensitization, patients find the idea of the 90-10 response more palatable than "overreacting." In educating patients, I find it helpful to contrast sensitization with *de*sensitization, in which *gradual* exposure to increasing levels of stress over time lessens reactivity. For example, a person can overcome a phobia of dogs by exposure to small and gentle dogs, working his way up to larger and potentially more intimidating dogs—provided that he doesn't get bitten in the process. In contrast to this desensitizing process, traumatic stress is anything but gradual; it is extreme as well as uncontrollable and unpredictable. Accordingly, instead of telling patients that they're making mountains out of molehills, I point out that there is a real mountain in the past and that their sensitized nervous system inclines them to react to molehills as mountains. They need to learn through treatment to mentalize in the sense of distinguishing molehills from mountains.

Foa's theory addresses the maladaptive nature of traumatic memory but does not account for the paradoxical combination of too much and too little memory. Brewin (2011) proposed a *dual-representation* theory, based on a long-standing distinction between explicit (declarative-verbal) and implicit (nondeclarative, perceptual-motor) memory. As discussed in the first chapter, I applied this implicit-explicit distinction from memory research to different levels of internal working models and mentalizing.

Along these lines, Brewin distinguishes explicit, *verbally* accessible memory from implicit, *situationally* accessible memory. When people think of memory, most have in mind explicit, verbally accessible memories, which take the form of narrative or stories. Such memories also have been called personal event memories (Pillemer 1998). Your friend sees you upset, asks what happened, and you tell her. You can retrieve these memories deliberately as needed, and they're integrated with your autobiographical memory and identity as a whole. Yet your capacity to establish such coherent memories can be undermined at times of traumatic stress.

In the midst of traumatic stress, someone may have difficulty constructing elaborate verbal memories, yet simultaneously be able to establish highly durable situationally accessible memories. These situational memories are the stuff of flashbacks, which occur with a sense of reliving the trauma. Rather than being deliberately recalled, flashbacks are triggered involuntarily by situational reminders. These nonverbal memories take the form of sensory-perceptual images, including not only sights (e.g., a looming, shadowy figure), sounds (e.g., a slamming door), and smells (e.g., alcohol), but also body sensations (e.g., pain). As noted earlier in this chapter (see section Definition of Trauma), these intrusive memories typically pertain to the hotspots or worst moments of the experience.

Naturally, PTSD sufferers learn to avoid thoughts and situations that trigger flashbacks. Yet avoidance inevitably fails; it is impossible to avoid being blindsided by reminders (e.g., an unexpected assault scene in a movie). Moreover, efforts to suppress memories backfire by worsening PTSD symptoms (Brewin 2011). In my view, the sheer ineffectiveness of experiential avoidance is a major reason for learning to think, feel, and talk about traumatic experience—that is, to mentalize rather than relive the experience.

We humans not only perceive far more than we can translate into language but also register unconsciously far more than we can attend to consciously. We automatically direct attention to the immediate source of threat (e.g., the gun, knife, fist, or enraged expression) to the exclusion of more peripheral details (e.g., the red shirt or cologne); nevertheless, we may encode these extraneous details in situational memory—and situational memory can be triggered by later exposure to these unattended details (Brewin 2005). The upshot can be a combination of too much memory—unconsciously and involuntarily triggered images and sensations coupled with overwhelming fear—and too little memory—inability to relate such images to a coherent autobiographical narrative. Accordingly, some memories for traumatic events are described as *fragmented*: isolated images that cannot be integrated into a meaningful personal event memory that fits into an autobiography. In this context, traumatic memories can be profoundly confusing. To make matters worse, traumatized persons are unable to communicate to others the reasons for their behavior—for example, being curled up into a ball in a corner or closet in a state of terror in conjunction with a vague image of a looming figure.

The prospect of translating fragmented, emotion-laden images into coherent narratives is fraught with the peril of *confabulation*—that is, imaginatively filling in memory gaps with plausible but inaccurate narratives, complete with images to match. Confabulation isn't confined to trauma; given normal limitations of memory, we're all liable to confabulate to varying degrees. Therapists' concern with confabulation arises particularly in conjunction with potentially suggestive memory-recovery techniques, such as guided imagery, dream interpretation, and the ill-informed use of hypnosis. In the worst-case scenario, patients may confabulate memories that are compatible with therapists' erroneous

assumptions about a traumatic basis for symptoms. Accordingly, therapists are counseled wisely "to concentrate treatment efforts on a patient's
memory *as it exists*" (Geraerts 2010, p. 82, emphasis added). My advice to
therapists and patients is simple but not easy: keep an open mind, tolerate
not knowing, and don't force it. *Work with what you know.* It's not uncommon for patients to be focused on vague memories or suspicions of
childhood sexual abuse while minimizing blatantly traumatic experiences
that they remember clearly (e.g., a combination of terrifying parental
fights, painful emotional neglect, bullying, and sexual assaults in adolescence).

Yet controversy reigns here as elsewhere. Dorthe Berntsen and colleagues take issue with the idea that traumatic memories are fragmented;
on the contrary, they propose that trauma is remembered all too well.
That is, traumatic memories are excessively processed and firmly en-
sconced in autobiographical memory. These memories become *landmarks*
in the autobiography: the traumatic memory "may be too dominant in the
organization of the life-story" (Berntsen et al. 2003, p. 679). That is, the
trauma becomes central in the life story—self-defining. These researchers
found that greater centrality of the traumatic event in the autobiography
was associated with more severe PTSD symptoms (Berntsen and Rubin
2007). Thus, they cautioned that reconstructing a life story centered on
trauma, as therapists and patients might be inclined to do, could be maladaptive. We therapists need to help patients construct more complex
narratives that give due weight to their strengths, successes, and resilience
and to relationships that involved trust and islands of security.

I worked with a patient who exemplified Berntsen's view dramatically. He had had all the symptoms of PTSD for over a decade, and this
was noteworthy because his landmark traumatic memory—which
formed the core of his identity—was *not* traumatic in the physically inju-
rious sense entailed by DSM criteria.

Case Example

Greg was hospitalized in his early 30s after his depression became inca-
pacitating. He felt utterly worthless. This feeling had deep roots: throughout much of his adolescence, his mother had compared him cruelly to his
father, for whom she expressed nothing but contempt. His mother had
dominated his father, who was passive, submissive, and depressed. She
told Greg that he was just like his father—for example, a "wuss" and a
"wimp" who would never amount to anything. His older brother, who was
physically strong, aggressive, and comparatively headstrong, was her favorite. Greg's slight build and more anxious, inhibited nature worked
against him. In high school he remained in his brother's shadow among his
peers; his brother was admired as a "jock."

Greg, like his father, was relatively introverted, showing aesthetic and intellectual interests. He buried himself in books. He excelled in school, which mattered little to his mother, who prized more "manly" pursuits. Greg looked forward to college and was delighted when he won an academic scholarship that allowed him to go away to school. He hoped he would find acceptance among more mature and academically oriented peers, and he did so for a time. He was delighted when he was accepted into a fraternity known for its academic leanings. But he suffered a major setback during a routine hazing ritual during which a relatively burly upperclassman berated and intimidated him; he was blindsided by an anxiety attack, lost control of his bladder, was laughed at by his peers, and felt utterly humiliated.

Greg withdrew from the fraternity and remained socially isolated, with the crucial exception of finding a devoted girlfriend, whose support helped him to finish college and graduate with honors. He and his girlfriend married after graduation; thereafter, he became a teacher and was well liked by his students. Yet all the while, he was haunted by intrusive memories of his fraternity brothers' hazing, with the image of his burly upperclassman's taunting never far from his mind. This experience confirmed his mother's view: he was a wimp. His feelings of humiliation were intertwined with fantasies of revenge, and he was mired in ruminations. Moreover, he frequently came into conflict with his female department head, whom he characterized as perfectionistic, critical, and bossy. He felt shamed and infuriated by her continual "hazing." In his mind, she became an amalgam of his earlier tormentors, his mother and the upperclassman. He was afraid to challenge or confront her for fear of losing his job, but his submissiveness only confirmed his feeling of being a wimp and added fuel to his resentment. But his torment was not confined to the memories of hazing or his superior's criticism; any slight or rudeness rankled him, particularly if he didn't stand up for himself.

As Greg's anxiety and depression increased, his performance at work deteriorated, further escalating the conflict with his department head. When he was at home, he tried to bury himself in one hobby after another to block the traumatic images and prevent himself from ruminating. These efforts were somewhat effective in suppressing intrusive memories, but they also led to his isolation from his wife. As he became more withdrawn, she became more frustrated. She was utterly bewildered by his preoccupation with the hazing experience and his department head, which overshadowed all his talents and accomplishments. Her reassurance carried no weight.

Greg's traumatic experience as a college freshman crystallized his identity and shaped his subsequent experience—not only his difficult relationship with his department head, which consumed much of his attention at work, but also his reactions to seemingly innocuous events, such as someone cutting ahead of him in line at the movie theater. Sadly, he had lived with depression and symptoms of PTSD for a decade without seeking treatment. Once he recognized the potential benefits of treatment, he put his energy into making use of it. He found the concept of mentalizing to be illuminating, enabling him to be more aware of his ruminative thought processes and their detrimental impact on his mood. He made use of mindfulness in becoming less entangled with intrusive images and vengeful fantasies. In tandem, he recognized that he'd given short shrift to his healthy relationships; he redirected his focus from traumatic relationships to his relationship with his wife as well as that with a close friend, a relationship he'd let slide as he became more depressed.

Greg's memory for the painful hazing experience was not fuzzy or fragmented; it was vivid and clear. It was indeed a developmental landmark that organized his subsequent experience: he could recount innumerable painful, intrusive memories of embarrassing submission. For others, however, whose traumatic experience is more terrifying or horrifying, the memory problems are more complex. Having fragmented memories does not exclude a life defined by trauma. To reconcile this seeming contradiction, Brewin (2011) proposes a third form of memory, in addition to verbal and sensory memory: *conceptual knowledge* concerning the self. As Brewin points out, it is possible to know that one has been traumatized in various ways—sexually abused as a child, for example— while being haunted by intrusive images and unable to remember details or to elaborate a meaningful narrative. This conceptual knowledge, in the form of a general memory of being abused, can play the role of a landmark memory, organizing identity and subsequent experience—for example, a life of isolation centered on a pervasive feeling of shame associated with a sense of self as dirty, disgusting, and degraded.

Plainly, traumatic memories take many forms, and many traumatic memories are not distinct from other memories associated with strong emotions. Yet, as Brewin's (2011) research has made clear, *in the context of PTSD* we're liable to see an amalgam of limited detail in verbal accounts of the events, intrusive images that come to mind unbidden, and identity formed around general knowledge of having been traumatized or victimized. Notwithstanding skeptics, fragmentation and disorganization of traumatic memories has been well demonstrated in careful research (Jelinek et al. 2009). However, well-organized memories based on general knowledge of a trauma history also can play a powerful role in trauma. As Greg's experience exemplifies, this development is especially problematic when such memories are established in the context of attachment relationships early in life: these memories form internal working models of self and others that can influence subsequent experience over much of a lifetime.

Identity

As just discussed, trauma can shape—or misshape—identity, and the impact of trauma on the self has been a major focus of treatment. In the framework of attachment theory, trauma shapes internal working models that include thoughts and feelings about the self, others, and relationships. Thus, trauma colors the sense of self and the sense of self-in-the-world. Ronnie Janoff-Bulman (1992) proposed that trauma shatters three fundamental assumptions: the world is benevolent, the world is meaningful, and the self is worthy. With trauma, the world can be viewed as dangerous and malevolent as well as meaningless, and the self can be viewed as worthless. In a similar vein, Foa and colleagues (2007) highlight two basic trauma-related beliefs that perpetuate PTSD: "The world is entirely dangerous," and "I am completely incompetent to cope with it" (p. 14).

Yet incompetence can be a gross understatement of the impact of attachment trauma on the self. Here are some examples from patients I have worked with: "I'm a dirty little whore," "a freak," "tainted and used garbage," "an inhuman monster that repulses everyone," "evil," "the anti-Christ," and "nonexistent" (Allen 2001, p. 91). For such patients with a lifelong history of trauma, traumatic events don't shatter benign assumptions but rather reinforce and strengthen long-held negative assumptions (Cahill and Foa 2007). According to Brewin (2003), "trauma does not have to shatter illusions when they have been shattered already" (p. 66).

Trauma aside, the unity of the self is a matter of degree. Typically, our self-concept is a hodgepodge of positive and negative attributes, although trauma and depression can bring the negatives into the foreground such that they obliterate the positives. Also, our sense of self changes with our moods and in different situations and social roles. Most important, as attachment theory attests, we develop a sense of self in relationships, and our working model of self varies from one relationship to another. Brewin (2003) offers a metaphor for the impact of trauma on the self that allows for far more complexity than a wholesale shattering of assumptions:

> This approach to identity rejects the simple idea of a monolithic structure that is flattened by trauma and has to be rebuilt. Identity may instead be thought of as more akin to an area of sand dunes that stands in the path of a tornado. When the tornado has passed, the configuration of the dunes will be different, with some being larger and others smaller than they were before.... While it will never be possible to restore the dunes exactly to the way they were before, there are opportunities to rebuild dunes that have been moved or destroyed and to level sand that has accumulated in unwanted places. (p. 86)

Brewin's metaphor regards identity as akin to continually shifting sands. Experiences of attachment trauma are like recurrent storms ranging in severity from stiff winds to overcast skies, menacing clouds, thunderstorms, hurricanes, tsunamis, and tornadoes—intermingled with periods of respite and clear weather with safe havens from the storms. The shifting sands represent shifting security in relationships and corresponding shifts in the sense of self and others.

Causes of PTSD

The obvious answer to the question of what causes PTSD is traumatic stress; however, this answer is surprisingly misleading. The partial truth in this answer fits with the well-documented dose-response relationship: the more severe and recurrent the stress, the greater the likelihood of PTSD. Yet, as I discussed earlier in this chapter (see section Definition of Trauma), there is a loose coupling between severity of stress and extent of trauma, and this looseness is consistent with highly complex developmental pathways eventuating in PTSD. The likelihood of developing PTSD is based on a host of vulnerability factors that can be separated in time: those that occur before, during, and after the traumatic stress. Table 2–2 provides an overview of these key contributors to the development of PTSD.

First, attesting to developmental vulnerability, a multitude of *pre-trauma* factors confer risk for PTSD. Genetic risk is twofold: risk for exposure to potentially traumatic events and risk for developing PTSD after exposure (Segman et al. 2007). For example, genetic factors can influence the likelihood of engaging in risky, impulsive, or reckless behavior that leads some persons to put themselves in harm's way. Notoriously, for example, substance abuse increases the risk of assault. In addition, genetic factors can contribute to distress proneness, which can increase the impact of traumatic events; temperamental anxiety acts like an amplifier for stress. In addition, gender bears a complex role in risk for PTSD (Kimerling et al. 2007). Men are more likely to be exposed to traumatic events, but women are more likely to develop PTSD after exposure. Also, gender and type of trauma exposure are intermingled. Women are more likely to be exposed to high-risk traumas such as sexual abuse and assault; moreover, such trauma often occurs repeatedly in attachment relationships—namely, in childhood sexual abuse or in violent relationships with an intimate partner in adulthood.

Beyond genetics and gender, many other developmental factors predispose a person to PTSD: young age at exposure, lower socioeconomic and educational levels, low intelligence, personal and family psychiatric history, impaired family functioning, and prior trauma exposure—most notably, when child abuse increases vulnerability to later trauma (Vogt et al. 2007). Moreover, as discussed in the first chapter, disorganized attachment in infancy renders children who are exposed to subsequent trauma more vulnerable to symptoms of PTSD.

TABLE 2–2.	Potential contributors to the development of posttraumatic stress disorder

Pretrauma factors

Genetic predisposition to engage in impulsive and risky behavior

Genetic predisposition to high levels of anxiety and distress

Being female

Disorganized attachment

Young age at exposure to trauma

History of prior trauma

Lower levels of socioeconomic status, education, intelligence

Personal or family history of psychiatric disorder

Impaired family functioning

Social disruption (loss, changing parental figures, changing residence)

Substance abuse

Antisocial behavior

Peritrauma factors

Objective severity of stress

Subjective level of emotional distress

Dissociation around the time of exposure to traumatic stress

Posttrauma factors

Continuing stressors

Lack of social and emotional support

Many studies on early experiences associated with PTSD are retrospective. For example, adults with PTSD or depression are asked about their childhood experiences in the family. Researchers raise concern that current symptoms influence what one remembers; someone who is depressed is more likely to remember painful experiences. Thus, we are on most solid ground with prospective longitudinal studies. Because longitudinal research on PTSD is extremely rare, the Dunedin, New Zealand, study in which participants were carefully assessed at multiple intervals from birth to age 32 is particularly valuable (Koenen et al. 2007). One set of risk factors is associated with the likelihood of trauma exposure; these factors include difficult temperament, antisocial behavior, hyperactivity, maternal distress, and loss of a parent in childhood. A second (somewhat overlapping) set of risk factors is associated with the likelihood of developing PTSD after exposure; these factors include low intelligence, difficult temperament, antisocial behavior, unpopularity, change of parental figures, multiple changes of residency, and maternal distress. Consistent with extensive developmental research, a cascade was plainly apparent: an accumulation of different categories of risk factors most powerfully predicted PTSD.

In addition to pretrauma factors, experiences around the time of the trauma—*peritrauma* factors—also play a role in the development of PTSD. As stated earlier, subjective responses of fear influence the likelihood of developing PTSD. Thus, the fact that women report substantially more distress than men in the midst of traumatic events may contribute to the gender difference in PTSD (Kimerling et al. 2007). Most notably, dissociative responses in the midst of trauma exposure and its immediate aftermath have been identified in numerous studies as a significant risk factor for subsequent PTSD, and one review found peritraumatic dissociation to be more strongly predictive of PTSD than a range of pretrauma and posttrauma factors (Ozer et al. 2003). I discuss reasons for this correspondence in the following section on dissociative disorders.

Underscoring the crucial role of mentalizing in attachment relationships, Brewin (2003) concluded, "What happens *after a trauma* has been shown consistently to have the *biggest impact* on whether a person develops PTSD" (p. 56, emphasis added). Not surprisingly, one prominent posttrauma risk factor is ongoing stress in the aftermath of the traumatic event (Vogt et al. 2007). Yet Brewin found the most powerful posttrauma factor to be *lack of social support*. Most problematic are *negative* responses to traumatized persons, such as coldness, lack of sympathy, and criticism. Of course, the PTSD syndrome itself can contribute to negative social responses, such as others' negative reactions to emotional volatility or such injunctions as "Why can't you just put the past behind you?!" I put great weight on such unempathic and nonmentalizing responses insofar as they are liable to resonate with those in earlier attachment experience, constituting reminders of past experiences of feeling alone in emotional pain.

Posttrauma social support has been explored in studies of others' reactions to the disclosure of traumatic events. From an attachment perspective, disclosure is ideal: obtaining comfort and restoring security entails confiding in a trusted companion. Much trauma stems from keeping abuse and assaults secret. Yet secrecy is not without basis, particularly in the context of insecure attachment relationships within which attachment trauma occurs. Disclosing sexual trauma—especially within the family—puts a person at risk of being disbelieved, blamed, shamed, punished, and excluded. All such responses reflect lack of mentalizing. Thus, disclosure can be further traumatizing, thereby increasing the risk of PTSD. Deciding when, to whom, and whether to disclose requires difficult judgments. These decisions are difficult enough for adults to make, and they are far more difficult for children to make. Consistent with Brewin's research, those whose disclosure meets with negative responses have worse outcomes than those who refrain from disclosing (Ullman et al. 2010). Plainly, disclosing sexual trauma is a double-edged sword, with benefits and risks dependent on the response. One recent study of adult women's experience of disclosing sexual assault was encouraging in showing that the vast majority disclosed to at least one person (most often friends and family members) and that positive responses far outweighed negative responses (Jacques-Tiura et al. 2010). A related study suggested that negative responses typically are inadvertent (Littleton 2010), resulting from the confidant's distress. That is, confidants may try to alleviate their own discomfort or anxiety by distracting the assaulted person or encouraging her to "move on."

I would underscore the fact that attachment relationships are one thread running through my synopsis of factors that influence the development of PTSD—before, during, and after the traumatic events. Family functioning and a history of early attachment trauma heighten vulnerability to subsequent trauma. As emphasized throughout this book, trauma occurring in the context of attachment relationships is a major concern and plays a significant role in dissociative responses. Finally, as Brewin's research highlights, the quality of attachment relationships—in effect, security and mentalizing or the lack of it—plays an important role in the likelihood of developing PTSD after exposure to traumatic events.

What We Can Conclude About PTSD

By the time a group of us clinicians at The Menninger Clinic started to appreciate the role of trauma in psychiatric disorders in the 1980s, PTSD had become an official diagnosis. In hindsight, I realize that—without thinking or knowing much about it—I took it for granted that PTSD was a well-defined illness. Now aware of decades of research just summarized, I'm skeptical—not about the extent of suffering but rather about the idea of boxing the suffering up into PTSD. None of us—therapists, patients, and researchers alike—doubts that exposure to horrifically stressful events can result in a cruel psychological process in which these events are reexperienced painfully in the mind, not only during waking hours but also in sleep. This reexperiencing is accompanied by anxiety and a host of other emotions and, understandably, by unconscious as well as deliberate strategies to avoid such painful reexperiencing. Particularly (but not only) in the context of adverse attachment relationships, the trauma extends beyond PTSD to affect profoundly the core sense of self, relationships, and the experience of being in the world.

Yet beyond the social-political controversy that surrounded the codification of PTSD into DSM-III, healthy scientific skepticism and inquiry completely undermine a simplistic view that discrete traumatic events result in a well-defined illness. Plainly, from a developmental perspective, identifying "the trauma" as a particular stressful event or set of events is arbitrary. Psychiatry has labored to specify what level of stress qualifies as objectively traumatic and is on the brink of giving up on defining traumatic subjective experience. Then we have the major problem of figuring out what constitutes a normal response to extreme stress as contrasted with a psychopathological response (i.e., a psychiatric disorder). Brewin (2003, p. 212) emphasizes the failure of normal adaptation as the key concern:

> The symptoms described in the DSM-IV are clearly not all pathological precisely because in the beginning they are part of a normal response to overwhelming threat. As in many other psychiatric disorders, the pathology lies not so much in the symptoms themselves as in their persistence and the amount of distress they cause.

Frueh and colleagues (2010) also focus on the persistence of symptoms but propose that rather than focus on the amount of time elapsing, the therapist should diagnose PTSD "when functional impairment becomes and remains significant" (p. 267). Of course, in making all these judgments, from levels of stress to degrees of disorder, we struggle with the lack of bright lines.

Moreover, the ostensible syndrome of PTSD is a moving target. No wonder: PTSD is not clearly separable from other diagnoses; furthermore, PTSD isn't the only psychiatric diagnosis associated with trauma—or even the most common one. Accordingly, on the basis of their findings in the Minnesota longitudinal study, Alan Sroufe and colleagues (2005) wrote the following comment about PTSD: "it is unfortunate that the consequences of trauma, and harsh experience more generally, are sequestered into such a category" (p. 275). Gerald Rosen and colleagues (2010) made a similar point: "the diagnosis of PTSD creates the illusion that a disorder in nature has been identified: a disorder that accounts for and even 'explains' an individual's problems" (p. 272). They conclude that on the contrary, "It is difficult to imagine that the enormous complexity of human reactions to adversity will ever be explained by a single disorder in nature" (p. 273). Finally, exposure to extreme stress is only one among many factors in the etiology of PTSD—and potentially not the most influential one.

We therapists should view diagnoses as stepping-stones for understanding individuals. The medical model has great utility in psychiatry, but we shouldn't be ensnared by it—trapped in the boxes. In the face of all the research that has informed psychiatric diagnoses, we shouldn't lose sight of the fact that they are the product of mentalizing: we construct them to categorize patterns of human problems in various ways. Because psychiatric diagnoses have shaped research and our knowledge, I have organized the balance of this chapter and much of the next chapter around them, notwithstanding their limitations. But I take pains to highlight the problems with the premier trauma-related disorder, PTSD, to advance my campaign of nudging therapists and patients into a developmental foundation for plain old therapy that places a premium on psychological understanding of individuality.

Dissociative Disorders

Collective perplexity about dissociation propelled me into a two-decades-long endeavor to educate patients about trauma (Allen 2005). When a group of us clinicians at The Menninger Clinic began developing a specialized inpatient program for traumatized patients (Allen et al. 2000), we were most captivated by multiple personality disorder—subsequently relabeled dissociative identity disorder. Patients with the disorder were bewildered and frightened by their experience; their peers and staff members were confused as well as intrigued. I conducted some educational sessions in the patient group to initiate some understanding. We all had much to learn, and we were caught up in working with the most controversial disorder in psychiatry. Controversy persists, along with considerable disagreement among specialists about how to understand dissociation. To a degree, dissociation remains on the fringes of psychiatry, with dissociative disorders significantly underdiagnosed (Bremner 2009). One telling example: the standard method for diagnosing psychiatric disorders for research purposes, the Structured Clinical Interview for DSM-IV Axis I Disorders (First et al. 1997), doesn't include dissociative disorders. To rectify this omission, Marlene Steinberg (1993) went to great lengths to develop a separate manual, the Structured Clinical Interview for DSM-IV Dissociative Disorders, along with specialized training for clinicians.

Paul Dell, one of the foremost scholars in the field of dissociation, commented that dissociation "has never suffered from an excess of clarity" (Dell 2009c, p. 712) and that "despite intense investigation during the final decades of the 19th century and the final decades of the 20th century, the concept of dissociation continues to be vague, confusing, and even controversial" (Dell 2009b, p. 225). Definitions of dissociation in the diagnostic manuals aren't a great help. DSM-IV-TR proposes, "The essential feature of the dissociative disorders is a disruption in the usually integrated functions of consciousness, memory, identity, or perception" (American Psychiatric Association 2000, p. 519). The draft DSM-5 criteria (www.dsm5.org) include a more elaborate definition, referring to "a subjective loss of integration of information or control over mental processes that, under normal circumstances, are available to conscious awareness or control, including memory, identity, emotion, perception, body representation, motor control, and behavior." Got that?

Integration is the operative word in these definitions. Dissociation implies that things that should be together (associated) are kept apart. For example, a traumatic memory could be dissociated—kept out of conscious awareness, not integrated with your personal history or sense of self. I find two terms in the literature on dissociation to be most helpful: *detachment* and *compartmentalization* (Allen 2001). These are descriptive metaphors, not explanations. *Detachment* includes feeling detached from yourself (e.g., as if observing yourself from the outside) and feeling detached from the outer world (e.g., as if in a dream). In its most stark form, *compartmentalization* pertains to dissociative identity disorder, a classic form of dissociation in which parts of the personality are separated from one another and alternately take control over behavior. Insofar as they interfere with a feeling of connection with self and others, dissociative detachment and compartmentalization exemplify a failure of mentalizing. To state the obvious, mentalizing trauma is painful, and mentalizing an abusive parent's indifference or malevolence can be downright terrifying (Fonagy and Target 1997). Thus, dissociation can serve a defensive function in blocking mentalizing.

Detachment and compartmentalization are fundamentally different psychological processes (Holmes et al. 2005a): detachment entails *altered* consciousness, whereas compartmentalization entails *divided* consciousness. I start this section with the wellspring of dissociation: the profound detachment that can occur in the midst of extreme danger. We humans share this instinctive response to danger with nonhuman animals. We can think of this response as *peritraumatic* dissociation—that is, dissociation around the time of the traumatic events. With this foundation, I next discuss posttraumatic detachment and then turn to compartmentalization. A discussion of the overlap between dissociation and PTSD follows, and I conclude this section with some comments on overcoming dissociation. Table 2–3 provides an overview of dissociation and related experiences. Because clinicians disagree on what counts as true dissociation, I'm casting a wide net. Traumatized patients struggle with all these experiences, and they find them confusing and frightening.

Dissociation in the Midst of Traumatic Events

I think of fight-or-flight responses as *trauma-prevention responses.* Plainly, fight and flight are not always effective reactions; predators capture prey.

TABLE 2–3. Overview of dissociative and related experiences

Animal defense responses

Freezing (immobility with heightened alertness to danger)

Tonic immobility (biological shutdown, diminished consciousness, "deep freeze")

Detachment

Absorption in fantasy or engrossing activity

Feeling spaced out, robotic, gone away

Depersonalization and derealization

Compartmentalization

Amnesia

Fugue (travel with loss of identity)

Dissociative identity disorder (identity alteration with amnesia)

In modern times, of course, tigers and panthers rarely threaten us; we threaten each other, potentially starting in childhood. Fight and flight are not options in traumatic childhood attachment relationships. When abused children are old enough to be capable of fighting back, doing so is liable to result in worse abuse. Although children sometimes run away when they're old enough, doing so merely substitutes one set of dangers for another. Of course, adults also are liable to be trapped in the same way, physically or psychologically. Only a minority of women, for example, report actively resisting physical and sexual assault, inasmuch as doing so is perceived to be useless or dangerous (Nijenhuis et al. 1998). Dissociation is an alternative option to the fight-or-flight response.

I start this heavy discussion on a lighthearted note. I was taken by the word *tharn* in Richard Adams's (1972) charming novel *Watership Down*. Adams tells the tale of a small band of rabbits and their harrowing adventures. Their warren was about to be destroyed and they had to escape and search for a new home. At one point, several rabbits were huddled in a burrow, crouching in fear of a thunderstorm. Yet a crucial battle was brewing. These lines caught my attention: "All were silent and frightened and one or two were close to the stupefaction of terror." Their leader, Bigwig, commanded, "This is no time to go tharn.... Your lives depend on doing as I say" (p. 351). In the book's rabbit language, Lapine, *tharn* is defined as "stupefied, distraught, hypnotized with fear" (p. 416). We're all familiar with the fight-or-flight response to threat, and many of us also recognize a third possibility: freezing—or going tharn. This last alternative takes us into the territory of dissociation.

We share with nonhuman animals not only two active forms of animal defense, fighting and fleeing, but also two passive forms of animal defense, freezing and tonic immobility (Fanselow and Lester 1988). *Freezing* involves a state of heightened alertness and tension, as the animal is prepared immediately to flee or fight if spotted. If the animal is caught, and fighting is ineffective in permitting escape, the animal may lapse into a state of *tonic immobility*, a form of surrender—in effect, a *deep freeze* response (Schore 2009). This deep freeze response of tonic immobility can be construed as our most primitive biological defense, a defense we share with reptiles and other mammals. Prepared by evolution, we use this animal defense to cope with grave danger. Tonic immobility is a complex response (Porges 2011) involving a prolonged biological shutdown reaction that conserves energy: heart rate and respiration slow down, and muscle tension decreases. In addition, the endogenous opioid (narcotic-like) system is activated, diminishing sensation and pain. In the extreme, the biological shutdown response can be fatal; in addition, by diminishing consciousness and pain, the response can make for a relatively painless death (Porges 2009). Gruesome? Indeed. So is attachment trauma, and we humans can employ these same animal defensive strategies when threatened by each other.

A patient in psychotherapy talked about her experience of "going limp" in the midst of being sexually abused by her father; she was "far away" in her mind and only slowly "came back" after he'd left, not remembering what had happened. Is this a counterpart of the animal defense response? Similarly, traumatized children appear numb, robotic, nonreactive, glazed, daydreaming, unresponsive—in effect, not there. In animals, this defense can be adaptive in some instances: the predator might let go of the animal in the state of tonic immobility, permitting escape (Fanselow and Lester 1988). Here I stretch your imagination: could the following example of disorganized attachment observed in the Strange Situation (Ainsworth et al. 1978) be analogous to tonic immobility followed by escape?

> Upon reunion, a mother picks up her very active son and sits down with him on her lap. He sits still and closes his eyes. His mother calls his name but he does not stir. Still calling his name, she bounces him on her knee and gently shakes him, but he remains limp and still. After several seconds he opens his eyes, slides off her lap, and darts across the room to retrieve a toy. (Main and Morgan 1996, p. 124)

Detachment

As just discussed, tonic immobility entails a profound alteration of consciousness and the most extreme form of detachment. At the other extreme is active *engagement*, with alert consciousness directed flexibly between self-awareness (i.e., awareness of what's going on in your mind and body) and awareness of the outer world. Thus, we can think of degrees of disengagement, as depicted in Figure 2–1. The mildest form of disengagement from the environment is *absorption* (Tellegen and Atkinson 1974). You can be so absorbed in an activity or in thought or a daydream that you're unaware of your surroundings—a child absorbed in a video game, for example, may not hear his mother calling his name. Thus, to be intensely absorbed in any one thing is to be detached from all others. Aptly, absorption is associated with absentmindedness—being absorbed in thought, for example. Absorption is not pathological; on the contrary, we must be able to become totally engrossed in what we do.

Absorption is relatively flexible: some stimulus—your name being called or a tap on your shoulder—snaps you back into outer reality. We enter the realm of dissociative disorders when detachment reaches the point of losing the feeling of reality—for example, feeling as if living in a dream. Patients who struggle with detachment use many different words to describe their experience: they feel spacey, foggy, or fuzzy; they feel as if they're floating or drifting; or they feel as if they are automata, robots, or on autopilot. This more extreme detachment takes two forms. *Depersonalization* is a sense of unreality associated with the self or the body. This would include feeling as if you're an actor in a play; out-of-body experiences such as looking down on yourself from above; feeling as if you're not in control of your speech or behavior; looking in a mirror and seeing yourself as unfamiliar; feeling disconnected from your thoughts or emotions; or lacking ordinary body feeling or sensation (e.g., feeling numb or as if you don't exist from the neck down). *Derealization* involves the outer world feeling unreal. For example, you might feel as if other persons are actors in a play, or as if you're looking at the world through glass, fog, or a tunnel. Derealization commonly accompanies depersonalization and rarely occurs in isolation.

Absorption in imagination is the fount of creativity; to live without imagination would be to be imprisoned in reality. Some of us are more capable of absorption or more talented at it than others, and capacity for absorption relates to hypnotic susceptibility, which also can be considered an aptitude (Dell 2009c). Absorption also relates to *fantasy proneness* (Wilson and Barber 1983). For some extremely fantasy-prone children, the inner world of imagination feels more real than the outer world. Notably, such detachment can serve a defensive function; escape into fantasy proneness sometimes is associated with a history of punishment, abuse, loneliness, and isolation (Lynn and Rhue 1988). Authors differ as to whether absorption should be considered a form of dissociation (Dalenberg and Paulson 2009; Dell 2009c). I think of an extreme propensity for

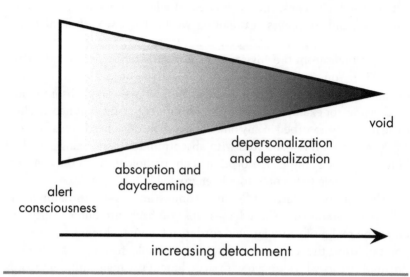

FIGURE 2–1. Degrees of dissociative detachment.

Source. Reprinted from Allen JG: *Coping With Trauma.* Washington, DC, American Psychiatric Publishing, 2005, p. 190. Used with permission.

absorption, whether triggered involuntarily or used defensively to avoid painful emotions, as a possible *predisposition* to dissociation. Plainly, absorption can be too much of a good thing.

Depersonalization is the third most common psychiatric symptom (after anxiety and depression), reported by 80% of the general population (Coons 1996). Although depersonalization experiences are common, depersonalization *disorder*—the chronic experience of depersonalization— is not. At worst, depersonalization and derealization can be severe and persistent; sufferers live a life without vitality, enlivenment, passion, or much of any emotion short of a pervasive sense of unease or ennui. One patient complained that he was among the "living dead." As Dell (2009c) wrote, *"every aspect of experience has been drained of its personal emotional immediacy"* (p. 781, emphasis in original).

Case Example

Harold was hospitalized in his mid-30s when his substance abuse and self-cutting had escalated to dangerous levels. He was referred to me for a trauma evaluation and psychotherapy, complaining that he was "not alive." He quickly acknowledged that his self-cutting enabled him temporarily to feel alive. He gave a history of extensive childhood trauma, including molestation by an uncle, physical abuse by his father, witnessing of parental violence in which his father occasionally threatened to murder his mother, and discovering his brother after he committed suicide by hanging. Dangerous and sometimes life-threatening fights and assaults in conjunction with substance abuse compounded this early trauma.

Harold said he never had a clear sense of identity. He said his mother doted on him, but he mainly remembered being dressed up as her "little prince" and paraded about "like a doll" to her friends. When he was in early adolescence, his father took him to bars and strip clubs, telling him it was time for him to "be a man." For Harold's eighteenth birthday, his father set him up with a prostitute, telling him not to reveal his age.

Harold described his whole life as consisting of "playacting." In school, he easily took on the role of "class clown." He was active in theater in high school and college. He said he lived in a "dream world" beginning in childhood; he immersed himself in fantasy, often taking on the attitudes of characters in books, plays, television shows, and movies. His profligate use of various drugs abetted his feelings of unreality, and regular use of marijuana buttressed his detachment. When we discussed "depersonalization" in psychotherapy, he said he was never "personalized."

To the extent that he felt real, Harold said he felt disgusted with himself; he said he was "a vile excuse for a person." He'd lived most of his life "in a dream—a nightmare," and he said he wanted to "wake up." He recognized that he'd "wasted" previous therapy by "playing the role of a neurotic patient," and he wanted to "get real." He used the therapy as an anchor in his hospital treatment, where he became conscious of "slipping into roles" and losing himself in the process. He did the same in therapy when it became evident that he was entertaining me instead of working with me. His participation in a 12-step group was enormously helpful because he wrote an autobiographical narrative that was "brutally honest," one that I also found hair-raising for its descriptions of dangerous behavior.

By the time he was ready for discharge from the hospital, Harold felt ambivalent about the therapy process, stating that he'd "replaced bad dreams with painful realities." Yet he was glad to feel more grounded, had no urges to cut himself, and said he was ready to start a "real life."

As Daphne Simeon (2009) reviewed, depersonalization disorder usually begins in mid-adolescence, and it is equally common in males and females. No doubt, depersonalization typically is a stress-related disorder, but it may develop suddenly or gradually, and its precipitants are many, including prolonged stress, other psychiatric disorders (e.g., panic, anxiety, or depression), or drug use (e.g., marijuana or hallucinogens). Compared with persons who have no psychiatric disorders, those with depersonalization disorder are more likely to have a history of childhood abuse (e.g., physical or sexual abuse) and are especially likely to have a history of emotional abuse and neglect—caregivers' mentalizing failures. As Simeon summarizes,

> We can safely say that chronic depersonalization can occur in the context of widely varying traumatic stressors, mainly chronic childhood trauma,

later severe life stress, and overwhelming states of other emotional illness. What all these have in common might be an overwhelming challenge to one's sense of self which, in individuals genetically predisposed, might trigger a chronic depersonalization state. (p. 438)

Depersonalization and derealization entail awareness with a feeling of unreality. Yet some patients report even more extreme detachment in which they lose any experience of awareness (or at least remember none). They report being "gone," "in the void," or "in the blackness." They may stare into space for minutes or even hours with no sense of the passage of time. It's as if they are unconscious or comatose—perhaps akin to tonic immobility. At some point, they "come to," but they're disoriented as to what time it is or even where they are. They have no memory for the gap in experience and report "lost time." Patients may have this profoundly detached experience in psychotherapy, triggered by a traumatic memory or other sources of anxiety or distress. I have worked with patients who have "gone away" to this extreme in a therapy session, and it's not easy to "bring them back," although I've never found it to be impossible. Once they regain some awareness, it's not easy for them to become reoriented and reconnected with themselves or the outer world. Sometimes they need to walk in the fresh air. Not uncommonly, patients have to sleep it off, becoming reengaged only after they wake up.

Because of its seeming self-protective function, we're inclined to think of dissociation as a defense. There is plenty of room for confusion here (Dell 2009c). In its bedrock extreme of tonic immobility, although it is protective, dissociation isn't so much an active defense as it is a manifestation of fear. It's a reaction, not an action. Subsequently, as individuals become sensitized to stress, dissociation can be triggered by less dire circumstances, including traumatic memories. It is common, for example, for patients to become detached—feeling spacey or unreal—when they're talking about traumatic experiences in psychotherapy. Sometimes they become downright sleepy. Such detachment is an expression of fear. Yet some patients can learn to shift more voluntarily and defensively into a state that was initially experienced as being out of their control.

Case Example

Irene was highly averse to any distressing emotions. She had grown up in an extremely violent household. She coped in a straightforward manner: when she could, she went up into her bedroom, shut the door, turned on music or—in desperation—shut herself in the closet and wrapped a pillow around her head. But she couldn't always go to her room. Sometimes she and her brother were forced to remain at the dinner table while her parents were screaming at each other, occasionally hitting or throwing things at each other. She had learned to tune them out. In a therapy group, when conflicts between group members started to erupt, she would do the same thing. She'd discovered a strategy for doing so: she would fix her gaze on a spot in the corner near the ceiling until she was no longer there, oblivious to what was happening in the group.

Compartmentalization

With compartmentalization, we come to the original sense of dissociation, and what some clinicians consider to be the only proper use of the term (Steele et al. 2009a). In this sense, rather than involving alterations of consciousness, true dissociation entails a division of consciousness such that one part of the mind is not aware of another part of the mind. This classic form of dissociation was discovered in the context of hypnosis, the checkered history of which began with Franz Anton Mesmer, a physician whose "animal magnetism" was purported to cure and prevent all illnesses. Resembling sleepwalking, hypnotic states also were construed as artificial somnambulism. This historical backdrop prepares us to appreciate dissociation in its stark form, as described by Henri Ellenberger (1970) in his classic *The Discovery of the Unconscious:*

> The first magnetizers were immensely struck by the fact that, when they induced magnet sleep in a person, a new life manifested itself of which the subject was unaware, and that a new and often more brilliant personality emerged with a continuous life of its own. The entire nineteenth century was preoccupied with the problem of the coexistence of these two minds and of their relationship to each other. (p. 145)

One striking feature of hypnotic states is the fact that upon return to the ordinary state of consciousness, the hypnotized person doesn't remember what transpired during the trance state. Moreover, when a subsequent trance is induced, the person remembers the previous trance experience, suggestive of dual consciousness (i.e., dissociation). Such amnesia suggests the metaphor *compartmentalization*—as if there were segregated compartments in the mind. Dell (2009c) rightly cautions, however, that

> so-called compartmentalization is an ongoing, active process; the mind does not possess an internal compartment that passively contains dissociated material. Although compartmentalization is a useful metaphor for dissociation, the reader is urged to keep in mind that this metaphor is also somewhat misleading (because it tends to veil the active process that almost certainly sustains dissociative amnesia). (p. 786)

The simplest form of compartmentalizing is dissociative amnesia, defined in DSM-IV-TR as "inability to recall important personal information, usually of a traumatic or stressful nature, that is too extensive to be explained by ordinary forgetfulness" (American Psychiatric Association 2000, p. 519). Albeit rare, dissociative amnesia can be so extensive as to include not only loss of memory but also, at the extreme, loss of identity in dissociative fugue states during which the person might travel to a distant place and be completely disoriented, not remembering who he or she is.

Lenore Terr (1994) gave a dramatic example of dissociative amnesia with origins in early attachment trauma. One evening, the police found her client, Patricia, in a car on the side of the highway. She was unresponsive and they assumed she was intoxicated. As they tried to arouse her and decided to arrest her, she became combative. When she awoke in jail the next morning, she had no idea who she was. By the time Terr was called in, Patricia had recovered her sense of identity, but she didn't remember the events leading up to her arrest. Through interviewing, Terr was able to reconstruct what happened: Patricia had discovered her boyfriend in her bed with another woman; a confrontation ensued, and then Patricia went blank. When being arrested, she remained in a dissociative state and thought the policeman was going to kill her. Notably, Patricia reported a history of other dissociative episodes dating back to age 9 when she saw her intoxicated mother burn to death in a fire. Patricia told Terr that after having witnessed this, she'd gone into the bathroom, drawn a bath, gotten into the tub, and "drifted into a weird shut-off never-never land" (p. 93). Perhaps this profound detachment reminiscent of tonic immobility constituted the developmental fault line for her later proclivity to dissociative amnesia.

Dissociative identity disorder, formerly multiple personality disorder, goes a step beyond amnesia in that different aspects of identity and experience are compartmentalized, excluded from ordinary consciousness. The change in terminology marks the difference between the patient's subjective and the clinician's objective perspectives. Multiple personality disorder fits patients' experience; to the extent that they become aware of it, they feel as if they are inhabited—or even possessed—by different personalities (or "alters"). As clinicians, we see a disorder of identity based on dissociation. In coarse terms, dissociative identity disorder entails amnesia for behavior that is out of character. More specifically, in DSM-IV-TR, dissociative identity disorder is diagnosed on the basis of "two or more distinct identities or personality states" that "recurrently take control of the person's behavior." This identity alteration is accompanied by "inability to recall important personal information" (p. 529). Hence, the person doesn't remember what he or she has done in the altered state.

No mental health professional questions that depression, bipolar disorder, schizophrenia, and panic disorder are valid diagnoses. But although dissociative identity disorder is codified in DSM-IV (and in the DSM-5 draft) and has been reported in the literature for two centuries (Ellen-berger 1970), a substantial minority of professionals don't consider it a valid diagnosis (Cormier and Thelen 1998; Pope et al. 1999). Some ob-servers attribute the disorder to zealous believers—therapists who talk suggestible patients into believing they have the disorder. I have worked with patients who have been misled in this way about their diagnosis, and I have educated these patients accordingly. Yet seeing is believing, and I'm a believer.

In my initiation, not only did I *not* talk the patient into it but—on the contrary—I was oblivious to obvious signs of the disorder, as I first de-scribed two and a half decades ago in a paper written with my colleagues Joyce Davidson and Bill Smith (Davidson et al. 1987). I simply didn't un-derstand what was happening.

Case Example

In one therapy session, Joan suddenly and uncharacteristically expressed anger; cursing, she pounded her fist on the arm of the chair. I was sur-prised but considered it a breakthrough, because she was usually timid about expressing anger. When I referred back to her angry outburst mo-ments later, Joan had no idea what I was talking about. As I persisted, she thought I was playing some kind of game to make her angry. I let it drop. Over the next couple of sessions, she referred to "blackouts"—that is, blocks of times for which she had no memory (e.g., in trips away from the hospital). She wasn't alcoholic, and I was puzzled.

Before too long, Joan hit me over the head with the problem: her alter identity, Mary, came rushing into the therapy session with a paper bag containing a bottle of alcohol and a stash of pills and commanded, "Take these—she [i.e., Joan] is going to kill herself with them!" I put the bag in a drawer in my desk and we sat down and talked. Mary implored me not to tell Joan about her! I agreed, and then Mary switched back to her usual state of mind, Joan. Joan, bewildered and disoriented, said this experience in my office was like one of her blackouts. Fortunately, she was hospital-ized, and I was able to walk her back to her inpatient unit. When I told the staff that I thought Joan might have multiple personality disorder, they thought I was out of my mind. Gradually, we all accepted this diagnosis, including Joan, and she eventually became more aware of her different dissociated states.

Believing in dissociative identity disorder does not translate into being able to explain it. Many great minds took on the task a century ago. Pierre Janet pioneered modern understanding of multiple personality disorder, but many others made significant contributions, including such lumi-naries as Alfred Binet, Morton Prince, and William James (Dell 2009c). Hypnotic susceptibility is a pathway to normal dissociation of the sort observed in dissociative identity disorder. Of greater interest here, as Janet recognized long ago, psychological trauma is another pathway (van der Hart and Dorahy 2009). In contemporary terms, dissociative identity disorder involves structural dissociation of the personality, wherein the sense of self "*alternates* and is *inconsistent* across time and experience" (Steele et al. 2009a, p. 160, emphasis in original). In the context of trauma theory, for example, an *apparently normal part of the personality* can be distinguished from an *emotional part of the personality*. The normal part is typically avoidant and numb, phobic of reminders of trauma; by contrast, the emotional part is fixated on traumatic memories. Moreover, there may be multiple emotional parts of the personality, each related to different kinds of traumatic experiences or emotions. At the extreme, there also may be different normal parts of the personality, developed, for example, to manage different social roles (Steele et al. 2009b).

Attachment Trauma and Dissociation

As I discussed in the first chapter, dissociation-like behaviors are evident in infancy in conjunction with disorganized attachment, and extensive research has documented an association between childhood maltreatment and risk of later dissociative disturbance. Such predisposing traumatic experience ranges from physical and sexual abuse to neglect, loss, and witnessing violence. There is a dose-response relationship insofar as risk of dissociation is associated with earlier age of abuse, greater severity, and longer duration. The most convincing evidence for the connection between early trauma and later dissociation comes from longitudinal research showing that disorganized attachment in infancy predicts dissociative symptoms in adolescence and early adulthood (Carlson et al. 2009b; Dutra et al. 2009). Although the relation between maltreatment and dissociation is well documented, we need to understand the psychological nature of the connection.

Compartmentalization of experience is normal in infancy in the sense that infants' experience consists of alternations among behavioral states— alternating not only between waking and sleeping but also between calm and distressed states. Thus, integration of disparate experiences is a developmental achievement, and such integration rests on a mentalizing infant-caregiver relationship in which the caregiver holds the infant's mind in mind. As Elizabeth Carlson and colleagues (2009b) stated in the context of their developmental research on dissociation,

> In infancy, the "self" consists of discrete behavioral states of consciousness. Early on, these states are modulated by the caregiver and her/his daily

routines. Over time, however, the capacity for self-regulation is internalized. Through repeated exchanges with a sensitive caregiver, the child comes to experience the self as a cohesive, unitary entity. (p. 47)

Such sensitive caregiving is the basis of secure attachment, in which mentalizing begets mentalizing: over the course of development, through mentalizing, the child is aware of a range of emotions and experiences—including painful experiences—and able to integrate them into a coherent sense of self with an autobiography.

In contrast, disorganized infant attachment represents a failure of integration associated with a profound conflict: the activation of attachment needs, such as a desire for comfort, creates a need for closeness with the caregiver; simultaneously, fear of the caregiver creates a need for distance. Lacking the capacity to integrate these contradictory desires, the disorganized infant demonstrates contradictory behavior, alternating dramatically between approach and withdrawal. As Giovanni Liotti (2009) proposed, the child's dramatically conflicting internal working models of self and other, and the associated alternations in behavior, bear resemblance to the compartmentalization of experience typified by dissociative identity disorder. Just as secure attachment promotes integration, disorganized attachment impedes it: "pathological dissociation, in infancy, is a primary failure in organizing unitary mental states and coherent behavioral strategies—a failure taking place in an interpersonal context of defective caregiving" (p. 56).

Infant disorganization is especially likely to lead to dissociative disturbance when coupled with ongoing trauma (Carlson et al. 2009b). Jennifer Freyd's (1996) *betrayal trauma* theory illuminates this connection. She proposes that traumatic experiences are compartmentalized to keep them from interfering with normal interactions: "Under this theory, the purpose of dissociation is not escape from pain, but the *maintenance of the attachment relationship* by not-knowing about information that would threaten it" (Barlow and Freyd 2009, p. 100, emphasis added). The sexually abused child, for example, cannot maintain a normal interaction with her parents at the dinner table with the sexual abuse in mind. She compartmentalizes the two kinds of relationships, dissociating the internal working models.

The developmental research on dissociation underscores the thesis of this book—namely, that mentalizing failures that leave the child psychologically alone in emotional pain comprise the core of traumatic experience. As Carlson and colleagues (2009b) wrote, "When experience is acknowledged and accepted, integration follows; to the extent that dissociation prevails, there is fragmentation of the self" (p. 44). On the heels of disorganized attachment, this dissociative fragmentation follows from "the severity and repetition of *empathic failures*" (p. 46, emphasis added).

Longitudinal research on the relation between disorganized attachment and later dissociation, summarized by Lissa Dutra and colleagues (2009), underscores the role of maternal psychological unavailability in the development of dissociation. These researchers conducted home observations of mother-infant interactions when infants were 12 months old and assessed infant attachment in the Strange Situation at 18 months. They measured dissociation and administered the Adult Attachment Interview when the children were 19 years old; in addition, they interviewed mothers at that later time. They found that disrupted maternal communication, rather than outright abuse, was the key factor in dissociative disturbance:

> Maternal hostile or intrusive behavior was not significantly related to later dissociation. Instead, lack of positive maternal affective involvement, maternal flatness of affect, and overall disrupted maternal communication were the strongest predictors of dissociation in young adulthood. What is notable about these types of maternal interactions is that they all serve to subtly override or ignore the infant's needs and attachment signals, but without overt hostility. (p. 87)

Dutra and colleagues (2009) describe observations of a research participant that show dramatic parallels between infancy and young adulthood. In the Strange Situation, the infant wandered aimlessly, as if lost and confused, rather than playing with the toys. When he attempted to show his mother a toy, she didn't respond. When his mother left the room, he enjoyed interacting with the stranger in a game with a ball. When his mother returned, she didn't approach or greet him; he lowered his gaze and moved toward the door. He refused to engage in any shared activity when she subsequently tried to engage him. Notably, in the second reunion, his mother made no effort to comfort his distress but rather asked for a kiss, suggesting that she gave priority to her attachment needs over his. This infant's aimless wandering in the Strange Situation was paralleled by his response at 19 years old to an assessment item implying dissociative detachment; he said he frequently had the experience of finding himself someplace and not remembering how he got there. In the Adult Attachment Interview, he described his early childhood as bouncing around from one place to another. He also said his mother was more of a friend than a mom; he consoled her after she fought with his father, and he said he brought himself up. When interviewed at this time, his mother stated that she had difficulty setting rules and was a friend for her child. Paralleling the interaction in the second reunion in the Strange Situation, she stated that the best moments with her children were those in which she felt wanted. As the authors conclude, this mother

> demonstrates a tendency to abdicate her parental role and ask for love and attention, rather than attending to her children's needs. Accordingly, in this vignette, it is notable that the affectively unavailable and withdrawn nature of the parent's involvement with the child was evident in the second-to-second interactive dialogue between mother and infant, after which the child eventually begins to focus on his mother's needs, as per her request, rather than attend to his own needs. (Dutra et al. 2009, p. 89)

To recap, attachment trauma represents the failure of parental mentalizing of the child, and this failure is especially dramatic in the context of dissociation when the parent's dissociative state is frightening to the child and then mirrored by the child's dissociative state. Research reveals a remarkable developmental cascade: the parent dissociates in the Adult Attachment Interview and in the Strange Situation; the child dissociates in the Strange Situation; and the child then continues to dissociate in later life, perhaps into parenthood. Dissociation is the antithesis of integrated awareness, within individuals and within relationships. Mentalizing is inherently integrative in bringing together multiple perspectives, grappling with emotional conflicts, and reflecting on experience and making sense of it. Through mentalizing, a person brings diverse experiences together into a coherent narrative—authoring and revising his or her life story. Accordingly, mentalizing is the antidote to dissociation. But overcoming the aversion to mentalizing—thinking the unthinkable—entails arduous and emotionally painful work. Plain old therapy might sound simple, but it's hardly easy.

Dissociation in PTSD

PTSD and dissociation are intimately associated. Dissociation around the time of the trauma is a strong predictor of PTSD (Ozer et al. 2003), especially when it persists in the aftermath of trauma (Waelde et al. 2009). Such persistent dissociation, like the avoidance symptoms of PTSD more generally, impedes the emotional processing of trauma—a failure of mentalizing.

As characterized in DSM, some symptoms of PTSD—flashbacks and amnesia—can be regarded as dissociative. Moreover, emotional detachment and numbing symptoms of PTSD also can be considered dissociative (Ginzburg et al. 2009). Going further, some specialists regard PTSD as a form of dissociative disorder. Kathy Steele and colleagues (2009b) assert that "PTSD always involves primary structural dissociation" (p. 247).

The intrusive symptoms of PTSD exemplify the experience that Dell (2009c) regards as central to pathological dissociation—namely, "recurrent, jarring, involuntary intrusions into executive functioning and sense of self" (p. 770). As he elaborated, such *split-off material is experienced as being odd, unfamiliar, not mine, belonging to another, and so on*" (p. 809, emphasis in original). Julian Ford (2009), however, cautions that flashbacks and amnesia in PTSD are dissociative only when they are discordant with the person's sense of self, that is, when the person "*cannot recognize the self who had those experiences and the relationships that formed the context for those experiences*" (p. 480, emphasis in original). In a similar vein, based on neurobiological differences, some authors propose a *dissociative subtype* of PTSD (Lanius et al. 2010). In part, this dissociative subtype can be viewed as a relatively severe form of PTSD associated with a history of childhood abuse (Waelde et al. 2009).

Diagnostic Challenges

As should be evident from this discussion, the challenges in diagnosing dissociative disorders parallel those in diagnosing PTSD. We therapists are faced with another version of the problem of identifying diagnostic boxes and deciding which symptoms go in which boxes. Clinicians disagree as to whether dissociative disorders should include only symptoms that reflect compartmentalization (structural dissociation) or whether they also should include symptoms reflecting detachment, such as depersonalization (alterations of consciousness). In addition, Dell (2009a) expresses dissatisfaction with the DSM-IV criteria for dissociative identity disorder, claiming that they place too much emphasis on alter personalities and amnesia; while overt switching among alter personalities is relatively rare, the intrusion of dissociative states into consciousness is common. Moreover, patients diagnosed with dissociative identity disorder typically experience the full array of dissociative symptoms—including high levels of absorption and detachment. Hence, Dell proposes that dissociative identity disorder be renamed *complex dissociative disorder.* Furthermore, Colin Ross (2009) makes the point that dissociative symptoms are common in conjunction with many different psychiatric disorders. Most notably, many symptoms of PTSD—if not the entire disorder—can be regarded as dissociative.

Overcoming Dissociation

I'll be discussing treatment at length in Part II of this book, but some thoughts about overcoming dissociation are in order here. I consider dissociation a blessing and a curse—at once self-protective and potentially self-defeating. Dissociation, ranging from detachment to dissociative identity disorder, might be thought of as an extreme form of experiential avoidance. Fundamentally, in the face of dire and even life-threatening danger, this avoidance is automatic and reflexive—indeed, instinctive from an evolutionary point of view. With sensitization to stress and the development of dissociative disorders, dissociative states can be prompted by increasingly less severe stress and, at worst, relatively ordinary levels of emotional distress. Moreover, to varying degrees, persons with a history of involuntary dissociation can learn how to dissociate deliberately to avoid conflict and distress.

Thus, overcoming avoidance is central to the treatment of dissociative disorders, just as it is to PTSD and other anxiety disorders. Dissociative detachment is the antithesis of mindful awareness and mentalizing; correspondingly, the antidote to dissociative flashbacks and detachment is *grounding*—that is, focusing attention mindfully on present experience. In the context of dissociation, strong stimuli are required. Calling a person's name and engaging in conversation might work. But more potent stimuli might be needed, such as getting up and walking around, splashing cold water on one's face, or holding crushed ice in one's hand. We must keep in mind, however, that such efforts go against the grain: the purpose of dissociation is disconnection, escaping reality. Thus, efforts to ground must be accompanied by assurances of safety in the present. Patients can learn how to prevent dissociation with grounding techniques, but doing so requires mentalizing—that is, being aware of dissociative detachment or switching as it is unfolding, in effect, nipping it in the bud. Beyond a certain point, voluntary control diminishes dramatically; with hyperbole, I refer to this problem as going beyond the point of no return. This is true of dissociation as it is with all else: anxiety can be regulated more easily than panic, irritation more easily than rage, and blue moods more easily than hopeless despair.

Overcoming experiential avoidance is nowhere more challenging than in relation to the most extreme of the trauma-related disorders, dissociative identity disorder. Treatment approaches abound (Michelson and Ray 1996), as does controversy. Regardless of technique, overcoming experiential avoidance is the goal. This endeavor will entail increasing awareness and acceptance of dissociated emotions, memories, and relationships. To use the metaphor of compartmentalizing, therapy entails gaining access to the compartments, in effect opening the doors so as to move around more fluidly with greater continuity of consciousness across time and different states of mind.

Case Example

Leroy was in the process of coming to terms with the diagnosis of dissociative identity disorder, and he was worried about engaging in behaviors
that felt out of his control. He had good reason to worry. Prior to his hospitalization, he had told his wife he was going on a hunting trip with a
friend, and his wife learned that Leroy had visited a former girlfriend instead. Leroy didn't remember doing this, but he believed his wife.

In talking through this event, Leroy realized that he had been anxious
about the hunting trip because he had been suicidal and had seriously contemplated shooting himself. Moreover, he was gradually able to acknowledge motivation for visiting his former girlfriend: he'd come to resent his
wife's "coldness" as his behavior had become more disruptive, and he became aware of conscious longings to reunite with his girlfriend, whom he
characterized as "exceptionally warm." He also realized that acknowledging these feelings—much less acting on them—threatened his marriage.

In effect, this work in therapy enabled Leroy to mentalize his discon-
certing behavior; the door to his compartmentalized experience was ajar,
setting the stage for greater awareness of dissociated desires and fears. But
opening these doors can be downright terrifying, especially as it brings
awareness: "This happened to *me*." I worked with a patient who had come to
terms with the knowledge that she had been sexually abused in childhood,
but she was extremely fearful of remembering the abuse in her ordinary
state of mind; by dissociating, it was as if this had not happened to her.

Given that dissociative identity disorder is an extreme response to extremely traumatic experience, the treatment is long and difficult. In principle, however, treating dissociative disorder is akin to other applications of
plain old psychotherapy, all of which can be construed as helping the patient
to encompass a broader range of experience into the sense of self and to
move from experiential avoidance to experiential acceptance. Above all,
such therapy requires a safe and trusting relationship. The paradox in all
treatment of attachment trauma is most glaringly evident here: the trauma
history and profoundly insecure attachment preclude the easy development
of such a relationship. I can only reiterate the words of Richard Kluft (1993),
a contemporary pioneer in the understanding and treatment of dissociative
identity disorder: "The slower you go, the faster you get there" (p. 42).

Key Points

◆ The essence of PTSD is an alternation between intrusive memories,
   triggered by reminders of trauma, and the avoidance of reminders,
   which includes avoidance of trauma-related situations as well as
   trauma-related thoughts and feelings. However, controversy continues
   to surround the PTSD diagnosis.

- Dissociative disturbance has been relatively neglected in psychiatry, despite its pervasiveness in conjunction with trauma. Two broad forms of dissociation are detachment (alteration of consciousness as in feeling spacey or unreal) and compartmentalization (division of consciousness as evident in amnesia and dissociative identity disorder).

- The diagnostic classification system can be misleading in implying that specific disorders represent discrete illnesses. We must employ diagnostic categories as a stepping-stone to understanding the adaptive efforts of individual persons in all their complexity.

- Extensive overlap exists between PTSD and dissociation, as well as between these disorders and other anxiety disorders and depression. PTSD and dissociation can have enormously complex etiologies that call for understanding of individual developmental trajectories. Attachment relationships play a major role in the development of these disorders—potentially before, during, and after exposure to traumatic events.

- Compromised mentalizing plays a role in PTSD and dissociation. Mentalizing failure is most glaring in posttraumatic flashbacks, where memories are conflated with current reality (i.e., in the nonmentalizing psychic-equivalence mode). Mentalizing failures are also evident in dissociative detachment, in which emotion is not mentalized and in which the feeling of unreality has the hallmarks of the nonmentalizing pretend mode. And mentalizing failures are apparent in dissociative compartmentalization, in which continuity across mental states is lost in a failure of integration. Accordingly, *reestablishing mentalizing in attachment relationships*—this aspiration of plain old therapy—is central in the treatment of both PTSD and dissociative disorders.

Complex Traumatic Stress Disorders

I've laid the groundwork for this chapter by emphasizing the point that traumatic stress is a nonspecific risk factor for a wide range of disorders and problems beyond posttraumatic stress disorder (PTSD), as illustrated in Figure 3–1. This point is particularly applicable to stress that is severe and prolonged, occurs early in life, and takes place in attachment relationships. Clinicians have been wrestling with diagnosing complex trauma for two decades; as has been true with PTSD, the issues are social and political as well as scientific. In this chapter, I discuss some of the additional disorders and problems to which attachment trauma makes a relatively prominent contribution: depression, anxiety, substance abuse, ill health, eating disorders, nonsuicidal self-injury, suicidal states, and personality disorders. Then I discuss proposals to lump this array of trauma-related problems into new diagnostic categories.

This list of trauma-related problems encompasses a fair chunk of the DSM, and I can hardly claim to do each of these problems justice. For example, I'm glossing over individual differences in genetic vulnerability and temperament, which influence the impact of trauma on development. I intend this survey merely to serve three purposes: first, to underscore the sheer breadth of problems stemming from attachment trauma;

91

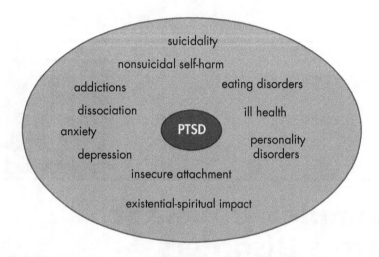

FIGURE 3–1.   Complex traumatic stress disorders.
Posttraumatic stress disorder (PTSD) is a disorder to which trauma is inappropriately reduced.

second, to link these problems to impaired mentalizing; and third, to disabuse you of any remaining illusion that trauma-related problems can be neatly diagnosed. In so doing, I'm continuing to set the stage for plain old therapy, an approach to treating attachment trauma that transcends diagnosis and respects the full complexity of individual development.

Depression

In the course of conducting educational groups on trauma, I gradually appreciated the need to give adequate attention to depression, because depression seemed to be the most pervasive and disabling problem for patients with a history of attachment trauma. I began conducting an educational group focused on depression in the Professionals in Crisis program at The Menninger Clinic, where I was particularly struck by the observation that patients with a history of attachment trauma had achieved enormous professional success and then plummeted into severe depression. Their success came at the price of an extremely stressful lifestyle, which contributed to the pileup of stress. I also came to appreciate how childhood trauma created a vulnerability to more recent stress that triggered depressive episodes, as depicted in Figure 3–2.

In focusing on attachment trauma, I pass over much of the complexity in the etiology of depression and the diversity of developmental pathways

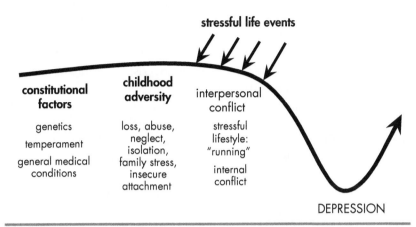

FIGURE 3–2. Stress pileup model of depression.

Source. Adapted from Allen JG: *Traumatic Relationships and Serious Mental Disorders.* Chichester, UK, Wiley, 2001, p. 107. Used with permission.

(Kendler et al. 2002). Just as in PTSD and a host of other disorders, genetic vulnerability and environmental stress interact over the lifetime. As Kenneth Kendler and colleagues (1995) put it simply, "Genes have an impact on the risk of major depression in part by altering the individual's sensitivity to the depression-inducing effect of stressful events" (p. 834). Attachment trauma is but one contributor to depression among many others in a developmental cascade. Constitutional risk factors include not only genetic predispositions and temperament (e.g., anxious temperament) but also general medical conditions and ill health, which contribute to vulnerability over the lifetime. Giving constitutional factors short shrift, I'll discuss precipitating stressors in adulthood and vulnerability from childhood trauma, concluding with the role of mentalizing in depression.

Precipitating Stress

The role of stressful life events in depressive episodes is well documented (Hammen 2005), as is the prominent role of interpersonal stress in particular (Joiner 2002). Depression was one of John Bowlby's (1980) main concerns; in his words, "loss of a loved person is one of the most intensely painful experiences any human being can suffer" (p. 7). Bowlby was echoing Sigmund Freud (1927/1961), who wisely proclaimed, "We are never so defenceless against suffering as when we love, never so helplessly unhappy as when we have lost our loved object or its love" (p. 33).

In the course of reviewing the extensive literature on the development of depression, I was particularly impressed with the landmark research of

British sociologist George Brown and colleagues (Brown and Harris 1978). This research is particularly valuable for its meticulous method, employing intensive interviews to illuminate the personal experience of depression. These researchers focused on depressive episodes in adult women, many of whom were living in impoverished circumstances and raising young children—often without partners. Brown and Harris showed that depressive episodes commonly were provoked by *stressful life events*, with loss a prominent theme: examples include separations, a life-threatening illness in an attachment figure, material losses, and being forced to change residence. Loss also can be accompanied by disillusion-ment, such as a woman's discovering her husband's infidelity. Feeling let down or betrayed at a time of need—alone in emotional pain—is a pow-erful precipitant. Moreover, depression also emerged in relation to *on-going difficulties* associated with unremitting stress. Examples include marital conflict, difficulties with children, problems at work, financial hardship, inadequate housing, and ill health. Such difficulties were pro-longed: Brown and Harris counted only those difficulties that went on for at least 2 years; the average was 4 years.

Unsurprisingly, the combination of stressful life events and ongoing difficulties was especially likely to provoke episodes of depression. In ed-ucating patients about stress pileup and depression, as depicted in Figure 3–2, I also include a stressful lifestyle (e.g., being a workaholic or com-pulsive caregiver; being continually on the go, or "running" as some pa-tients put it). Sometimes, such a stressful lifestyle can serve the defensive function of distraction, keeping past trauma out of mind. I also include in-ternal stress (e.g., perfectionism that spawns a continual sense of failure and shame; suppressed resentment intermingled with dependency, as is characteristic of ambivalent attachment). Brown and colleagues also paid careful attention to the *meaning* of life stress, which included themes of humiliation and entrapment (Brown et al. 1995). Humiliating events, for example, included being rejected or devalued in attachment relation-ships. Such events assault self-esteem. Entrapment involved ongoing dif-ficulties with relationships, housing, employment, or health. Suffering loss as well as feeling humiliated and trapped can lead to feelings of defeat and hopelessness, which then can lead to a sense of futility and giving up the struggle.

Insecure attachment is associated with depression, from childhood and adolescence into adulthood (Luyten et al. 2012). Sidney Blatt's (2004) clinical work with depressed patients led to his focus on the polarities of re-latedness and self-definition that I highlight throughout this book. Blatt identified two distinct patterns of depression, labeled dependent and self-critical. *Dependent depression* "is characterized by feelings of loneliness, helplessness, and weakness; the individual has intense and chronic fears of being abandoned and left unprotected and uncared for. These individuals have intense longings to be loved, nurtured, and protected" (p. 156). Lacking psychological security, persons with dependent depression are solely reliant on others for comfort: "Because of their failure to have adequately internalized experiences of gratification or the qualities of the individuals who provided satisfaction, others are valued primarily for the immediate care, comfort, and satisfaction they provide" (p. 156).

In contrast, *self-critical depression* "is characterized by self-criticism and feelings of unworthiness, inferiority, failure, and guilt. These individuals engage in constant and harsh self-scrutiny and evaluation and have a chronic fear of criticism and of losing the approval of significant others" (Blatt 2008, p. 156). As many patients in The Menninger Clinic's Professionals in Crisis program exemplify, to guard against feelings of failure, persons vulnerable to self-critical depression are driven to succeed and, at the extreme, become perfectionistic: "They strive for excessive achievement and perfection, are often highly competitive and work hard, make many demands on themselves, and often achieve a great deal, but with little lasting satisfaction" (p. 156). Their criticism goes outward as well as inward: their competitiveness leads them also to be critical of others. Hence, their relationships often are infused with hostility, jealousy, and envy, leaving them feeling alienated and alone.

As Brown and colleagues (1995) proposed, life events and difficulties that precipitate episodes of depression do so by virtue of their meaning, and Blatt's (2004, 2008) work underscores the two overarching psychological themes: loss and failure. Vulnerability to stressors signifying loss and failure is tied to personality development: excessive dependency confers sensitivity to loss, and self-criticism confers sensitivity to failure. In turn, these two patterns are linked to insecure attachment: ambivalent attachment is associated with greater vulnerability to dependent depression in the context of feelings of neglect or abandonment, whereas avoidant attachment is associated with greater vulnerability to self-critical depression in conjunction with experiences of humiliation or failure. Patterns of insecurity are not static, however, and some depressed individuals show a mixture of dependent and self-critical depression. For example, it's not uncommon for relentless striving for success and recognition to be ways of masking longings for closeness and comfort.

Attachment Trauma

Brown and Harris (1978) found that episodes of depression commonly were preceded by stressful life events and ongoing difficulties, yet only about 20% of women exposed to stress developed episodes of depression. Thus began the search for vulnerabilities. Although early loss of a parent is a widely recognized risk factor for depression, Bowlby (1980) stressed the "enormous importance of a child's experience after the loss" (p. 312). Confirming Bowlby's point, Brown and colleagues (1990) found that maternal loss conferred vulnerability only when followed by lack of adequate care—that is, either neglect or parental rejection. More specifically, subsequent research showed that the vulnerability was associated with lack of maternal care prior to the loss, lack of paternal or substitute care after the loss, and the child's experience of helplessness in the aftermath of the loss (Bifulco et al. 1992). In short, early loss in the context of insecure attachment creates vulnerability to later depression.

Further investigating developmental antecedents of adulthood depression, Brown's colleague Antonia Bifulco developed a systematic, interview-based method for assessing and classifying childhood maltreatment. Bifulco and Moran (1998) found that all forms of maltreatment— physical, sexual, and psychological abuse, as well as neglect—were associated with increased risk of depression in adulthood. Subsequent research has shown that childhood maltreatment not only increases the risk of episodes of depression but also contributes to the severity of episodes (Harkness and Monroe 2002), the likelihood of suicidal behavior (Brodsky et al. 2001), and the likelihood of recurrence (Bernet and Stein 1999). Subsequent longitudinal research studying participants at 11 points from age 3 to age 32 revealed that major depressive episodes were associated with a history of maltreatment but not with a history of parental loss (Moffitt et al. 2010).

Depression and Mentalizing

Like all other psychiatric problems, depression and mentalizing interact in a vicious circle: depression impairs mentalizing capacity, and impaired mentalizing contributes to depression (Luyten et al. 2012). Although you aren't aware of your own mentalizing when you're doing well, mentalizing is an extremely complex process that requires considerable mental effort. Feeling depressed, you may not have the mental energy to make the effort to mentalize. You may be so withdrawn and self-absorbed as to be relatively oblivious to others' experience. And you may not be able to make much sense of your own experience. Alternatively, you may be mentalizing too much in the sense of obsessing about your problems and feelings or obsessing about what others are thinking. Such preoccupation is another form of impaired mentalizing, better labeled *rumination*. Effective mentalizing involves thinking flexibly and seeing things from different perspectives. Rumination involves going around in circles, thinking inflexibly. Depressive rumination also involves impaired mentalizing in the sense that the depressed person has the illusion of engaging in problem solving while actually only digging a deeper hole of depression (Nolen-Hoeksema 2000).

Distorted mentalizing also plays a role in the development of depression. Cognitive therapy (Beck et al. 1979) puts an emphasis on distorted thinking—that is, unreasonably negative thoughts about oneself ("I'm a complete failure"), the world ("Everyone hates me"), and the future ("No one ever will love me"). Such negative thinking can be viewed as part and parcel of internal working models stemming from insecure attachment. No doubt, such pernicious working models of the self (e.g., as being a failure and unlovable) play a major role in depression. Yet distorted working models of others as uncaring or unduly critical also contribute to depression by interfering with relationships—not only by creating stress but also by undermining interpersonal problem solving (Luyten et al. 2012). An obvious example would be misinterpreting a partner's anxious preoccupation as cruel indifference and then berating the partner for neglect and thereby inflaming conflict in the relationship. Such impaired mentalizing can result from applying the internal working models stemming from past trauma to current attachment relationships.

These observations attest to the importance of improving mentalizing in treating depression. As I view it, plain old therapy promotes a mentalizing stance: you learn not to take your negative thoughts and feelings too seriously, recognizing the influence of depression on your thinking and remaining mindful that your mental state will change. Concomitantly, mentalizing actively and accurately is essential in restoring a feeling of connection and security in attachment relationships—the antidote to depressive isolation and alienation. After recovery from depressive episodes, this mindful stance can prevent relapse, heading off the prospect of ruminating yourself into a persistently depressed mood (Segal et al. 2010).

Anxiety

DSM-IV-TR (American Psychiatric Association 2000) classifies PTSD among the anxiety disorders, notwithstanding its significant overlap with depression. PTSD, however, is not the only anxiety disorder associated with trauma. In this section, I first note research relating childhood trauma to generalized anxiety; then, I revisit the overlap between depression and anxiety, as well as the relation between trauma and anxiety. To conclude, I summarize the differences between depression and anxiety and the nature of their overlap.

Anxiety, Depression, and Trauma

The challenge of disentangling depression and PTSD is exceeded only by that of disentangling depression from generalized anxiety disorder, which is characterized by uncontrollable worry in conjunction with chronic symptoms of anxiety that include restlessness, fatigue, difficulty concentrating, irritability, muscle tension, and sleep disturbance. Major depression and generalized anxiety share genetic susceptibility and proneness to distress; in addition, the two disorders often respond to the same medications (Moffitt et al. 2010). Most pertinent to our concerns, childhood abuse, neglect, and loss contribute to both disorders (Kessler et al. 2010), and the combination of generalized anxiety and major depression is associated with the highest level of developmental risk (Moffitt et al. 2010).

In disentangling depression and anxiety, Brown (2010) distinguishes two meanings associated with stressful events: "*Loss*…involving either a person, role, or cherished idea has been associated with depression, and *danger* defined as the possibility of some future loss has been associated with anxiety" (p. 311, emphasis in original). Blatt's two polarities of relatedness and self-definition also apply to anxiety: danger applies not only to anticipated loss but also to anticipated blows to self-esteem and potential humiliation. Thus, ambivalent and avoidant attachment confer susceptibility to each kind of danger (i.e., loss of love or loss of self-esteem). Many stressful events—including childhood maltreatment—entail both loss and danger. Accordingly, Brown (2010) points out that the common co-occurrence of depression and anxiety results from their common causes in childhood maltreatment as well as adulthood stressors that involve *both* loss and danger.

One Disorder or Two—or Three?

Although they frequently go together, acute anxiety and depression occur in *episodes* over the lifetime. Either one is equally likely to precede the other (Kessler et al. 2010); moreover, the occurrence of one is likely to increase the likelihood of the subsequent occurrence of the other (Fergusson and Horwood 2010). Anxiety begets depression, and depression begets anxiety. Thus, a cascade of episodes occurs: as time goes on, an individual who has a lifetime history of either disorder is increasingly likely to have a history of the other (Goldberg 2010).

Extensive psychological research has clarified the overlap between depression and anxiety as well as the differences between them (Watson 2009), as diagrammed simply in Figure 3–3. Anxiety and depression overlap in their high level of negative emotionality, for which psychologists have proposed many different labels. *Neuroticism* is the most venerable

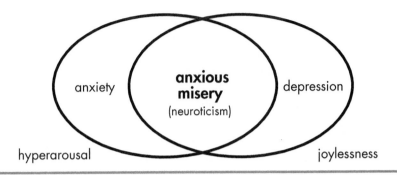

FIGURE 3–3. Relations between depression and anxiety.

term for this overlap, but my favorite label is *anxious misery*. Anxious misery also comprises many symptoms of PTSD. Depression is somewhat distinctive from anxiety in its *low level of positive emotionality*—that is, lack of capacity to experience interest, excitement, pleasure, joy, and love. On the other hand, anxiety is somewhat distinctive from depression in its *high level of anxious arousal*, which might be evident in accelerated heart rate, shortness of breath, or dizziness. In short, anxiety is distinguished from depression in being rooted in fear (G. Andrews et al. 2009).

In tandem with depression, high levels of anxiety and attunement to threat are the enemy of mentalizing. Threat activates the fight-or-flight response, which shuts down mentalizing (Arnsten 1998). Someone threatened with dire harm doesn't take time to think, but takes action by fighting or fleeing. Anxiety tends to focus all attention rigidly on threat, thus constraining mentalizing. Accordingly, if you're anxious, you are more likely to misinterpret others' actions as being hostile or ill intentioned—and to see yourself as being incompetent and helpless. It's easy to see how anxiety and depression conspire to distort mentalizing by interfering with *what* you think (i.e., misinterpretations) as well as *how* you think (i.e., rigidly).

Substance Abuse

I find it impossible to overstate the significance of substance abuse in the development and treatment of psychiatric disorders—even apart from considering trauma. Having worked in a psychiatric hospital for over three decades, I've come to think of substance abuse as a potential developmental disaster. And I feel disheartened when I see patients who've worked hard in treatment and benefited significantly from it relapse into substance abuse, potentially undermining all the work they've done—not least undermining the attachment relationships that had been strained and then partially rebuilt. The flip side of this coin, which I've also seen repeatedly, is the sheer benefit of effective treatment and hard work on substance abuse problems in tandem with psychiatric treatment, which establishes a foundation for enduring recovery.

From the start of this book, I have emphasized the core function of attachment as emotion regulation. When high levels of distress are coupled with insecure attachment, substance abuse provides an alternative method of emotion regulation. Consistent with this supposition, insecure attachment (preoccupied and unresolved) in adulthood, as assessed by the Adult Attachment Interview, is associated with heightened risk of drug abuse (van IJzendoorn and Bakermans-Kranenburg 2008).

When we consider the research on anxiety and depression reviewed in the previous section of this chapter, addictive substances may seem akin to miracle drugs. Alcohol, narcotics, and antianxiety medications dramatically decrease negative emotion and potentially increase positive emotions. Stimulants such as amphetamines and cocaine, by activating reward circuits in the brain, dramatically increase positive emotion. The problem, of course, is the temporary nature of these salutary effects. Alcohol, narcotics, and antianxiety agents are depressants, thus contributing to depression, and withdrawal from these agents can lead to rebound anxiety, which then must be quelled by more of the same. Stimulants not only evoke positive emotion but also activate stress circuitry, fueling anxiety and fear as well as exacerbating PTSD symptoms. Also, withdrawal from stimulants can provoke depression. Not uncommonly, patients use *both* stimulants *and* depressants to manage these complex emotional effects—alternately elevating and dampening emotional arousal, aspiring to achieve some stability while unwittingly destabilizing their emotions and associated brain chemistry.

In this section, I begin by discussing the complex relations between substance abuse and trauma. Next, I review some literature on the relations between substance abuse and key trauma-related disorders: PTSD, dissociation, and depression. I make the obvious point that integrated treatment is best for combined substance abuse and trauma-related problems. And I conclude by relating substance abuse to impaired mentalizing.

Trauma and Substance Abuse

Substantial research indicates that the accumulation of traumatic experiences in childhood dramatically increases the odds of alcohol and drug abuse (Felitti and Anda 2010). In combination with genetic risk, childhood sexual abuse has been associated with substance abuse in adolescence (Kendler et al. 2002); in part, childhood sexual trauma is associated with adult substance abuse by virtue of contributing to PTSD, which, in turn, contributes to substance abuse (Epstein et al. 1998).

We shouldn't overlook the other direction of causation: intoxication associated with substance abuse also increases the risk of exposure to traumatic stress (McFarlane 1998). A few examples illustrate. Drunk driving is an obvious case in point, because motor vehicle accidents are a prominent source of PTSD (Norris 1992). Drug abuse and drug dealing are associated with a heightened risk of exposure to violence and assaults (Brady et al. 1998). Also, a substantial minority of women report alcohol intoxication in conjunction with rape (Resnick et al. 1997). Alcohol intoxication increases vulnerability to sexual assault in many ways, such as by impairing judgment and mentalizing, blunting awareness of risk, decreasing capacity for self-protection, and contributing to being perceived as sexually available (Ruzek et al. 1998).

PTSD, Dissociation, Depression, and Substance Abuse

PTSD and substance abuse are commonly co-occurring disorders. Consistent with its emotion-regulation function, substance abuse more commonly follows than precedes PTSD (Stewart et al. 1998). Accordingly, substance abuse can be viewed as an experiential avoidance symptom of PTSD (Friedman 1990). Moreover, substance abuse might also be considered analogous to dissociation. Eli Somer (2009) construed narcotic addiction as a form of chemical dissociation: in effect, when psychological dissociation is insufficient to alleviate distress, narcotics can provide additional help. Interviews with persons who had a history of addiction underscored the similarities between dissociation and the narcotic high (pp. 514–515): "Heroin helps me forget the pain in my life." "When I'm high I don't care about the horrors of my childhood.... I can't remember my nightmares." "After I shoot up, the anger doesn't bother me anymore. It's like I disconnect it. I turn it off. Maybe it's still there, but I'm elsewhere." A former prostitute stated, "When I was on the drug, they could take my body and do what they f**king pleased with it. I wasn't home." Other interviewees' experiences were consistent with the link between addiction and attachment: "I'm cold from the inside.... When I shoot up, I have this great rush of warmth.... It's so comforting." "Nothing beats the feeling I got from heroin...like a gentle blanket that was lovingly wrapped around my shoulders." "There was something sweet about the seduction of the stuff...imagine being caressed from inside."

Many persons use substances to manage the distress and low level of positive emotion associated with depression. As diagrammed in Figure 3–4,

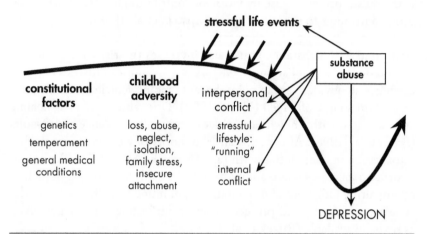

FIGURE 3–4. Substance abuse as a catalyst for depression.

Source. Adapted from Allen JG: *Traumatic Relationships and Serious Mental Disorders.* Chichester, UK, Wiley, 2001, p. 107. Used with permission.

in working with this problem, I have come to view substance abuse as a *catalyst:* in the face of stress pileup, substance abuse will speed up the slide into depression (Allen 2006). That is, substance abuse increases the likelihood of stressful life events (e.g., being arrested for drunk driving or losing a job); leads to chronic interpersonal conflict that further undermines attachment security; contributes to a stressful lifestyle (e.g., being preoccupied with procuring drugs and hiding the addiction); fuels internal conflict (e.g., feelings of guilt and shame); and, in a direct path to depression, stresses the nervous system (e.g., through intoxication and withdrawal).

Regardless of which comes first, the addiction or the psychiatric disorder, both must be treated together. Lisa Najavits and colleagues (2009) developed an integrated approach to treating trauma-related substance abuse, aptly called Seeking Safety. This present-focused, cognitive-behavioral approach employs psychoeducation and skills training to help patients achieve greater safety in their lives. The program has been employed with men and women recovering from all kinds of trauma and with a history of all kinds of substance abuse. The focus on safety resonates with the experience I had with my colleague AnnMarie Glodich in developing a psychoeducational group for traumatized adolescents to promote mentalizing (Glodich et al. 2006). We quickly learned that the first priority was not processing previous trauma but rather preventing future trauma; substance abuse loomed large as a focus of our group.

Mentalizing and Substance Abuse

When we educate patients about the relation between psychiatric disorders and mentalizing impairments, we start with substance abuse because the vicious circle is so clear-cut (Allen et al. 2012). We hardly need to take pains to explain how intoxication impairs mentalizing! Beyond intoxication, however, addiction undermines mentalizing by means of the sheer preoccupation it involves, such as preoccupation with obtaining drugs and obsession with concealing addictive behavior.

Yet the other side of the vicious circle may be more important: impaired mentalizing can play a major role in substance abuse. Compromised mentalizing and insecure attachment go hand in hand; both are implicated in problems with emotion regulation. Simply put, as I noted earlier, substance abuse affords an alternative to secure attachment relationships in regulating emotional distress. Attachment and addictive substances activate the same brain circuits; thus, they overlap in providing feelings of pleasure and soothing (Insel 2003). Of course, seeking substitutes for attachment relationships further undermines these relationships, not only cutting the addicted person off from the relationship but also communicating rejection to the partner: the addictive substance becomes the other lover. Given the potentially close links between substance abuse, mentalizing impairments, and insecure attachment relationships, clinicians are developing and researching mentalizing-enhanced substance abuse treatments (Philips et al. 2012).

Ill Health

Extensive research attests to the potential adverse impact of attachment-related traumatic stress on the developing brain and the potentially enduring compromise in capacity for stress regulation (Schore 2009). At worst, childhood trauma has been linked to heightened risk of serious disease, including liver disease, chronic obstructive pulmonary disease, coronary artery disease, and autoimmune disease (Felitti and Anda 2010). Fortunately, however, stress-related physical symptoms often are *not* associated with diagnosable disease but rather with many forms of generalized ill health (Weiner 1992). Symptoms associated with childhood maltreatment include pain in the back, chest, face, pelvis, genitalia, breasts, abdomen, and stomach; headaches; bruising; problems with urination; diarrhea and constipation; appetite disturbance; choking sensations; and shortness of breath (McCauley et al. 1997).

Moreover, as a chronic stressor, PTSD accounts for a substantial amount of the risk of physical health problems (Andreski et al. 1998).

PTSD is associated with problematic health-related behaviors, including alcohol, drug, and nicotine use; poor diet, sleep problems, and lack of exercise; and failure to obtain regular health care and poor adherence to treatment recommendations. We see glaring vicious circles: chronic stress undermines resilience; health-compromising behavior such as addictions and eating-disordered behavior are employed as strategies to decrease stress; and such behavior further undermines resilience.

Notably, posttraumatic avoidance and dissociative symptoms impair the ability to mentalize emotion—that is, to express emotions openly and to process traumatic experience. Again, a vicious circle occurs: nonmentalized emotions can contribute to symptoms of ill health, and ill health—fatigue and pain—can undermine mentalizing. Conversely, expressing emotional reactions to traumatic experience and putting the feelings into words improves physical health (Pennebaker 2004). Accordingly, regardless of whether impaired mentalizing is the cause or the effect of ill health—more likely both—effective treatment must restore mentalizing. In this vein, Patrick Luyten and Boudwijn Van Houdenhove (in press) identified the importance of embodied mentalizing in restoring health in patients with chronic fatigue syndrome and fibromyalgia. *Embodied mentalizing* refers to the ability to link mental and bodily states—for example, understanding that accelerated heart rate reflects feelings of anxiety. Similarly, a person struggling with chronic fatigue would benefit from being attuned to his or her energy levels so as to tailor activity levels accordingly (e.g., to avoid overdoing it).

Embodied mentalizing exemplifies the more general process of explicating the psychological meaning of symptoms. I worked with a patient, for example, who was utterly perplexed by her conversion disorder, which took the form of paralysis. She'd had extensive medical workups that ruled out any neurological basis for her paralysis. Thus, when she came for psychiatric treatment, she had accepted the idea that her symptoms had a psychological basis, yet she couldn't make any psychological sense of her paralysis. Through a course of intensive psychotherapy, with attachment trauma as a focus, we were able to understand that she'd been *paralyzed by fear,* and she gradually gained more freedom of movement (Allen and Fonagy, in press).

In our educational groups on mentalizing, we engage patients in an activity wherein each group member offers a symptom for consideration, and then we ask the question, "If your symptom could talk, what would it say?" With this framework in mind, group members speculate about what the symptom might be communicating. For example, a patient offered the symptom of agitation and trembling for the group's consideration, and group members speculated that the symptom might be communicating either "Help me!" or "Leave me alone!" The patient who offered the symptom let the group know that they had identified his conflict when he's anxious: he desperately wants help, but he's afraid to allow anyone near him.

Eating Disorders

We might think of eating disorders as analogous to substance abuse: like addictions, eating-disordered behavior is an effort to regulate emotional distress. Anorexia (restricting food intake) can be an effort to take control, including controlling what goes into one's body. Bingeing is akin to addiction in providing emotional comfort, and both bingeing and purging provide powerful distractions from emotional distress while also affording some sense of control.

Unfortunately, as with substance abuse, the positive effects of eating-disordered behavior are short-lived, and the behavior ultimately undermines control (Swirsky and Mitchell 1996). Bingeing provides a feeling of soothing or dissociative detachment, but bingeing is followed by guilt, shame, disgust, and self-hatred, which then must be relieved by purging. Purging then provides temporary relief and a sense of being back in control, but the same cascade of negative emotions follows purging. Hence, bingeing and purging recur in a vicious cycle: for example, purging relieves the shame and guilt resulting from bingeing, and bingeing soothes the shame and guilt resulting from purging.

Attachment trauma is prominent among a wide range of factors that contribute to the development of eating disorders. Thus, eating disorders have been related to a history of sexual, physical, and emotional abuse as well as neglect in childhood (Fischer et al. 2010). The particularly adverse effects of emotional abuse are noteworthy, because emotional abuse implies a lack of mentalizing. Moreover, eating disorders are more likely to develop when women with a history of abuse also have problems with attachment and social support (Mallinckrodt et al. 1995).

As is the case with substance abuse, eating disorders may complicate the treatment of trauma, and vice versa (Becker and Zayfert 2008): processing trauma evokes distress that eating-disordered behavior strives to relieve, and refraining from eating-disordered behavior can heighten trauma-related symptoms. Thus, as with substance abuse, both disorders must be treated in an integrated fashion. Like substance abuse, starving, bingeing, and purging are nonmentalizing ways of managing emotional distress that can substitute for attachment relationships. Accordingly, Finn Skårderud has developed a specialized treatment program for patients with eating disorders that he designed to enhance mentalizing (Skårderud and Fonagy 2012). This program, called Minding the Body, goes beyond holding mind in mind to holding body in mind. Like the mentalizing approach to ill health described in the previous section of this chapter, Minding the Body aims to enhance embodied mentalizing. Such mentalizing is a middle ground between hyperembodied experience (i.e., undue focus on the body) and disembodied experience (i.e., lack of awareness of the body). Mentalizing failures are evident in equating a psychological aspiration, such as a feeling of self-worth, with the physical condition of one's body (e.g., being thin) or in attempting to control one's emotional state by controlling what one eats. Embodied mentalizing entails seeing the body not only as a physical reality but also as a metaphorical or symbolic representation of the self (e.g., as strong) rather than a literal embodiment of the self (e.g., equating fat with being a repulsive person). In addition, as stated in relation to ill health, embodied mentalizing entails awareness of the relation between emotional states and bodily sensations. In sum, the mentalizing approach to eating disorders fosters the patient's addressing psychological problems and conflicts in attachment relationships directly, rather than trying to solve them indirectly and concretely via food and the body.

Nonsuicidal Self-Injury

For most of us, it's not obvious that self-injury can be a potent means of relieving distress. I remember my introduction to this mechanism many years ago when a patient who regularly cut herself told me how seeing the blood beading on her arm and feeling the warm sensation made her feel as if she were taking a soothing bath. I didn't doubt her sincerity; I was simply uncomprehending. I had no idea that she was immersed in a venerable tradition. Armando Favazza (2009) chronicled the cultural history of self-injury, noting that the behavior has been recorded "in all cultures since the earliest days of humankind" and making the bold point that it "might be seen as tapping into traditions that attempt to foster healing spirituality" (pp. 28–29). From this perspective, the term *self-injury* reflects the clinician's perspective; for the patient, the behavior can be experienced as self-healing to the degree that it provides dramatic relief from distress.

In this section, I start out with a description of self-injury, summarize research on its relation to childhood abuse and neglect, and then consider the multiple functions it serves as well as its adverse impact on attachment relationships.

Description

Terminology for self-injurious behavior varies; the terms *deliberate self-harm* (Morgan et al. 1975), *parasuicidal* (i.e., falsely suicidal) *behavior* (Linehan 1993a), and *self-mutilation* (Favazza 1987) have been employed. I prefer *nonsuicidal self-injury*, a term used by Matthew Nock (2009) to underscore its difference from suicidal behavior. Nock defines nonsuicidal self-injury as "the direct, deliberate destruction of one's own body tissue in the absence of suicidal intent" (Nock and Favazza 2009, p. 9) and stipulates that "the intent to die must be completely absent" (p. 13). Nock's definition doesn't include nonsuicidal overdosing, which can serve a similar function: rather than intending to die, many patients who overdose are, in effect, striving merely to seek relief from emotional pain by knocking themselves out for a time. Although it was new to me many years ago, nonsuicidal self-injury is not rare: 8% of preadolescents, 14%–21% of adolescents and young adults, and 4% of adults engage in the behavior (Nock and Favazza 2009). Nonsuicidal self-injury takes innumerable forms:

> Cutting, burning, slapping, punching, scratching, gouging, skin-piercing, hair-pulling or plucking, harmful enemas and douches, interfering with the healing of wounds, inserting dangerous objects into the vagina or rectum, head-banging, picking at cuticles and nails until they bleed, poking the ear, pulling out eyelashes or teeth, digging into the gums, choking, hitting oneself with objects, chewing the inside of the mouth/cheeks, ingesting sharp objects (such as razor blades, staples, needles, and pins), using an eraser to "burn" or tear the skin, and biting oneself. (Connors 1996, pp. 199–200)

Among these methods, skin cutting is by far the most common, followed by banging or hitting, and then burning; moreover, many individuals employ more than one method (Rodham and Hawton 2009).

Karl Menninger (1938) underscored the difference between self-injury and suicidal behavior by characterizing self-injury as *antisuicidal* behavior. Self-injury might be viewed as behavior intended to make life bearable. Many persons engage in both: 50%–75% of persons who engage in nonsuicidal self-injury also attempt suicide at some point (Nock and Favazza 2009). For example, when efforts to cope through nonsuicidal self-injury and other means fail, the traumatized person may give up and attempt suicide in desperation. Moreover, the line between nonsuicidal self-injury and suicide can be blurred. For example, patients have told me that their primary goal in overdosing was to escape pain temporarily, but if they were to die, that was OK too. Therapists and patients should keep ambivalence and blurry boundaries in mind: "Clinically, it's wise to assume that all [deliberate self-harm] sufferers want at some level to die and that all 'serious' suicidal people want, somewhere in their deepest being, to live" (Holmes 2011, p. 154).

Development

Nonsuicidal self-injury has been related to sexual, physical, and emotional abuse (Yates 2009) as well as emotional neglect (Dubo et al. 1997). A reexperiencing of neglect (i.e., mentalizing failure) often serves as the trigger for self-injury; as Louise Kaplan (1991) observed, it is "often precipitated by an unanswered phone call, the departure of a friend or lover or therapist, a caring face that turned away" (p. 384). In the Minnesota longitudinal study, Tuppett Yates (2009) found that, consistent with its roots in trauma, disorganized infant attachment was associated with more than a threefold increase in the odds of engaging in nonsuicidal self-injury. Given the role of attachment trauma in its development, Yates proposes that nonsuicidal self-injury can have origins in internal working models of the self as defective, others as malevolent, and relationships as dangerous. Thus, the coupling of a high level of emotional reactivity to distress with the inability to rely on attachment relationships for comfort and soothing leads to desperate measures to regulate emotion, nonsuicidal self-injury among them.

One important factor that comes into play—often in *initiating* nonsuicidal self-injury—is social contagion: individuals learn about it from their peers who can serve as models (Prinstein et al. 2009). Of great current concern is the phenomenon of contagion through media. Janis Whitlock and colleagues (2009) reported a dramatic increase in the number of movies and songs with self-injury content over the previous two decades. Moreover, they reported how social media come into play in Internet message boards devoted to self-injury that are increasingly prevalent, easily accessed, and highly frequented. Social networking has a positive side insofar as individuals share strategies for ceasing the behavior and obtaining help; yet, worryingly, they also share strategies for "avoiding detection, treating severe wounds, and even for injuring in new or different ways" (p. 144).

Functions

No one would cut, bang, or burn to relieve distress if other means were equally effective. Fundamentally, I view nonsuicidal self-injury as a nonmentalizing emotion-regulation strategy stemming from a failure of attachment. Elucidating its complexity in a fashion that can help therapists and patients mentalize this potentially bewildering behavior, Nock and Cha (2009) identified four basic functions of self-injury, each of which reinforces the behavior, albeit in different ways.

First and most commonly, self-injury provides relief from emotional pain—in short, tension reduction. In my view, its primary function is escape from unbearable emotional states, which include feelings of terror, rage, shame, despair, and the like. Cutting also can trigger dissociative detachment and thereby blunt emotional pain.

Second, self-injury provides rewarding sensations, for example, as in my patient's likening the effects of cutting to being in a soothing bath. Persons who feel sensory pain can find this effect reinforcing in the sense that the sensation of physical pain is more tangible and controllable than is un-fathomable (i.e., nonmentalized) emotional pain. Yet, when coupled with analgesia, these rewarding effects may result from the activation of endog-enous opioids (Sher and Stanley 2009). Alternatively, cutting also can bring the person out of a painful state of dissociative detachment—that is, produce a rewarding feeling of being alive. In this sense, self-injury is a form of grounding, by virtue of anchoring the person in the present.

Third, self-injury can be reinforcing in eliciting concern and help from others. This potential function is the reason that persons who self-injure can be criticized as being "manipulative" and "just trying to get attention." Such responses are way off the mark in overlooking the more prominent function of relief from emotional pain. Hence, Ellen Leibenluft and col-leagues (1987) cautioned therapists: "Our experience leads us to believe that professionals are prone to attribute primarily hostile or manipulative intent to the behavior, and that they pay insufficient attention to the in-ternal experience of the client" (p. 323). In my view, getting attention—comfort and concern—is a *desirable* attachment-related goal, especially in view of the fact that self-injury is associated with a history of emotional neglect. Here's an account of positive social reinforcement:

> After an overdose attempt that leads to hospital admission, the estranged parent or partner is often—*but, sadly, not always*—to be found at the pa-tient's bedside. The…episode has worked its magic, and normal attach-ment relations…may well have been restored. (Holmes 2011, p. 155, emphasis added)

Such a positive effect of restoring attachment security has the poten-tial to *decrease* the need for self-injury. Yet the problem with self-injury in this respect is not the desire but rather the sheer *ineffectiveness* of such ef-forts to get attention (Linehan 1993a). One example of ineffectiveness is eliciting criticism (e.g., for being manipulative), which only reinforces the person's experience of emotional neglect (i.e., being misunderstood).

Fourth, self-injury potentially can result in escaping social demands, avoiding punishment, or staving off further abuse. Injuring oneself, for ex-ample, might prompt others to back off. Hurting oneself and making oth-ers aware of extreme suffering also might temporarily prevent them from causing more hurt.

Vicious Circles in Attachment Relationships

Self-injurious behavior has a powerful expressive or communicative function (Prinstein et al. 2009). Unable to mentalize their emotions, many traumatized persons are at a loss for words. Moreover, they're liable to feel that words cannot possibly express the depth of their emotional pain; only actions will do. There's often an aggressive or even vengeful quality to this expression, for example, when blood, burns, or scars shockingly convey, "See how much you've hurt me!" Like substance abuse and eating disorders, self-injurious behavior boldly reflects the developmentally early teleological (action-oriented) mode of nonmentalizing that I introduced in the first chapter ("Attachment, Mentalizing, and Trauma").

In educating patients in groups about self-injury, I use the diagram in Figure 3–5 to highlight its connections to attachment relationships. I construe tension relief as the behavior's main effect: the cascade goes from feeling stressed in the context of disrupted attachment, then to unbearable emotional states, then to self-injury, and finally to tension reduction. I invite patients to enumerate emotions under the rubric of unbearable emotional states; such emotions include fear, terror, panic, frustration, rage, shame, guilt, disgust, helplessness, hopelessness, despair, and so forth. I describe the interpersonal consequences as side effects, while recognizing that sometimes the primary intent can relate to its interpersonal effects (e.g., seeking care or communicating vengeful feelings). As already noted, the side effects can be positively reinforcing when the behavior elicits concern and help.

To the extent that the behavior is severe and persistent, however, the effects on attachment relationships are powerfully negative. I invite patients to enumerate the emotions their partners feel, and it becomes evident quickly that the partner is liable to feel *all* the same unbearable emotions as the patient. Moreover, I emphasize that self-injurious behavior not only evokes unbearable emotional states in the partner but also undermines the partner's attachment security in the relationship. Thus, in this cascade, the patient's insecurity dramatically fuels the partner's insecurity. The partner's emotions and insecurity can lead the partner to engage in similarly self-destructive behavior (e.g., the patient cuts and the partner drinks). In these vicious circles, neither the patient nor the partner is able to mentalize, leaving each psychologically unavailable to the other. At best, the partner is liable to alternate between withdrawing and becoming coercive and controlling. At worst, confirming the patient's worst fear of being abandoned, the partner becomes fed up. Sometimes, anticipating abandonment, patients will drive their partners away, taking control over what they consider to be inevitable (i.e., getting it over with). This process can become mutually traumatizing, heaping present trauma upon past trauma, as each member of the pair is left painfully alone in increasingly unbearable emotional sates. This escalation of insecurity and emotional pain reaches its peak in suicidal behavior.

PATIENT   PARTNER

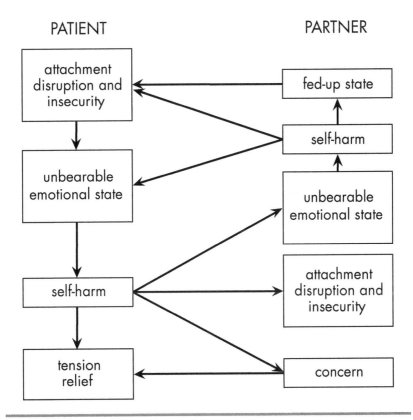

FIGURE 3–5. Self-harm and vicious circles in attachment relationships.

Source. Adapted from Allen JG: *Traumatic Relationships and Serious Mental Disorders.* Chichester, UK, Wiley, 2001, p. 229. Used with permission.

Suicidal States

Nock and Favazza (2009) distinguish suicidal behavior not only from nonsuicidal self-injury but also from a suicide threat or gesture—that is, "a statement or behavior in which people lead others to believe they intend to kill themselves when they really have no intention of doing so" (p. 12). In contrast, suicidal behavior is a result of a relatively unambivalent intent to die; such behavior includes suicidal thoughts, suicide plans, preparation for suicide, and suicide attempts. The essential contrast between nonsuicidal self-injury and suicidal behavior is the difference between a desire for temporary and for permanent escape from pain.

Development of Suicidal States

Many factors predispose persons to suicidal states: psychiatric disorders; genetic vulnerability; family history of suicidal behavior; maladaptive personality traits such as perfectionism, impulsivity, and isolation; lack of social support; and a chaotic family life (Blumenthal 1990; Harris and Barraclough 1997). Of course, many of these factors also are intertwined with trauma. Unsurprisingly, childhood abuse and neglect are widely recognized as risk factors for suicide, especially in conjunction with an accumulation of developmental adversities (Felitti and Anda 2010). Bifulco and colleagues (2002), for example, found a dose-response relationship between childhood maltreatment and suicidal behavior in adulthood. That is, the higher the number of types of maltreatment (i.e., psychological, sexual, and physical abuse, as well as neglect), the higher the likelihood of suicidal behavior. Moreover, psychological abuse (i.e., tormenting, terrorizing, and humiliating behavior) bore a stronger relation to suicidality than did other forms of maltreatment.

Feeling alone in emotional pain serves as a trigger for much of the behavior discussed in this chapter: alcohol and drug abuse; bingeing, purging, and starving; and the various forms of nonsuicidal self-injury. But perhaps nowhere is the feeling of being alone in emotional pain more prominent than in suicidal states (Allen 2011). In this vein, Thomas Joiner (2005) identified two key contributors to suicidal states: a *lack of belongingness* as well as a sense of *burdensomeness*—that is, a person's belief that others would be better off if he or she were dead. This combination leaves the person feeling alienated and alone. The present resonates with the past: current experience of feeling isolated, excluded, rejected, let down, betrayed, and unworthy of care resonates with past trauma, such that feelings of disconnection can lead to the most excruciatingly unbearable emotional states.

No doubt, committing suicide goes against the grain of the basic instinct to survive. To overcome this basic instinct requires what Joiner (2005) called an *acquired capability*—namely, becoming accustomed to pain and fear as a result of repeated painful experiences. I've worked with patients who were practicing for suicide by means of increasingly lethal attempts, thereby working up to suicide. Practicing is one way of acquiring capability, as are repeated episodes of nonsuicidal self-injury. Sadly, being subjected to abuse also can contribute to acquired capability for suicide. Consistent with this supposition, Joiner and colleagues (2007) found that compared with less physically painful forms of childhood abuse, physical abuse and violent sexual abuse created an especially high risk for adulthood suicide attempts.

Nonmentalizing in the Suicidal Mode

We commonly associate suicide with depression, and for good reason, although anxiety also plays a prominent part. But it's not enough to focus treatment on depression and anxiety; the specific reasons for suicidal states also must be addressed directly. Thus, cognitive therapists have developed effective suicide-specific treatments (Wenzel et al. 2009). The cognitive model of suicide dovetails with the mentalizing perspective insofar as suicidal states involve dramatic mentalizing failures that commend a mentalizing approach to treatment (Allen 2011).

The cognitive model holds that developmental vulnerabilities render the individual liable to enter a suicidal state of mind—*the suicidal mode*—in the face of stress (Rudd 2006). Importantly, these vulnerability factors, which include insecure attachment, also contribute to the generation of interpersonal stress; that is, insecure attachment fuels conflicts in emotionally intense and unstable relationships. At the same time, impaired mentalizing interferes with interpersonal problem solving, and impaired interpersonal problem solving plays a significant role in suicidality (Rudd and Brown 2011). Moreover, in thinking about impaired mentalizing and problem solving, we shouldn't overlook the role of alcohol intoxication, which is a notoriously significant contributor to suicide (Jamison 1999). The same goes, of course, for other forms of substance abuse. Fueled by substance abuse or not, as the stress escalates while mentalizing and problem-solving ability plummets, two critical suicide-specific cognitive vulnerabilities come into play: a perception of emotional pain as being unbearable and a state of hopelessness. The suicidal person thus believes, "I can't take this anymore" and "This will never get better" (Wenzel and Beck 2008, p. 194).

Crucially, this cognitive model includes not only *what* the person is thinking but also *how* the person is thinking (or not thinking): the suicidal state entails cognitive constriction or rigidity characterized as *attentional fixation:* all problem-solving efforts are focused on suicide, including making plans and obtaining potential methods (Wenzel et al. 2009). In this mode, the individual considers suicide as the only solution to escaping the unbearably painful emotional state, and the person is thinking only about reasons for dying and not reasons for living (Jobes 2006).

Attentional fixation is the antithesis of mentalizing (i.e., flexible and reflective thinking in the context of emotional arousal), and the suicidal state as characterized in this cognitive model exemplifies the nonmentalizing mode of *psychic equivalence:* suicidal persons lose the sense that their thoughts and feelings *represent* reality in a particular way; equating the mental with the real, for example, they equate *feeling* hopeless with actually *being* hopeless. As Jeremy Holmes (2011) also emphasizes, mentalizing entails having in mind the distinction between thinking and acting; that is, mentalizing, a person is aware that he or she can think about doing something without actually doing it. From this vantage point, Holmes states flatly that "in all cases, albeit in differing ways, suicide can be seen as a failure of mentalizing—that is, of the capacity to differentiate thoughts and feelings from the reality of what is objectively the case" (p. 151). In short, in Holmes's view, full mentalizing is incompatible with suicide. Edwin Shneidman, a pioneer of suicide research, made a point that is consistent with this view: "a person who could write a meaningful suicide note would not be in the position of completing suicide" (quoted in Jobes and Nelson 2006, p. 37).

Holmes (2011) normalizes thinking about suicide: "Thinking about suicide at difficult moments in one's life is existentially normal and at times even helpful" (p. 150). Boldly, he proposes that "it may be a mark of narcissism never to have at least contemplated suicide, and, conversely, to be able to mentalize one's suicidality may be an indication of a degree of psychological health" (p. 160). Accordingly, the capacity to mentalize— thinking about suicide without acting on the thoughts or desires—is crucial in prevention: "Underpinning the mentalizing perspective is the implicit paradox that the capacity to think and talk about suicide is likely to reduce its occurrence" (p. 150). Consistent with Holmes's view, many patients with whom I have worked find the possibility of suicide to be comforting, which, paradoxically, can help them refrain from it. Holmes quotes the following quip: "Whenever everything else fails, all I have to do is consider suicide and in two seconds I'm as cheerful as a nitwit. But if I could *not* kill myself—ah, then I would" (p. 150, emphasis in original). Taking suicidal thinking for granted, Holmes does not inquire *if* the person has thought about suicide; rather, "'How suicidal are you?' is a question that every depressed, sad, or bereaved person needs to be asked" (p. 160).

Suicidal states exemplify the need for plain old therapy—that is, a mentalizing relationship (Allen 2011) in which a therapist's empathy allows the patient to no longer feel alone in emotional pain (Orbach 2011). Of course, a patient's suicidal state of mind poses a great challenge to the therapist, who is liable to feel threatened and anxious, which will interfere with his or her mentalizing capacity (Bateman and Fonagy 2006a). Israel Orbach (2001) articulated the therapist's aspiration: "a basic, empathic, and compassionate attitude (not pity) toward the suffering individual that cannot be faked" (pp. 172–173). As he elaborated,

> Being empathic with the suicidal wish means assuming the suicidal person's perspective and "seeing" how this person has reached a dead end

without trying to interfere, stop, or correct the suicidal wishes. This means that the therapist attempts to empathize with the patient's pain experience to such a point that he/she can "see" why suicide is the only alternative available to the patient.... Instead of working against the suicidal stream and trying to instantly increase the patient's motivation to live by persuasion or commitment to a contract, the therapist takes an empathic stance with the suicidal wish and brings it to full focus. As a tactic, I ask the suicidal person to actually "convince" me that suicide is the only solution left and communicate with him or her from that empathic focus. I try to participate in the consideration of suicide as an actual alternative without pressing against the suicidal decision. This, of course, does not connote agreement with the suicidal intention, but rather a way of connecting with the patient's experience and offering myself as a listener and companion at a time of crisis. (pp. 173–174)

In empathizing with the patient's suicidal state, the therapist must not *join* with the patient's hopelessness. As Holmes (2011) explains, mentalizing in this context "requires the therapist to have, as it were, one foot in this world of fantasy, one firmly planted in reality's camp" (p. 161). This aspiration is no small feat: the therapist must maintain hope, which often entails maintaining a conviction that the patient's life can become bearable and valuable even when the pathway by which this might occur is completely obscure. As long as the patient remains alive, the potential exists to discover pathways that cannot be imagined at the peak of hopelessness.

In sum, the antidote to nonmentalizing is mentalizing: as the developmental research attests, empathy from others begets empathy for the self. I foreshadow the discussion of plain old therapy here because suicidal states pose the greatest therapeutic challenge for patients and therapists. But the solution is basic: developing a collaborative mentalizing relationship in which the patient can feel understood and thereby understand himself or herself. To put it technically in the language of the Adult Attachment Interview, therapists who treat suicidal patients are aiming for narrative coherence (Michel and Valach 2011)—in simpler words, they are enabling the patient to tell the story as well as to create alternative stories.

My colleague David Jobes (2006) developed a structured assessment of contributors to suicidal states that I find extremely useful in initiating a mentalizing stance. Sitting beside the patient, the therapist assists him or her in filling out some rating scales and answering a series of questions. Patients are invited to rate their levels of psychological pain, stress, agitation, hopelessness, and self-hate; they also articulate the reasons for each of these experiences. They estimate their overall risk of dying by suicide in the future. They consider how much their suicidal states relate to feelings about themselves versus feelings about their relationships. Then they list their reasons for living and reasons for dying, and they rate separately the extent to which they wish to live and wish to die. Some patients rate themselves as having been unambivalent at the time of an attempt (i.e., rating wishing to die at the high end of the scale and wishing to live at the low end), whereas others rate themselves as having been ambivalent (e.g., wishing to live and wishing to die at equal strength). The assessment concludes with a particularly evocative question: What is the one thing that would help you no longer feel suicidal? This collaborative assessment of the basis of the suicidal state establishes the platform for suicide-focused treatment that addresses the driving forces for the suicidal state. I use this assessment early in the therapy with all suicidal patients.

Case Example

Natalie sought intensive hospital treatment after a serious and seemingly impulsive suicide attempt, which was not her first. We addressed this attempt immediately in psychotherapy, and she presented it as being mysterious. She said she had been out to lunch with a friend and had a good time, laughing and joking. After lunch, she decided not to return to work but—uncharacteristically—didn't let her coworker know she wouldn't be coming back in. Two hours later, she drank a pint of whiskey, took a stash of pills, and attempted suicide by carbon monoxide poisoning in her garage. Her coworker knew that Natalie had been struggling with depression and became concerned when she didn't return for work and didn't answer her phone, and Natalie was rescued.

By the time Natalie began therapy, she said she was feeling "OK," as she said she felt 90% of the time. She said her suicidal states came out of the blue and there was no reason for them. Yet the suicide assessment, focusing on her state of mind at the time of the attempt, quickly revealed chronic problems. Indeed, the first issue, psychological pain, got to the heart of her suicidality. What she found most painful was worrying about her father's anxiety and feeling helpless to do anything about it. She said her father always had been a "nervous wreck" and that she had been very close to him throughout her lifetime. Her mother had been "the rock of the family" and had maintained the stability of the family as she and her father as well as her brother had leaned on her mother. Her mother had been killed in a car accident a few years earlier, at which point her father became even more anxious and depressed. About a year after her mother's death, her father became involved in a romantic relationship with a woman Natalie considered to be "unstable," thus adding to his stress rather than relieving it. Meanwhile, Natalie was struggling to support herself and felt guilty for consequently "abandoning" her father. Moreover, when she did attempt to comfort him, he brushed her off and she felt her efforts were "useless."

Several other contributors were intertwined with the family situation. Natalie felt stressed by the combination of a demanding job that she had just started after graduating from college; she felt agitated when she was pressured by the demands of her boss while worrying that she could not help her father; she felt hopeless about changing the psychological pain and stress; and she hated herself for what turned out to be a crucial factor in her chronic suffering: substance abuse. She was caught up in amphetamine and cocaine abuse during the day, along with intermittent alcohol abuse and regular use of marijuana to "wind down" at night. She felt guilty and ashamed, particularly as she aspired to live up to her parents' high standards, which she had internalized. Although she had occasionally abused alcohol and "flirted" with drugs in adolescence, she recognized that her substance abuse became more problematic after her mother's death and then escalated dramatically after the breakup of a romantic relationship in which she had put great stock. She had been concealing the extent of her substance use and minimizing the severity of it; ironically, her feelings of guilt and shame about substance abuse in relation to failing to live up to her parents' ideals only added fuel to her substance abuse. Moreover, Natalie felt exquisitely guilty about her suicide attempts, which contributed to her father's anxiety and distress. In a further irony, she said that one incentive for suicide was her guilt feelings about her father's worry about her suicidality. Along with substance abuse, suicide was her "escape hatch."

Natalie first stated that the one thing that would help her no longer be suicidal would be if her mother were alive, attesting to the pivotal role of her family relationships in her suicidality. Invited to think about a realistically possible alternative response, she said the one thing that would enable her to live would be to have a healthy lifestyle. In the aftermath of the loss of her mother and her boyfriend, Natalie had moved into an avoidant stance; she had come to pride herself on being self-reliant. She confessed that she had a hard time accepting her need for treatment, because she looked down on people who relied on psychiatry and therapy. Yet she had a history of security in her family that enabled her to overcome her avoidance, particularly with her peers in treatment, with whom she could identify. By the time she was ready to move to outpatient treatment, she was keenly aware of her vulnerability to suicidal states and accepting of her need for ongoing professional help. Because she had become more self-aware in treatment, she realized that her previous view that she had been OK for 90% of the time was an illusion. On the contrary, she said she had actually been "in despair, 100% of the time."

Finally, I want to underscore the obvious fact that suicidal states are especially threatening to attachment relationships. The vicious circles I discussed in relation to nonsuicidal self-injury are magnified dramatically in the context of suicide. The threat of loss leads to extremely unbearable emotional states in the partner or caregiver that parallel those of the suicidal person—potentially including terror, rage, helplessness, hopelessness, shame, guilt, and despair. Concomitantly, the threat of loss dramatically escalates attachment insecurity. Parents, partners, friends, or therapists can lose the capacity to mentalize and then withdraw or become coercive.

Such responses then leave the suicidal person feeling all the more distressed and alone.

Personality Disorders

As emphasized throughout this book, attachment relationships play a key role in personality development. To a large degree, individual differences in personality are evident in relationships—attachment relationships and others. Extroversion and introversion are prime examples. Individual differences in attachment play a central role in our closest relationships— those in which our emotional needs are at stake. And attachment relationships shape our sense of self and identity. In short, attachment trauma leads to disturbances in identity and relationships; in psychiatry, such enduring disturbance is diagnosed as personality *disorder.*

Of all the psychiatric diagnoses, personality disorders are the most emotionally loaded. Being told that you have a personality disorder can feel like being told you have a "bad personality" or, worse, that you're a "bad person." The diagnosis can add insult to injury. In educating traumatized patients about personality disorders, I strive to dispel three myths:

1. *The myth of bad personality:* Personality disorders relate to problematic aspects of personality; they don't characterize the whole person. For example, many patients with personality disorders are engaging, kind, compassionate, and considerate much of the time.
2. *The myth of permanence:* Personality disorders aren't immutable. On the contrary, over a year's time, the majority of patients diagnosed with a personality disorder might be expected no longer to meet full criteria for the disorder (Shea et al. 2002). Like clinical syndromes, personality disorders can be episodic to a degree; symptoms wax and wane with stress, anxiety, and other factors such as substance abuse and abusive relationships (Allen 2003). Thus, although basic personality *traits* are relatively stable, *disorders* are less so (Oldham 2007).
3. *The myth of untreatability:* An increasing range of treatment approaches tailored to personality disorders have been developed and demonstrated to be effective. The caveat: the treatment takes time; long-term psychotherapy is a mainstay of treatment for personality disorders (Leichsenring 2009).

In this section, I define personality disorder more specifically and then note findings that relate trauma to various personality disorders. I conclude the section with discussion of borderline personality disorder

(BPD), which has been most extensively understood in relation to attachment trauma.

Diagnosing Personality Disorders

Roughly speaking, many personality disorders take the form of exaggerated personality traits that create difficulty in relationships. Examples are being paranoid (suspicious), narcissistic (arrogant and self-centered), dependent (relying too much on others), avoidant (sensitive to rejection), obsessive-compulsive (preoccupied with details, perfectionistic, and duty bound), and antisocial (being deceitful, showing disregard for others, breaking the law). Despite current controversy about diagnosing personality disorders (Livesley 2010), it is important to keep in mind that these diagnoses did not come out of nowhere: some individuals display them in prototypical form (Yudofsky 2005). Yet when it comes to the challenge of putting a number of symptoms into neat boxes, personality disorders take the prize: many persons show more than one personality disorder or a large number of traits scattered across a wide range of personality disorders. Personality traits, normal and maladaptive, are matters of degree and are intermingled in all of us. Thus, I came to think of a continuum of *personality disorderedness* (Allen 2001). John Oldham, chief of staff at The Menninger Clinic, and his colleagues found that personality-disordered patients met criteria for an average of 3.4 different personality disorders; they recommended that patients meeting criteria for multiple diagnoses be diagnosed with *extensive personality disorder* (Oldham et al. 1992). All of us fall somewhere on the continuum of personality disorderedness; few of us can be neatly typecast.

Consistent with Blatt's (2008) view of personality development as being based on relatedness and self-definition, the broad criteria for personality disorder being developed for DSM-5 entail significant impairment in interpersonal functioning and sense of self. Key aspects of self-functioning are *identity* (i.e., experiencing oneself as unique with clear boundaries between self and others; coherent sense of time and personal history; stability and accuracy of self-appraisal and self-esteem; capacity for a range of emotional experience and its regulation) and *self-direction* (i.e., pursuit of coherent and meaningful short-term and life goals; utilization of constructive and prosocial internal standards of behavior; ability to self-reflect productively). Key aspects of interpersonal functioning are *empathy* (i.e., comprehension and appreciation of others' experiences and motivations; tolerance of differing perspectives; understanding of the effects of behavior on others) and *intimacy* (i.e., depth and duration of connection with others; desire and capacity for closeness; mutuality of regard reflected in interpersonal behavior). As these criteria attest, problems in attachment and mentalizing play a fundamental role in personality disturbance.

Contribution of Attachment Trauma to Personality Disorders

As Judith Herman (1992b) made plain, it's little wonder that prolonged trauma leads to personality disturbance and disrupted attachment relationships:

> Social judgment of chronically traumatized people…tends to be extremely harsh. The chronically abused person's apparent helplessness and passivity, her entrapment in the past, her intractable depression and somatic complaints, and her smoldering anger often frustrate the people close to her. (p. 115)

Research supporting the relation between childhood trauma and adulthood personality disorders can be illustrated by Johnson and colleagues' careful study of the relation between abuse and neglect in childhood, as documented in an official U.S. state registry, and personality disorder in adulthood (Johnson et al. 1999). The findings were clear: persons with a documented history of childhood maltreatment were four times more likely to have an adulthood personality disorder than those without a trauma history. Yet, as you might surmise from all the foregoing, the effects of childhood trauma are nonspecific: although there were some differences among personality disorders depending on the type of maltreatment, the range of trauma-related personality disorders was extensive: antisocial, borderline, dependent, depressive, passive-aggressive, narcissistic, avoidant, paranoid, schizoid (interpersonally detached), and schizotypal (odd and eccentric). Employing psychological testing to assess personality functioning in women hospitalized for psychiatric disorders related to childhood maltreatment, we found a similarly wide array of disturbance (Allen et al. 1999). Yet, of all the personality disorders, BPD has been most systematically linked to attachment trauma and impaired mentalizing.

Borderline Personality Disorder

BPD exemplifies complex traumatic stress disorders. In brief, core problems in BPD include identity disturbance, unstable close relationships marked by insecurity and sensitivity to abandonment, intense emotional reactivity, and impulsive self-damaging behavior. Not only is the symptomatology of BPD multifaceted, but also BPD typically is intertwined with a range of co-occurring disorders. I've worked with a number of patients diagnosed with BPD who have *all* the problems discussed so far: PTSD, dissociative symptoms, depression, generalized anxiety, substance abuse, ill health, eating disorders, nonsuicidal self-injury, and suicide attempts.

Childhood abuse and neglect are well established as contributors to the development of BPD (Ball and Links 2009). Childhood maltreatment, however, is only one of many contributing factors; moreover, maltreatment is neither necessary nor sufficient for the development of the disorder (Gabbard 2000). Although childhood sexual abuse may play a particularly prominent role in the development of BPD, it's often intertwined with a broader pattern of family disturbance: "childhood sexual abuse reported by borderline patients may represent a *marker of the severity of the familial dysfunction* they experienced, as well as being a traumatic event or series of events in itself" (Zanarini et al. 1997, p. 1104, emphasis added). Moreover, neglect also puts the child at risk for sexual abuse outside the immediate family, "by making it clear to the potential perpetrators that no one will notice or care if the child is abused" (p. 1105).

Much of the research on the relation between BPD and childhood maltreatment has relied on retrospective reports, but recent prospective studies are providing more solid footing for developmental conclusions. All these findings are consistent with my focus on attachment and mentalizing. Jeffrey Johnson and colleagues (2006), for example, conducted a series of assessments of family members and their offspring spanning ages from 6 to 33. These researchers found that low levels of parental affection and nurturing, as well as aversive parental behaviors such as harsh punishment, were associated with later BPD (as well as other personality disorders). Karlen Lyons-Ruth and colleagues (2005) found that disrupted maternal communication in infancy correlated significantly with symptoms of BPD assessed at age 18; notably, total amount of abuse over the lifetime reported in adolescence also contributed to symptoms. As developmental research repeatedly shows, the accumulation of adversities increases the risk of disorder; in this instance, disrupted maternal communication combined with later abuse resulted in the highest level of symptoms of BPD (Melnick et al. 2008).

Elizabeth Carlson and colleagues (2009a) reported results from the Minnesota longitudinal study that correlated extensive assessments from infancy onward with BPD symptoms at age 28. The following early developmental observations related to symptoms of BPD: attachment disorganization (12–18 months), maltreatment (12–18 months), maternal hostility and boundary problems (42 months), family disruption related to father presence (12–64 months), and family life stress (3–42 months). Several harbingers of BPD were evident at 12 years of age: attention disturbance, emotional instability, behavioral instability, and disturbed relationships. The findings also suggested that maltreatment led to disturbances in self-representation (i.e., internal working models) that, in turn, put the individual at risk for BPD. As these authors noted, "representations and related mentalizing processes are viewed as the carriers of experience" (p. 1328) that link early insecure attachment to later personality disturbance.

Peter Fonagy and colleagues (1996) established the link between mentalizing and BPD more directly, based on assessments of mentalizing capacity in the Adult Attachment Interview: 97% of the patients with a history of maltreatment coupled with impaired mentalizing capacity met criteria for BPD, whereas only 17% of the patients reporting abuse in the group with preserved mentalizing met criteria for the disorder. As Fonagy and colleagues concluded,

> If children are maltreated but have access to a meaningful attachment relationship that provides the intersubjective basis for the development of mentalizing capacity, they will be able to resolve (work through) their experience, and its outcome will not be one of severe personality disorder.... If, however, the maltreated child has no social support of sufficient strength and intensity for an attachment bond to develop that could provide the context for the acquisition of a reliable capacity to envisage the psychological state of the other, even in intense interpersonal relationships, then the experience of abuse will not be reflected on or resolved. Naturally, the unresolved experience of abuse diminishes the likelihood of meaningful relationships, which, in a self-perpetuating way, further reduces the likelihood of a satisfactory resolution of the disturbing experience through the emergence of reflective processes. (Fonagy et al. 1995, p. 261)

Consistent with Fonagy's research on mentalizing failure, Alan Sroufe and colleagues (2005) commented that an unanticipated finding in their longitudinal study "was the devastating consequences of 'psychological' maltreatment. The pattern of parental psychological unavailability had wideranging consequences from early childhood into adulthood" (p. 301). This finding is particularly apt for the development of BPD. As my colleagues and I concluded previously, "the central factor that predisposes the child to BPD is *a family environment that discourages coherent discourse concerning mental states*" (Allen et al. 2008, p. 274, emphasis in original). As Fonagy and Bateman (2008) elaborated, trauma plays a prominent role in shaping the development of BPD by undermining mentalizing; however, "the impact of trauma is most likely to be felt as part of a more general failure of consideration of the child's perspective through neglect, rejection, excessive control, unsupportive relationship, incoherence, and confusion" (p. 14).

Going beyond the findings on broadly impaired mentalizing, Fonagy and Luyten (2009) spelled out the relation between multiple facets of mentalizing, which I discussed in the first chapter, and the core symptoms of BPD (i.e., affective dysregulation, impulsivity, unstable interpersonal relationships, and identity disturbance). Specifically, the core problem in BPD is a collapse of explicit, internal, and cognitive aspects of mentalizing when attachment needs are activated by emotional distress resulting from automatic, implicit, emotion-driven mentalizing. For example, in the face of emotional distress and in need of comfort, the person with BPD is likely to misperceive facial cues (e.g., seeing a quizzical expression as a condemning and hostile scowl) and to misinterpret the other person's state of mind (e.g., as rejecting). Emotional contagion prevails over accurate understanding and effective communication. Such disturbance in interactions is most likely to occur in response to experiences of rejection, misattunement, or abandonment in attachment relationships. Such failures of mentalizing in contemporary interactions are a reflection of the core failure of caregiving that lays the foundation for the development of BPD: the absence of mentalizing in the context of the child's heightened need or distress. This mentalizing failure on the part of the caregiver can take the form of emotional withdrawal or emotional contagion. This failure is the context for disorganized and anxious-ambivalent attachment, both of which are associated with BPD (van Ijzendoorn and Bakermans-Kranenburg 2008).

Coupled with such psychological unavailability, other forms of trauma, such as frightening and hostile-intrusive behavior in early and later attachment relationships, may lead to chronic, unresolved activation of attachment needs. Notably, avoidant attachment provides greater capacity to preserve mentalizing under conditions of emotional arousal. Avoidance, however, offers only limited protection: it not only limits the development of secure attachment relationships but also is associated with vulnerability, insofar as increasingly intense levels of arousal are liable to eventuate in a collapse of mentalizing with potential flooding of emotion (Patrick Luyten, Linda C. Mayes, and Boudewijn Van Houdenhove, unpublished manuscript, December 15, 2011). The centrality of attachment conflicts and associated mentalizing impairments in BPD provided the impetus for Anthony Bateman and Peter Fonagy (2006a) to develop Mentalization-Based Treatment, which I'll discuss in Chapter 4 ("Evidence-Based Treatments").

Diagnosing Complex Traumatic Stress Disorders

The preceding review has made it abundantly clear that no single DSM category encompasses the range of problems associated with attachment trauma. In this section, I first review efforts to create suitable diagnostic categories for complex trauma pertaining to adulthood and childhood, and then I present my conclusion that we should give up this aspiration to find one gigantic diagnostic box.

Complex PTSD

Herman (1992b) was blunt in her antipathy for diagnostic labels that stigmatize persons who have been traumatized. She asserted that survivors of childhood abuse "are likely to receive a diagnosis that carries strong negative connotations." Of diagnoses "charged with pejorative meaning," she identified BPD as "the most notorious," stating that "this term is frequently used within the mental health professions as little more than a sophisticated insult" (p. 123). Herman (1992a) proposed the alternative diagnosis of *complex PTSD*. Complex indeed. She characterized the traumatic stress leading to this disorder as having been subjected to a prolonged period of domination and control, which includes such experiences as having been a prisoner of war, a victim of domestic battering, or a survivor of childhood abuse. The associated problems include alterations in emotion regulation, consciousness, identity, perceptions of perpetrators, relationships with others, and systems of meaning.

Herman (1993) proposed that this constellation of problems be diagnosed in DSM-IV (American Psychiatric Association 1994) as disorders of extreme stress not otherwise specified (DESNOS). This proposal led to what has been characterized since as a "spirited discussion" (Friedman and Karam 2009, p. 18) within the DSM-IV task force. The task force reasoned that the vast majority of persons meeting the proposed criteria for DESNOS would qualify for a diagnosis of PTSD, rendering the new diagnosis superfluous. Accordingly, the wide-ranging symptoms of complex PTSD were included in the text of DSM-IV as associated descriptive features. The task force's decision, however, continues to be challenged. Julian Ford (2009), for example, reviewed research indicating that nearly half of a group of traumatized persons meeting criteria for DESNOS did not meet criteria for PTSD; he concluded that "DESNOS is a complex variant of PTSD that is comorbid with, but distinct from PTSD itself" (p. 480). Consistent with Herman's research, DESNOS is associated with attachment trauma in early childhood and with severe problems in adulthood, including problems in relationships; consistent with the severity of their disturbance, persons diagnosed with DESNOS require high levels of psychiatric care.

Developmental Trauma Disorder

Bessel van der Kolk (1986) pioneered the understanding of attachment trauma and recently proposed a childhood counterpart to the diagnosis of complex PTSD: *developmental trauma disorder* (van der Kolk and d'Andrea 2010). As with the original diagnosis of PTSD, the impetus for the new diagnosis is partly social and political: "Despite the fact that the consequences of adverse childhood experiences constitute the single largest public health problem in the USA...and likely worldwide, there is enormous resistance to placing the care of developing humans where it belongs: at the forefront of our attention" (van der Kolk and d'Andrea 2010, p. 58). Echoing the history of PTSD, the diagnosis of developmental trauma disorder is based on the premise that complexly traumatized children "currently do not have a diagnostic home" (p. 59), which precludes coherent research. The proposed diagnosis is based on a comprehensive review of extensive research literature documenting the contribution of childhood attachment trauma to a range of disorders diagnosed in childhood, such as conduct disorder, bipolar disorder, and attention-deficit/hyperactivity disorder. This research raises the possibility that the standard diagnoses are "stand-ins" for a proper diagnosis; such stand-in diagnoses are employed "to the detriment of traumatized children to whom such diagnoses are applied" (p. 63).

The traumatic stress contributing to developmental trauma disorder includes prolonged exposure to interpersonal violence as well as disruptions of protective caregiving, including changes in primary caregiving, separations, and abuse. The wide-ranging symptoms encompass the realms of physiology, emotion, attention, behavior, identity, and relationships with caregivers and others. Van der Kolk and d'Andrea (2010) propose that the constellation of symptoms associated with attachment trauma is "best understood as a single coherent pathology" (p. 61), in contrast to the current practice of diagnosing multiple childhood disorders (typically three to eight).

Beyond Diagnoses

The diagnoses of complex PTSD and developmental trauma disorder ring true and indeed provide more coherence than a long list of psychiatric disorders. Yet I am doubtful about the usefulness of these huge boxes of symptoms, given the pervasive problems with the comparatively small box of symptoms diagnosed as PTSD. PTSD is complex enough! I have no doubt about the range of problems associated with attachment trauma; I'm dubious only about the prospect of adding more diagnostic categories.

Recognizing the absence of bright lines and the inadequacy of boxes to contain symptoms, I find it more helpful to conceive of broad *domains* of traumatic stress and developmental consequences. Attachment trauma covers a broad domain of traumatic stress and traumatic consequences. In a similar vein of referring to broad domains, I find terminology proposed by Julian Ford and Christine Courtois (2009) to be helpful. They define *complex psychological trauma* as "resulting from exposure to severe stressors that 1) are repetitive or prolonged, 2) involve harm or abandonment by caregivers or other ostensibly responsible adults, and 3) occur at developmentally vulnerable times in the victim's life, such as early childhood or adolescence" (p. 13). Then they define *complex traumatic stress disorders* as "changes in mind, emotions, body, and relationships experienced following complex psychological trauma, including severe problems with dissociation, emotion dysregulation, somatic distress, or relational or spiritual alienation" (p. 13).

For now, we must employ the language of psychiatric diagnosis and symptoms to identify the various problems within the broad domain of complex traumatic stress disorders. Yet, as these recent formulations of complex stress aspire to do, we must endeavor to attain some psychological coherence in understanding the complex relations among symptoms and disorders.

Toward Diagnostic Understanding

I have complained about the difficulty of packaging neat groups of symptoms into tidy boxes. Starting with DSM-III in 1980 (American Psychiatric Association 1980), this endeavor has been enormously helpful in organizing systematic research, including the research reviewed here. As we are on the threshold of developing DSM-5, however, the entire enterprise of diagnosis is being questioned. DSM-III was purposefully descriptive and atheoretical—that is, entirely open-minded about discovering causes for various disorders. PTSD is a notable exception in linking the syndrome to trauma exposure; thus, it's ironic that some researchers are proposing that the cause be deleted from the criteria. This open-minded attitude toward causality, however, might have outlived its usefulness: we need to make some psychological sense of psychiatric disorders. Moreover, diagnosing multiple disorders can be bewildering. Not infrequently, I see traumatized patients diagnosed with 10 ostensibly different disorders, including several anxiety disorders. I can only wonder, What's the real problem here?

To sum up, I see five fundamental problems with our current way of diagnosing disorders—none unique to trauma-related problems, but all most glaringly evident in this context:

1. There is no clear boundary demarcating normal from pathological levels of disturbance.

2. The various clinical syndromes such as anxiety and depression are not clearly distinct from one another.
3. Clinical syndromes aren't distinct from personality disorders, but rather personality organization is the context for development of clinical syndromes develop and gives them psychological meaning.
4. The different disorders—including PTSD—do not have distinct etiologies (causal pathways).
5. Distinct disorders do not consistently lead to distinct treatment approaches—even with medication, much less with psychotherapy.

Given that treatment ultimately is our primary concern, the last point is crucial, and it's one reason for my commitment to plain old therapy.

One common complaint about existing psychiatric diagnoses is this: we haven't carved nature at its joints—that is, we haven't discovered natural kinds. Thus, we might hope to base psychiatric diagnoses on research in developmental neuroscience. Thomas Insel and colleagues (2010), for example, propose the development of research domain criteria that would focus on "neural circuitry, with levels of analysis progressing in one of two directions: upwards from measures of circuitry function to clinically relevant variation, or downwards to the genetic and molecular/cellular factors that ultimately influence such function" (p. 749). This neurobiological approach does not exclude the domain of influence central to this book—namely, attachment trauma. On the contrary, the family environment and social context have profound influences on neurobiological development, as we have seen. Hence, "all these levels are seen as affecting both the biology and psychology of mental illness" (p. 749). But this approach envisions carving nature's joints at the biological level.

Pointing to major psychological joints in nature, Blatt and Luyten (2010) advocate a new approach to diagnoses that holds promise in making full use of developmental understanding and research on personality development and attachment relationships. This approach is based on the two-polarities model, in which development is organized around relationships and self-definition. From this standpoint, psychiatric disorders reflect failures in either domain (i.e., relatedness or self-definition) as well as significant imbalance between domains (i.e., exaggerated focus on relationships or self-definition).

Here is the premise for the two-polarities approach to diagnosis:

> Such a perspective facilitates an appreciation of the continuities between normal and various forms of psychopathology. In other words, this approach emphasizes the continuity between normal personality develop-

ment and various forms of psychopathology and provides the basis for understanding psychopathology not as a series of separate diseases, each assumed to derive from some hypothetical but as yet often undocumented neurobiological abnormality, but as distorted modes of adaptation that emerge from disruptions of normal psychological development. (Blatt 2008, p. 171)

Reflecting compromised relatedness and self-definition, insecure attachment relationships are a primary source of disruption in normal psychological development. This approach has the advantage of infusing diagnoses with psychological meaning based on developmental understanding. Although DSM emphasizes threat to physical integrity in the diagnostic criteria for PTSD, traumatized persons report *psychological* threat as being more prominent (Grey and Holmes 2008; Holmes et al. 2005b); moreover, this danger can take the form of threat to relationships or to sense of self. When thinking about anxiety disorders more generally, we therapists need to go beyond symptoms to understanding what the anxiety is *about*—it will be tied to relationships, sense of self, or both. As discussed earlier in this chapter (see section Precipitating Stress), Blatt's (2004) research on depression also has illuminated the fundamental distinction between dependent and self-critical depression: this distinction is linked to problems in relationships and self-definition and, in turn, linked to ambivalent and avoidant attachment. Similarly, Blatt and Luyten (2010) distinguish personality disorders as involving difficulty predominantly with relatedness (e.g., dependent or borderline personality disorder) or with self-definition (e.g., antisocial, narcissistic, and avoidant personality disorder).

As I've emphasized throughout, all forms of insecure attachment are associated with problems in emotion regulation: substance abuse, ill health, eating disorders, deliberate self-harm, and suicidal states are potentially linked either to problems in relationships or problems with self-definition—or both. In the context of the relatedness pole, suicidal states, for example, are likely to relate to feelings of neglect and abandonment in conjunction with a high level of dependency; in contrast, in the context of self-definition, suicidal states relate to the experience of failure and humiliation, vulnerability to which is associated with self-critical perfectionism (Blatt 2008).

We therapists are far short of redoing DSM in relation to distinct neurobiological abnormalities, and we are hardly in a position to redo DSM along the two-polarities model and the associated patterns of insecure attachment. But we need to move away from focus on symptom clusters to true diagnostic understanding, wherein personality development and attachment history will play a prominent role. This understanding is the basis for my advocating the move from a disorder-specific to a person-centered approach to treatment—that is, "a life history perspective" (Luyten et al. 2008, p. 41) that aspires to "map the myriad complex pathways from early childhood to later adaptive or maladaptive development which can then form the basis for interventions for both preventing and treating disorders" (p. 29).

In describing trauma-related problems, I started with the current state of the art: research based on DSM diagnoses. I do the same in the next part of the book ("Treatment and Healing") by beginning with a chapter on evidence-based treatments for PTSD—a disorder-specific approach. We have much to learn from this approach. But I devote the subsequent chapter to plain old therapy rooted in attachment and mentalizing, two common factors that cut across different diagnoses and brands of therapy.

Key Points

- ◆ The current diagnostic system inclines therapists to think in terms of symptoms and symptom clusters and to target treatments accordingly. Yet a psychotherapeutic approach to treatment requires that we think about diagnoses psychologically—that is, seek to understand the development and meaning of symptoms.

- ◆ Impaired mentalizing contributes to a wide range of symptoms, and mentalizing is the process by which we understand the meaning of symptoms (e.g., as illustrated by the collaborative assessment of contributors to suicidal states).

- ◆ Attachment trauma is a nonspecific risk factor in the development of a wide range of psychiatric disorders. Yet these disorders themselves exacerbate conflicts in attachment relationships, in vicious circles. Self-destructive behaviors (e.g., substance abuse, eating disorders, nonsuicidal self-injury, suicidal behavior) are examples of this process. Fueled by mentalizing impairments, attachment insecurity, and unbearable emotional states, self-destructive behavior elicits unbearable emotional states in the partner or caregiver, undermining the patient's attachment security and mentalizing capacity, and potentially leaving each member further traumatized—alone in emotional pain.

- ◆ For all their flaws, psychiatric diagnoses have made a monumental contribution to research, including extensive research on the impact of attachment trauma. Merely diagnosing multiple disorders, however, does not lead to coherent understanding of individual patients. Identifying a broad domain of complex traumatic stress has some appeal, but it doesn't get us very far.

◆ Psychotherapy requires a person-centered, developmental approach
to diagnostic understanding. Mentalizing—in the context of therapeutic attachments—is the process in plain old therapy through which we
therapists and our patients achieve such diagnostic understanding.

PART

II

Treatment and Healing

CHAPTER

4

Evidence-Based Treatments

In the three decades since the diagnosis of posttraumatic stress disorder (PTSD) was formalized, a wide range of treatment interventions have been developed, and their effectiveness has been researched systematically to varying degrees. I start by reviewing the more common treatments for PTSD, noting the extent of research support for their effectiveness. Next, I review the foremost treatments for borderline personality disorder (BPD), given its basis in attachment trauma. Two decades ago, Judith Herman (1992b) identified the need for specialized treatment of complex traumatic stress disorders, but research on these treatments is relatively new (Courtois and Ford 2009), and I briefly summarize current strategies. Lastly, I illustrate some approaches to parent-child therapy that hold promise for interrupting the development of complex traumatic stress disorders; these interventions are particularly pertinent to my main agenda insofar as they provide experimental evidence for the benefits of enhancing mentalizing in attachment relationships.

This chapter is illustrative rather than exhaustive, hitting some of the highlights. Notwithstanding my arguments for plain old therapy, I believe that therapists and patients should be aware of the array of specialized treatment approaches and the research support for them. Although I'll

133

strive for objectivity, my bias already is glaringly evident: I tend to see everything through the lenses of attachment and mentalizing, and here I apply these lenses to the specialized treatments, emphasizing areas of overlap with plain old therapy.

Treatments for Posttraumatic Stress Disorder

The PTSD Treatment Guidelines Taskforce (Foa et al. 2009b, p. 16) graded the quality of evidence for specialized treatments from A ("based on randomized, well-controlled clinical trials") to E ("based on recently developed treatment not subjected to clinical or empirical tests"). Here, I use these standards in reviewing popular evidence-based individual approaches: prolonged exposure, cognitive therapy, and Eye Movement Desensitization and Reprocessing (EMDR). Then I comment on the role of other clinically valuable but less well researched treatment modalities: group psychotherapy and couples and family therapy.

Prolonged Exposure

Exposure therapy is a commonsensical approach to coping with fearful avoidance associated with traumatic experience: After being thrown from a horse, you climb back on rather than giving up riding. If you've learned to be terrified of all dogs after being bitten, such that you can't visit your friend who has a dog (or can't risk going to a home where there might be a dog, or even risk going out on the street), you must gradually expose yourself to dogs. With repeated exposure, you will learn that you can manage the frightening situation, and your fear is likely to diminish—provided you are not hurt again in the process of exposure (i.e., thrown off the horse or bitten by another dog). PTSD complicates this natural desensitizing process enormously, because you can become frightened not only of various situations but also of remembering past trauma. Thus, PTSD calls for a structured exposure treatment.

Edna Foa and colleagues (Foa and Rothbaum 1998; Foa et al. 2007) pioneered exposure therapy for PTSD; their treatment approach has the advantages for therapists of being relatively simple to learn and to conduct as well as having the most extensive research support for its effectiveness. The treatment is time limited, typically concluded in a dozen sessions. The therapist educates the patient about common reactions to trauma and symptoms of PTSD as well as the way in which natural efforts to avoid reminders of trauma backfire, such that systematic exposure is required for healing. Notably, part of this education, and a crucial part of the healing process, entails what we call mentalizing: the patient learns to distinguish the present from the past—that is, to differentiate remembering trauma (the mental state) from being traumatized (reality). In addition to education, patients are coached in emotion regulation; for example, they are taught to use calming breathing techniques to help master fear.

To address both situational avoidance and experiential avoidance, the treatment involves both in vivo (in life) exposure and imaginal exposure (revisiting traumatic memories). Situational avoidance can be circumscribed, such as avoiding the scene of an assault, or downright life constricting, such as being afraid to leave the house alone. Thus, exposure therapy involves identifying specific situations that are avoided and—after ensuring safety—going into the situations and remaining there for a sufficient amount of time for the fear to be mastered (e.g., 30–45 minutes). Leaving the situation quickly to escape fear only reinforces the avoidance because it rapidly decreases distress.

Imaginal exposure requires relatively clear memories of traumatic events and the ability to tell and retell the story repeatedly. If possible, it's best to start with a memory that is especially frightening or haunting; if this prospect seems too daunting, the patient can start with less frightening memories and work up to more frightening memories. Traumatic hotspots, the most frightening or painful aspects of the traumatic events, might be addressed multiple times in a single session. To enhance the exposure, the therapist tape-records the recounting of trauma in sessions so the patient can listen to the recordings later as homework. In each session, after the patient tells and retells the story, the therapist assists him or her with processing the exposure—that is, discussing the meaning of the events as well as the associated emotions of anger, sadness, grief, guilt, and shame. I don't conduct prolonged exposure by the book, but I've had many occasions to talk through, in detail, patients' experience of traumatic events, in the course of which the sheer complexity of the painful emotional experience is evident.

Case Example

Olivia narrowly escaped from an apartment fire with her young son Patrick. She talked about the events leading up to their escape: she gradually became concerned (i.e., smelled smoke but believed initially that it was coming from nearby woods) and ultimately became alarmed (i.e., recognized that the building was on fire). In hindsight, she was grateful that her initial concern was sufficient that she took Patrick from his room into the living room as she sought to determine where the smoke was coming from. Olivia became agitated as she talked about her apartment starting to fill with smoke and beginning to feel the heat on her face. Then she came to the point where she panicked: she heard her neighbor screaming in the hallway outside Olivia's door, "We can't get out!" At that moment, Olivia thought she and Patrick were going to die. She felt trapped and froze, saying that her mind went blank. All she could remember was clutching Patrick, hearing sirens, and being grabbed and pulled by the firefighter, struggling to maintain her balance. She cried as she talked about her gradual relief when she and Patrick were out on the lawn, remembering the firefighter telling her over and over, "It's OK, you're safe now."

But Olivia also talked about other emotions. She felt ashamed and "stupid" for her slow reaction to smelling the smoke. She sobbed as she recounted the worried look on Patrick's face when he asked her if the fireman had saved Gloria and Elmo, his pet guinea pigs, and how he burst into tears when he realized they'd died in the fire. She had a hard time forgiving herself for not getting out sooner and saving the pets, even though she remembered clearly that all her attention had been riveted on Patrick.

Olivia said that when she realized she and Patrick were safe on the lawn, that was just the beginning of the stress. She lost her belongings and her home, and she felt guilty about imposing on her brother after he invited her and Patrick to live with him temporarily. She was frustrated with her insurance company regarding the paperwork and delays in reimbursing her losses. Yet, apart from grief and guilt feelings, her most intense feelings in the aftermath stemmed from learning afterward that the fire was related to negligence: the building was not constructed in accordance with city codes and had not been properly inspected. As she talked about this negligence, she was outraged; Olivia was "livid" every time she read something about the fire and apartment management in the local newspaper or heard anything about it on the TV news. Yet she consoled herself with Patrick's presence, her gratitude toward the firefighter who saved them, and her brother's caring and generosity from the moment he learned of their plight.

The effectiveness of prolonged exposure is solidly supported by extensive research, and it is considered an A-level treatment (Foa et al. 2009a), yet it's not uniquely effective. A systematic comparison of prolonged exposure with other treatments for PTSD (Powers et al. 2010) is noteworthy in combining the data from many studies encompassing 675 patients. Prolonged exposure was substantially more effective than a wide range of control treatments (including relaxation training, supportive counseling, and time-limited psychodynamic psychotherapy). The effects remained significant at follow-up (up to 12 months). Moreover, the effects were evident not only for PTSD symptoms but also for generalized anxiety, depression, quality of life, and social functioning. Although the review did not include medication treatment, the authors noted that based on previous research, prolonged exposure had stronger effects than the most effective medication for PTSD—that is, selective serotonin reuptake inhibitors (e.g., Prozac). Notably, the authors had predicted on the basis of previous research that prolonged exposure would *not* be more effective than other treatments focusing specifically on PTSD symptoms (i.e., Cognitive Processing Therapy, cognitive therapy, stress inoculation therapy, and Eye Movement Desensitization and Reprocessing), and this combined sample from many studies confirmed this prediction. The authors concluded that *exposure is common to all these treatments.*

Prolonged exposure has been demonstrated to be effective for treating PTSD stemming from a wide range of traumas, including motor vehicle accidents, criminal victimization, sexual assaults, and torture, as well as attachment trauma such as domestic violence and childhood abuse. Yet, consistent with my view, Foa and colleagues (2007) state flatly that prolonged exposure is *"a treatment for PTSD, not a treatment for trauma"* (p. 21, emphasis added). To expand this point as it applies to complex traumatic stress, Foa and colleagues (2009b) acknowledge that the practice guidelines have somewhat limited applicability: "Relatively little is known about the successful treatment of patients with these trauma histories. There is a growing clinical consensus, with a degree of empirical support, that some patients with these histories require multimodal interventions, applied consistently over a longer time period" (p. 2).

Also limiting their applicability somewhat, exposure therapies are inherently stressful owing to their emphasis on facing rather than avoiding fear and anxiety. Not surprisingly, a substantial percentage (20%–30%) of patients drop out (Foa et al. 2007). Nonetheless, clinicians may be unduly wary of employing exposure-based treatments; evidence suggests that they're generally well tolerated and do not detrimentally exacerbate PTSD symptoms, even for patients with complex traumatic stress disorders (Welch and Rothbaum 2007). Underscoring this point of tolerability, exposure therapy can be effective for treating PTSD even in patients with psychotic disorders, provided that it is conducted with a great deal of preparation and support (Frueh et al. 2009).

How does exposure therapy work? To demonstrate that it is effective is one thing; to understand why it is effective is another. Exposure therapy appears commonsensical; yet the extinction of fear is anything but simple (Craske et al. 2008). Ideally, over the long term, two things happen. First, *fear tolerance increases;* that is, one moves from situational and experiential avoidance to experiential acceptance. Accordingly, the fear of anxiety decreases. Paradoxically, accepting anxiety rather than fearing it tends to diminish it, in part by providing confidence that one can continue to function adequately while feeling anxious; a sense of control supplants feelings of helplessness in the face of the anxiety. Second, *new associations inhibit the fear response.* For example, a patient might be afraid when she hears a raised voice that reminds her of screaming that led to violent attacks when she was growing up. With repeated exposures (e.g., in malls or

restaurants or in her current family home), she can build new associations: raised voices are not dangerous in many environmental contexts.
Similarly, the safe context of the therapist's office can inhibit fear to a degree while the patient remembers traumatic events. There is a crucial
point here: the original learning is not erased but rather *overlaid* by new
associations. The cues (raised voice or memories) evoke competing responses: fear associated with the memories competes with inhibition of
fear associated with feeling safe with the therapist. Unfortunately, with
the passage of time or a change of context (e.g., outside the therapist's office), the original learning may trump the inhibition, and the fear returns.
Here is where mentalizing (keeping in mind the distinction between the
present and the past) and mindfulness (accepting the feelings with an attitude of self-compassion) can help.

Recognizing the complexity of the learning process, Foa and colleagues (2006) proposed that the core elements of treatment are 1) sustaining emotional engagement with the trauma memory; 2) modifying
unrealistic beliefs that the world is completely dangerous and the self is
totally incompetent; and 3) developing a coherent narrative of the traumatic experience. I find Foa's theory remarkably compatible with attachment theory in striving to modify internal working models of self and
others (i.e., the self as incompetent and others as dangerous) and in promoting mentalizing in the context of attachment relationships (i.e., engaging with the emotion and developing narrative coherence).

Although consistent with cognitive-behavioral approaches in general,
Foa's theory underplays the significance of attachment. This omission
from the theory is glaring, given the centrality of attachment relationships
in emotion regulation. Foa, however, is aware of the importance of the patient-therapist relationship in practice. She and her colleagues point to
the cardinal importance of building trust and a therapeutic alliance as
well as the need for the therapist to be nonjudgmental, accepting, calm,
and supportive while listening attentively to the patient's narrative. This
approach is consistent with mentalizing in the context of secure attachment. In addition, the therapist may offer additional support, such as being available to talk with the patient between sessions. The therapist also
may rally additional social support, such as encouraging the patient to invite a friend or family member to accompany the patient during in vivo
exposures or to drive the patient to and from therapy. Although recognizing that patient-therapist touch is potentially problematic, Foa and
colleagues (2007) note, "Infrequently, we have had clients who coped
with distress during exposure by continuously holding the therapist's
hand" (p. 121)—a demonstrably effective way of regulating emotional
distress in secure attachment relationships (Coan et al. 2006).

I find it heartening that the need for greater attention to the patient-therapist relationship in prolonged exposure therapy has not gone entirely unrecognized. Jay Morrison (2011) goes beyond addressing the importance of the therapeutic alliance to comment, "The systematic facilitation of the reexperiencing of what is often among the most profound events in patients' lives, can, in fact, be one of the most deeply personal ways of engaging with patients" (p. 25). He goes on to note that more therapists might be inclined to employ this method if more attention were given to the "rich humanity inherent in exposure procedures" (p. 25).

If the patient-therapist relationship were not typically downplayed, and if Morrison's (2011) viewpoint were taken into account, prolonged exposure could be viewed as highly compatible with attachment and mentalizing: the patient explores painful emotional experience in the context of a safe relationship and thus comes to find it more meaningful and bearable, no longer feeling so alone. Yet, in my view, prolonged exposure and other highly structured approaches to treating PTSD have a significant advantage over plain old therapy: they ensure that the patient and therapist stick to this difficult task of exploring traumatic memories and feelings. In less structured therapies, it's all too easy for patients and therapists to avoid this extremely stressful work by focusing on innumerable other pressing matters in the patient's life. Yet, as Morrison implies, the structured techniques of prolonged exposure are superimposed on plain old therapy. Some of the complexities of prolonged exposure are summarized in Table 4–1.

Cognitive Therapy

Exposure therapy and cognitive therapy differ from one another in emphasis, and the overlap bears noting. As Foa and Kozak (1991) acknowledged, "In effect, we practice informal cognitive therapy during exposure, in that we help clients to examine ways in which they evaluate threat and to develop inferential processes that lead to more realistic conclusions" (p. 45). Conversely, cognitive therapies entail exposure insofar as they entail bringing traumatic memories to mind and talking about them.

Cognitive Processing Therapy, developed initially by Patricia Resick and colleagues as a group intervention for rape-related trauma (Resick and Schnicke 1992; Resick et al. 2008), is a well-researched A-level treatment with empirical support second only to prolonged exposure therapy (Foa et al. 2009a). The exposure component entails writing a detailed narrative of the trauma and then reading it aloud to the therapist. The cognitive component entails educating the patient about the role of mal-

---

TABLE 4–1.   Complexities of exposure therapy

- Exposure entails facing what one fears and feeling the fear.
- Exposure can lead to greater acceptance of anxiety (and other painful feelings), thus diminishing fear of anxiety and fostering greater anxiety tolerance.
- Exposure does not eliminate old associations but rather builds new associations to anxiety-provoking stimuli (i.e., associating these stimuli with safe contexts) and thus inhibits anxiety responses.
- Remaining old associations can reinstate old fear responses (i.e., outside safe contexts).
- Exposure and greater anxiety tolerance can open the door to changing negative beliefs about the self and the world.
- Ideally, exposure takes place in a safe relationship wherein painful experience is understood and mentalized.

---

adaptive thinking in PTSD along with systematically exploring and challenging unrealistic negative beliefs so as to help the patient develop a more balanced view of the trauma, particularly in relation to self-blame and guilt feelings. Common cognitive themes include negative beliefs regarding safety, trust, power, control, self-esteem, and intimacy. Substantial research support (Cahill et al. 2009) includes an adaptation for treating complex traumatic stress related to childhood sexual abuse, an intervention that combines individual therapy (for processing trauma) with group therapy (to address cognitive distortions) and also addresses developmental history, communication skills, and social support.

A closely related approach is Cognitive Therapy for PTSD, developed by Anke Ehlers and David Clark (Ehlers et al. 2005). The treatment includes different forms of exposure (i.e., in vivo, writing a trauma narrative, and imaginal reliving of the trauma), although the balance of exposure and cognitive processing is different from that in prolonged exposure (i.e., only a quarter of the sessions are devoted to imaginal reliving). In addition to addressing cognitive distortions (e.g., self-blame and views of the world as completely unsafe), the cognitive processing is compatible with mentalizing in emphasizing the elaboration of fragmented trauma memories into a coherent autobiographical narrative. As I discussed in relation to PTSD (see Chapter 2, "Posttraumatic Stress and Dissociative Disorders"), this elaboration entails transforming involuntary and intrusive sensory memories into voluntary, verbally accessible memories. A small number of high-quality (A-level) controlled trials provide support for the effectiveness of cognitive therapy for PTSD (Cahill et al. 2009), although patients with complex trauma (e.g., BPD, active substance abuse, severe depression, suicidality) were excluded (Ehlers et al. 2005).

As is true of exposure therapy, the role of the patient-therapist relationship remains in the background when it comes to accounting for the effectiveness of cognitive approaches to treating PTSD. This relative neglect of the treatment relationship is true of cognitive therapy more generally, although there are some exceptions (Safran and Segal 1990), including some recent attention to incorporating attachment theory and research in the conduct of cognitive therapy (McBride and Atkinson 2009). To reiterate my point about exposure therapy, these cognitive approaches, albeit to varying degrees, also entail mentalizing painful emotional experience in the context of a safe relationship—the essence of plain old therapy.

Eye Movement Desensitization and Reprocessing

EMDR is an effective yet controversial—and, in my view, downright quirky—treatment for PTSD. Francine Shapiro (1996) developed and began researching the treatment after she made a fortuitous observation: when she was thinking disturbing thoughts while walking in a park, her rapid eye movements reduced her emotional distress. Thus, EMDR incorporates rapid eye movements in conjunction with exposure and cognitive processing techniques. In brief, the patient brings to mind images associated with traumatic experiences while simultaneously moving his eyes from side to side, following the therapist's finger moving back and forth in front of his face. After a series of eye movements, the patient is instructed to let go of the images and to say whatever comes to mind. Often, surprising thoughts and memories emerge that are associated with the trauma. The cognitive component includes identifying negative beliefs associated with the trauma (e.g., self-blame) and formulating more realistic alternative beliefs. In comparison with prolonged exposure, the exposure component of EMDR is relatively brief, in part because the eye movements interfere with the patient's capacity to visualize the trauma.

Well-controlled research has shown EMDR to be effective in treating symptoms of PTSD (Wilson et al. 1995), and improvement is maintained at follow-up (Wilson et al. 1997). Hence, EMDR is counted among the A-level treatments for PTSD (Foa et al. 2009a), although research fails to show superiority for EMDR in relation to prolonged exposure (Powers et al. 2010) or cognitive-behavioral approaches more generally (Seidler and Wagner 2006). Ironically, no consistent evidence indicates that the eye movements (or any other bilateral stimuli) contribute significantly to the effectiveness of the treatment (Spates et al. 2009). As one critic put it, "what is effective in EMDR is not new, and what is new is not effective" (McNally 1999). Some research suggests, however, that the distracting effects of the eye movements may promote distancing and detachment and thus facilitate processing of trauma for some patients (Lee et al. 2006). Regardless, a straightforward conclusion is that EMDR is effective by virtue of combining exposure and cognitive interventions; as with other cognitive-behavioral approaches, the patient-therapist relationship remains in the background in the theoretical accounts of EMDR's effectiveness.

Group Psychotherapy

Group psychotherapy is widely employed in the treatment of trauma, and group treatments are noteworthy for their sheer diversity (Ford et al. 2009): some groups focus on processing traumatic experiences, whereas others are more educational; some groups focus on present functioning and interpersonal relationships without processing trauma; and groups vary in theoretical orientation from psychodynamic to interpersonal and cognitive-behavioral. Group therapy for trauma survivors can be especially powerful in promoting a feeling of universality (Yalom 1970)—that is, a feeling of commonality with others and, crucially, a sense of not being alone in relation to trauma. Hence, groups can be especially powerful in overcoming shame and guilt feelings. Groups also can be highly stimulating: one member's recounting of traumatic experience can evoke reminders of trauma in other members, at worst leading to emotional contagion. For this reason, as Herman (1992b) recommended, processing traumatic experience in individual psychotherapy may be necessary before doing so in a group. Moreover, as in individual therapy, the group can be tailored to the stage of recovery: the focus of the group can move from establishing safety to remembering and talking about traumatic experience and then to developing sustaining relationships.

As Stacy Welch and Barbara Rothbaum (2007) lament, given its widespread use, group therapy is woefully understudied. The studies that have been done, however, are encouraging in revealing positive effects, albeit of varying magnitude (Shea et al. 2009). Unfortunately, insufficient evidence exists to support recommending any one type of group over another (e.g., trauma-focused versus present-focused); no evidence supports group therapy as superior to individual therapy; and there's no way to predict who might benefit most from group therapy. Nonetheless, unspecific as they may be, treatment guidelines recommend group therapy "as a useful component of treatment for PTSD related to different types of traumatic experiences" (Foa et al. 2009a, p. 578). From my perspective, a cohesive group can be invaluable in promoting a greater capacity to rely on attachment relationships as a first-line means of emotion regulation.

Couples and Family Therapy

Individual and group therapies provide *indirect* routes to enhancing attachment security. That is, both types of therapy meet attachment needs to some extent; they offer an opportunity to learn to relate in a more secure manner (e.g., to express painful feelings); and they provide a forum for examining problems in attachment relationships. However, compelling reasons exist for working *directly* with traumatized patients' key attachment relationships. PTSD and other trauma-related problems can lead to profound disruptions and conflicts in relationships. For example, sexual assaults and childhood sexual abuse can interfere with intimacy with romantic partners. More generally, fear, anxiety, irritability, and rage can lead to emotional contagion in close relationships, which then can lead to distancing on the part of partners and family members, perpetuating the core traumatic experience of feeling emotionally distressed and alone. Hence, couples and family interventions may be needed not only to ameliorate conflict and distress in relationships but also to enhance social support that is essential to recovery.

Sue Johnson's Emotionally Focused Therapy for couples and families warrants attention inasmuch as it is solidly based on attachment theory and research. The following is a prototypical example of the relationship problems potentially engendered by PTSD:

> When a husband withdraws from his wife and numbs himself with alcohol to blunt his PTSD symptoms and to avoid his feelings (in general and about the relationship), paradoxically, his nightmares and flashbacks may worsen, and his sense of efficacy may deteriorate. Needless to say, his wife is affected by both the withdrawal and numbing, and by the intrusive reexperiencing. The partners usually become increasingly *estranged and unavailable as comfort to each other.* (Johnson and Courtois 2009, p. 372, emphasis added)

I highlight emotional unavailability in this example, because the central goal of Emotionally Focused Therapy is creating a safe haven and secure base in attachment relationships. Interventions enhance expression of emotion while promoting mutual emotional attunement and responsiveness—as well as comforting touch. The therapist legitimizes and validates attachment needs, while encouraging acknowledgment of vulnerability and promoting effective emotional dependence. Insecure internal working models of attachment are identified as they play out in self-perpetuating patterns in couple relationships. For example, anxious clinging by one member promotes detached avoidance in the other in an escalating cycle. In brief, key elements of this approach are developing a collaborative treatment alliance, validating attachment needs and fears, privileging emotional responses, promoting accessibility and responsiveness, facilitating self-definition through emotional communication, shaping relationships in the direction of secure attachment, and healing relationship injuries associated with betrayal and abandonment at times of need (Johnson 2008).

Johnson rightly criticizes the "overuse of individual therapy at the expense of couple or family work" (Johnson and Courtois 2009, p. 374). As she contends, the therapist is a *surrogate* attachment figure; thus, couples and family therapy focuses on the real thing, capitalizing on the potential for full-strength emotion regulation in the natural environment (Johnson 2009). Although Johnson (2008) cites evidence for the effectiveness of emotionally focused couple therapy more broadly, the evidence for its effectiveness in relation to PTSD and complex trauma is preliminary (Johnson and Courtois 2009). Reviews of research on couples and family therapy for trauma are consistent in emphasizing the stark contrast between the solid theoretical rationale for this work and the limited evidence to support it (Riggs et al. 2009). Thus, current treatment guidelines recommend using couples and family therapy as an *adjunct* to evidence-based individual therapy for PTSD (Foa et al. 2009a). While we wait for more evidence, I don't think we should wait to make full use of enhancing security in key attachment relationships in the treatment of PTSD.

Comment

Reviewing the evidence, Elizabeth Hembree and Edna Foa (2010) draw a straightforward conclusion: "No patient diagnosed with PTSD should go without the benefit of evidence-based treatments" (p. 200). Their survey, however, showed that only a minority of therapists (27%) are trained in using prolonged exposure, and a smaller minority (9%) use it routinely in treating patients with PTSD. Foa consistently has made a strong case for exposure as being central to PTSD treatment and, as I've demonstrated, she has ample research evidence to support her view. Yet, while her treatment uses exposure in its purest form, exposure is embedded in other cognitive procedures, and the entire process is embedded in a therapeutic relationship. Although we all might agree on the value of exposure, there are many possible ways to implement it. Anthony Roth and Peter Fonagy (2005) conclude that exposure invariably must be integrated with other techniques and that "there are not clear research indicators as to how this is best done, or whether there are conditions under which efficacy is reliant on combinations of exposure and other approaches" (p. 235). As they also maintain, there is no substitute for clinical judgment and, especially for patients with the complex problems addressed in this book, "specialist knowledge of this population may therefore be more critical to outcome than the choice of any specific exposure-based treatment" (p. 235).

More generally, Matthew Friedman and colleagues (2009) concluded the following from their review of current research: "We have not reached the point where we can predict which treatments are most suitable for which patients under which conditions" (p. 617). Moreover, many patients appear to require combined treatments, and "at present, the integration of treatment techniques remains the art of the clinician" (p. 618). Consistent with the person-centered approach I have been advocating, they added, "It's not a generic 'PTSD' that one treats, but a particular patient" (p. 619). Research evidence inevitably will lag behind clinical practice and innovation; we therapists and patients need to be informed by research but not enslaved by it.

Treatments for Borderline Personality Disorder

Treatment of BPD is highly germane to the concerns of this book insofar as attachment trauma is a significant contributor to BPD for many patients. Core problems in BPD include identity disturbance; unstable close relationships marked by insecurity and sensitivity to abandonment; intense emotional reactivity; and impulsive self-damaging behavior. Fortunately, several treatment approaches lead to substantial improvement in patients with BPD (Bender and Oldham 2005). As the first well-researched treatment for BPD, Dialectical Behavior Therapy (DBT) seems to have a corner on the market of evidence-based treatments; however, it's important for patients and therapists to be aware of alternatives. Accordingly, I next highlight two other approaches supported by experimental research that are directly pertinent to the concerns of this book: Transference-Focused Psychotherapy (TFP) and Mentalization-Based Treatment (MBT).

Dialectical Behavior Therapy

Marsha Linehan (1993a) construes BPD as arising from a combination of difficulty regulating emotional arousal and an invalidating (in my terms, nonmentalizing) environment. The child's intense emotional distress isn't

contained by emotional attunement but rather is exacerbated when natural emotional reactions are dismissed or punished. With these developmental problems in view, DBT interventions build skills in emotion
regulation. Given the history of invalidation, empathic validation of perceptions and emotions is a core intervention in DBT. Yet the treatment as
a whole involves an ongoing *dialectic* between acceptance and validation,
on the one hand, and the need for challenge and encouragement to
change, on the other hand: "The treatment calls for a therapist to interact
with a patient in a flexible manner that combines keen observation of patient reactions with moment-to-moment changes in the use of supportive
acceptance versus confrontation and change strategies" (Linehan 1993a,
p. 77).

Linehan cautions that the problems are complex and the work of
treatment is arduous. She emphasizes that problematic behavior is an understandable effort to cope with overwhelming feelings, and she aims to
help patients find more effective and less self-injurious ways of coping.
DBT's first priority is to decrease self-destructiveness, including suicidal
behavior and nonsuicidal self-injury—the primary problems for which
DBT originally was developed (Linehan et al. 1991). The second priority
is to interrupt behavior that interferes with therapy, such as failing to attend treatment sessions, not cooperating in the work required, or not ad-
hering to the therapist's limits. These problematic behaviors, like any
others, become the focus of active problem solving. The third priority is
to decrease behavior that interferes with the quality of life, such as substance abuse, high-risk or criminal behavior, or problems in managing fi-
nances. The fourth priority is to increase behavioral skills—not only
enhancing interpersonal skills but also building tolerance for distress and
learning techniques for emotion regulation. Patients are encouraged to
adopt a stance of *radical acceptance*—accepting as part of life tragic realities that one cannot control. This philosophy is far easier to advocate
than to implement, and the means by which one might do so are not
abundantly clear. Radical acceptance is consistent with an emphasis on
experiential acceptance (Hayes et al. 1999), and mindfulness skills are included in DBT treatment.

DBT is noteworthy for its emphasis on *actively teaching and reinforcing
adaptive behavior.* The patient is encouraged to be highly active in concrete problem solving, carefully analyzing in step-by-step fashion the
chain of events leading to problematic feelings and self-destructive behaviors and then identifying new ways of thinking and acting to avert such
difficulties in the future. Patients use role-playing to practice different
ways of handling troublesome situations. DBT combines individual psychotherapy with educational groups that teach coping skills, including

mindfulness, emotion regulation, and distress tolerance. Patients also are encouraged to make use of telephone contact between sessions for on-the-spot consultation regarding hitches in problem solving. Especially pertinent to containment is DBT's emphasis on emotion-regulation training (Linehan 1993b), which involves learning to identify and label emotions, analyzing the functions of emotions, preventing negative emotional states, increasing emotional hardiness, increasing positive emotions, letting go of negative emotions by paying attention to them and accepting them, and changing painful emotions by acting in a manner opposite to the feeling. Because DBT skills are so practical and helpful in day-to-day coping with emotional distress, DBT skills groups are a mainstay of treatment at The Menninger Clinic.

Although DBT is a behavioral approach, the therapeutic relationship plays a central role, with the patient's history of emotional invalidation in the forefront. Linehan (1993a) put it starkly: "My emphasis on the therapeutic relationship as crucial to progress in DBT comes primarily from my work in interventions with suicidal individuals. At times, this relationship is the only thing that keeps them alive" (p. 21). The sheer complexity and flexibility of the therapist's manner of relating to the patient bears emphasis. Research shows that DBT therapists' affirmation and caring is associated over time with patients becoming less self-attacking and more self-loving. However, therapists also must vary their stance in relation to patients' behavior and functioning. Decreases in self-harm are associated with patients' perceptions of therapists as being alternately affirming, protecting, autonomy granting, instructive, and controlling (Bedics et al. 2011). This complexity captures the dialectic—that is, interweaving validation with influence for change. Sensitive responsiveness in psychotherapy takes many forms, just as it does in parenting.

DBT is the most extensively researched treatment for BPD and has accrued substantial evidence for long-term effectiveness in many studies (Kleim et al. 2010). DBT repeatedly has been shown to reduce suicidal behavior and nonsuicidal self-injury, its primary goals. Concomitantly, DBT reduces emergency room visits and hospitalizations. Also as intended, DBT yields improvements in symptoms of BPD as well as improvements in mood and interpersonal functioning. Accordingly, Linehan and colleagues (2006) regard DBT as the current standard of care for BPD. Nevertheless, although DBT has demonstrated superiority over usual care, it has not shown consistent superiority over other BPD-specific treatments (Kleim et al. 2010).

Research on adapting DBT to the treatment of PTSD is preliminary. Crucially, DBT requires that patients learn skills for coping with painful emotional states that lead to self-destructive behavior before delving into traumatic experience in therapy (Robins et al. 2001). Given DBT's obvious relevance to trauma, clinicians have shown interest in employing DBT interventions prior to trauma-focused therapy and incorporating them into multifaceted treatments for trauma (Follette et al. 2009). Moreover, using DBT interventions to help patients develop competence in emotion regulation may help *therapists* feel more comfortable in employing exposure treatment (Welch and Rothbaum 2007). Evidence for the potential benefits of combining DBT with cognitive-behavioral interventions for PTSD is encouraging but preliminary (Foa et al. 2009a).

Transference-Focused Psychotherapy

In contrast to the behavioral theory guiding DBT, TFP (Clarkin et al. 1999) is a psychodynamic treatment approach to BPD and, as such, it overlaps substantially with MBT (Allen et al. 2008), especially insofar as both approaches aspire to improve mentalizing in relation to attachment relationships (Kernberg et al. 2008). In my view, the difference between transference-focused and mentalizing approaches is a matter of emphasis as well as theoretical language. As its name implies, TFP emphasizes the patient-therapist relationship, given the assumption that the patient will transfer past attachment experiences into the treatment, where they can be explored and understood (mentalized): "The therapist's interpretation of the patient's direct affective experience of the therapeutic relationship is viewed as the route to increased integration of the representational world, to the shift from insecure to secure attachment, and to improvements in the capacity for mentalization" (Kernberg et al. 2008, p. 179). Consistent with its ties to psychoanalysis, TFP places a relatively great emphasis on exploring and understanding *unconscious* repetitions of past experiences in current relationships.

Although far less extensive than for DBT, controlled research has demonstrated the effectiveness of TFP. For example, TFP was shown to be more effective than psychotherapy provided by experienced therapists interested in working with patients with BPD (Doering et al. 2010). TFP was associated with comparatively greater decreases in symptoms of BPD, fewer suicide attempts, fewer inpatient admissions, and improved overall level of functioning.

One major study of TFP (Clarkin et al. 2007; Levy et al. 2006) made a substantial contribution to understanding the impact of psychotherapy on attachment and mentalizing in patients with BPD. Importantly, this study directly compared TFP with two other manual-based treatments for BPD—namely, DBT and supportive psychotherapy for BPD. All treatments were conducted for 1 year. The three treatments were generally equivalent with respect to broad improvements in the symptoms of BPD, although there were some differences: TFP showed effects across a broader range of outcome measures; TFP and DBT were more effective than supportive psychotherapy in reducing suicide attempts; and TFP led to more improvements than the other two treatments in anger and aggressive behavior (Clarkin et al. 2007). Especially pertinent to my concerns are additional findings related to attachment and mentalizing: based on comparisons of Adult Attachment Interviews administered before and after treatment (Levy et al. 2006), results showed that compared with DBT and supportive psychotherapy, TFP was associated with increases in the proportion of patients showing secure attachment as well as increases in narrative coherence and mentalizing. Notably, however, consistent changes in resolution of loss and trauma were not observed.

Mentalization-Based Treatment

Anthony Bateman and Peter Fonagy (2009) described MBT succinctly as

> a psychodynamic treatment rooted in attachment and cognitive theory. It requires limited training with moderate levels of supervision for implementation by generic mental health professionals. It aims to strengthen patients' capacity to understand their own and others' mental states in attachment contexts in order to address their difficulties with affect, impulse regulation, and interpersonal functioning, which act as triggers for acts of suicide and self-harm. (p. 1355)

Bateman and Fonagy (2006a) first implemented MBT in a day-hospital program, which patients attend initially 5 days per week; the maximum length of time patients remain in the day-hospital program is 18–24 months. The primary treatment intervention combines individual and group psychotherapy, but the day treatment also includes crisis management, medication management, and structured activities such as expressive writing and art that are intended to foster mentalizing. More recently, Bateman and Fonagy (2009) developed an intensive outpatient implementation of MBT, which consists of one 50-minute individual psychotherapy session and one 90-minute group psychotherapy session weekly over the course of 18 months.

MBT is distinguished by a *consistent focus on strengthening patients' mentalizing capacities* by exploring mental states of self and others in key attachment relationships, in the patient-therapist relationship, and in interactions with other patients in activities and group psychotherapy. The combination of individual and group psychotherapy (with the addition of group activities in the day-hospital program) is especially valuable in helping patients appreciate how the same situation (e.g., an argument) can be viewed and experienced from multiple perspectives.

Initial outcome research compared the day-hospital implementation of MBT to treatment as usual in the community at 18 months (Bateman and Fonagy 1999) and 36 months (Bateman and Fonagy 2001) after the initiation of treatment. The results showed significant advantages for MBT over usual treatment in the community. Most noteworthy, however, is Bateman and Fonagy's (2008) 8-year follow-up study in which patients in the two treatments were evaluated 5 years after completing treatment (and 8 years after starting it). This is by far the longest follow-up study of treatment for BPD, prompting researcher Ken Levy (2008) to characterize it as "destined to become a seminal study in the annals of psychiatry" (p. 556). In the 5-year period following the end of active treatment, patients in the MBT group made fewer suicide attempts (23% versus 74%); they made fewer visits to the emergency room and had fewer inpatient admissions; they used less outpatient treatment and medication; fewer met diagnostic criteria for BPD (13% versus 87%); and they showed less impulsivity and better interpersonal functioning, as well as greater capacity to maintain employment. The improvement in interpersonal functioning is especially noteworthy in implying amelioration of insecure attachment (although attachment patterns were not assessed directly): patients in MBT showed significant improvement in two core criteria for BPD, intense unstable relationships and frantic efforts to avoid abandonment. Especially noteworthy is the continued improvement after the conclusion of treatment, prompting Levy (2008) to comment that "the findings clearly support the notion that developing behavioral control need not be skill based but can occur through the *development of mental skills*" (p. 557, emphasis added). The long-term effectiveness of MBT led Herman (2009) to remark, "I believe this study may ultimately define a new standard of care for BPD. It leads me to wonder about developing similarly intensive, multimodal treatment models for complex PTSD" (pp. xvi–xvii).

To investigate the benefits of mentalizing-focused treatment in less intensive and more pure form than exists in a multifaceted day-hospital program, Bateman and Fonagy (2009) compared the effectiveness of the 18-month intensive outpatient treatment (individual and group psychotherapy) with that of structured clinical management, another active intervention based on guidelines for treating BPD. As expected, both treatments were associated with substantial improvements after 18 months. Nonetheless, MBT proved superior in effects to clinical management, especially in the last 6 months (i.e., after 12 months of treatment). Specifically, MBT was associated with fewer incidents of suicidal behavior and nonsuicidal self-injury as well as fewer hospitalizations and less use of medications. Moreover, the MBT group improved more in global functioning as well as in symptoms of depression and social adjustment. The differences between the MBT and clinical management groups are particularly note-worthy: patients in both groups received comparable amounts of therapy, but the clinical management therapy focused on support and problem solving, whereas MBT focused on enhancing mentalizing.

Treatments for Complex Traumatic Stress Disorders

As emphasized in the previous two chapters, problems stemming from attachment trauma potentially go far beyond PTSD and even BPD. Naturally, research on treatment of such complex problems lags behind research on more circumscribed disorders. Yet the need for treatment that addresses these complex problems has been apparent for many years, as evidenced by Herman's (1992b) pioneering work. Christine Courtois and Julian Ford (2009) made a major contribution in synthesizing subsequent work on understanding, assessing, and treating complex traumatic stress.

Current best practices for treating complex traumatic stress require that the treatment be individualized and focused on the whole person, as contrasted with treatment of distinct disorders. A core principle of Courtois and Ford's approach is consistent with this book's focus on mentalizing in the context of attachment: "The therapist seeks to create relationship conditions in which the client is emotionally validated and is 'seen' and appreciated, to counter the invalidation experiences typically associated with attachment trauma and subsequent victimization, and to encourage emotional expression and development" (Courtois et al. 2009, pp. 86–87). Following Herman (1992b), Courtois and colleagues advocate a three-phase approach to treating complex trauma. Phase I, which focuses on *safety and stabilization,* involves education about trauma; establishing a safe environment (i.e., free from ongoing abuse and violence); learning to regulate extremes of emotional arousal; maintaining safety from suicidal behavior and nonsuicidal self-injury; and developing supportive relationships. Phase I is neither merely preliminary nor quickly completed; these agendas are a mainstay of long-term treatment. Phase II consists of *processing traumatic memories* and creating a coherent narrative of the trauma; hence, this phase is the analog to exposure therapy. Phase III entails *reintegration,* that is, moving ahead in life with respect to establishing trusting relationships and intimacy, establishing healthy sexual functioning, developing effective parenting practices, and pursuing vocational and career interests—in sum, thriving in love and work.

Clinicians debate the extent to which treatment of complex stress disorders should focus on processing traumatic memories. Herman's (1992b) cautionary statement bears heeding: "Though the single most common therapeutic error is avoidance of the traumatic material, probably the second most common error is premature or precipitate engagement in exploratory work, without sufficient attention to the tasks of establishing safety and securing a therapeutic alliance" (p. 172). As I have construed it (Allen 2001), treatment requires a balance between processing and containment, where the two main pillars of containment are secure attachment relationships and individual capacities for emotion regulation—that is, being able to rely on others to provide a feeling of security in the face of distress as well as being able to manage distress on one's own when necessary. Finding this balance is a major challenge in trauma treatment for therapists and patients; as Herman identified, the dangers are avoidance on the one hand and overwhelming immersion in trauma on the other hand. The right balance will differ from one individual to another and, for any given individual, from one point in treatment to another. Moreover, we would be mistaken to believe that the goal of containment is to permit processing of traumatic memories. I argue the reverse: the goal of processing traumatic memories is to foster containment—that is, the capacities for secure attachment and emotion regulation. It is counterproductive to focus on processing traumatic memories as an end in itself; the ultimate goal is not to remember trauma, but rather to live well.

As I've only hinted here, we are blessed with a rich clinical literature on treating complex traumatic stress that includes not only individual psychotherapy but also group therapies (Ford et al. 2009). Yet the research support for various treatment approaches is limited, and we lack formal treatment guidelines; moreover, "No approach to memory reconstruction work has been definitively validated for clients with complex traumatic stress disorders" (Courtois and Ford 2009, p. 95). As Christie Jackson and colleagues (2009) reviewed, however, several controlled studies are encouraging in showing improvements associated with multifaceted treatment approaches that adapt cognitive-behavioral techniques to the treatment of patients with complex traumatic stress disorders. All these approaches balance containment and support with processing of traumatic memories.

Parent-Child Interventions

In this chapter, I have documented the range of treatment approaches to treating trauma and the varying levels of research support for them. Various treatments have been shown to lead to substantial gains, but there is ample room for improvement in the level of outcomes as well as the extent of research support—evidenced especially in the dearth of long-term follow-up studies. In particular, the limitations in outcomes indicate the need for prevention and early intervention—most importantly, the alleviation of traumatic interactions in early attachment relationships. Here we have much reason to be encouraged, particularly because parent-infant and parent-child interventions that promote mentalizing and attachment security have been shown to be effective.

Minding the Baby

Arietta Slade and her colleagues developed interventions explicitly directed toward enhancing parents' capacity to mentalize with regard to infants' and children's mental states as well as with regard to the parent-child relationship (Slade 2006). The aim is simple: "What we attempt to do, in a variety of direct and indirect ways, is to help the parents hold the child in mind" (Slade 2008b, p. 307). Slade begins by helping the parents contemplate the child's basic mental states (e.g., feelings); then she helps them appreciate the relation between mental states and behavior (e.g., appreciating that the child's fussiness is not due to being "mean" but rather to being "hungry and tired"); finally, she helps parents comprehend the mutual influences of the dyad's mental states (e.g., how the parent's anger frightens the child and the child's fearful behavior further frustrates the parent). Slade's approach focuses primarily on mentalizing the child and the parent-child relationship and only secondarily on the origins of problems in the parent's history (Slade 2008b).

Slade and colleagues (Sadler et al. 2006; Slade et al. 2004) developed the mentalizing-based parenting program, aptly named Minding the Baby, for high-risk first-time inner-city parents and their infants. Mothers in this program typically have a significant trauma history as well as a range of psychiatric disorders, often including substance abuse. With their own history of insecure attachment, the mothers typically have problems in mentalizing with respect to their own mental states as well as those of their children. The intervention extends from the pregnancy to the child's second birthday, and home visitors provide extensive practical help (e.g., providing parents with educational materials and other necessities as well as offering help in obtaining housing, social services, and health care). Throughout the program, the therapist models mentalizing. Initial mentalizing interventions during pregnancy are intended to help the mother articulate concerns about pregnancy and delivery, a form of help that's especially crucial for mothers with a history of sexual abuse and fears of childbirth. After giving birth, the mother is helped to appreciate her infant's mental states: "Understanding that the baby *has* feelings and desires is an achievement for most of our mothers" (Sadler et al.

2006, p. 280, emphasis in original). The therapist also videotapes mother-infant interactions and reviews the tapes with the mother, speaking for the baby in the process and enabling the mother to reflect on her own feelings and intentions as well as those of her baby; mentalizing one step removed can be easier than in the heat of a problematic interaction. In addition, the home visitors assist mothers in playing with their babies, thus promoting the secure base side of attachment security.

Slade (2008a) gives examples of parental mentalizing as follows:

> The development of the reflective or intentional stance is marked by the capacity to see behavior *as a function* of underlying mental states or intentions. We can think of a parent as reflective *once they manifest the capacity to link the child's (or parent's own) internal state to behavior or to other internal states.* "He threw a tantrum in the store (behavior) because he was tired and hungry (physical state), and I'd been dragging him around all day and he was sick of it (mental state)." "She didn't sleep all night because she'd been so frightened by how angry I'd gotten at her." When work with parents in child psychotherapy is going well, we begin to see such shifts from a behavioral to a reflective stance. For instance: "Oh, so maybe he's been running away from me when I pick him up at school because he can't bear for me to know how much he's missed me!" rather than "How can I get him to stop running away when I'm trying to get him in the car after school?" (p. 317, emphasis in original)

Research reviewed in Chapter 1 ("Attachment, Mentalizing, and Trauma") provides support for the theoretical basis of Minding the Baby: parents who show higher mentalizing capacities have more securely attached children; parental mentalizing is associated with more effective parenting practices; and parental mentalizing is associated with the development of child mentalizing (Slade 2006). Accordingly, initial outcome research suggests that the Minding the Baby program enhances parental mentalizing, improves infant health, and averts disorganized attachment while enhancing attachment security (Sadler et al. 2006).

Circle of Security

The Circle of Security project also bears attention in its aim to promote attachment security by means of enhancing parents' sensitivity to infants and children (Marvin et al. 2002; Zanetti et al. 2011). Parents are educated about the safe haven and secure base of attachment, with the idea that children circle between the two: with the secure base, they venture forth to explore the environment; when distressed, they circle back to the safe haven to seek comfort and restore security. Parents are coached to provide support for exploration by watching over the child, providing help as needed, and taking joy and delight in the child's activities and successes. They're also coached to be attentive to the child's distress signals and to respond with attunement and comforting. With John Bowlby's work in mind, the formula for parenting is as follows: "*Always* be Bigger, Stronger, Wiser, and Kind. Whenever possible follow your child's need. Whenever necessary, take charge" (Zanetti et al. 2011, p. 322, emphasis in original).

The intervention is a 20-week group program designed for six participants (typically mothers) with children ranging in age from 11 months to 5 years (Zanetti et al. 2011). The program begins with filming of each mother and child in the Strange Situation, paying particular attention to reunions. Then the parent is filmed while responding to a Circle of Security Interview in which she is asked about her experience with her child in the Strange Situation as well as about the parent's relationship with her own caregivers in childhood. These assessments are employed to discern where on the circle the parent is having particular difficulties (i.e., with supporting exploration or providing comfort). The therapist identifies a *linchpin struggle* between the parent and child—that is, "the key defensive strategy represented both in the parent-child interaction and in each partner's internal working model" (p. 327). This struggle becomes the focus of the intervention. The videotaped interactions are reviewed in the group so that parents can reflect on what they observe as well as support and learn from each other.

The following example of Marie and her 3-year-old son Samuel illustrates a linchpin struggle and the intervention. Marie had suffered from postpartum depression after Samuel's birth, and she experienced overwhelming anxiety after the birth of Samuel's sister, who was 2 months old when Marie sought treatment. She described Samuel as clingy and difficult in his first year and as a sensitive child in relation to whom she had difficulty exerting her authority. Marie was struggling with a history of unresolved losses, and she showed several manifestations of attachment and caregiving disorganization: fear of Samuel's aggression, feelings of helplessness, and loss of control of her anger. Because Marie had little experience of being comforted, comforting did not come easily to her: she provided comforting behavior (e.g., holding and patting) but not comforting emotional attunement (mentalizing). Accordingly, Marie was teaching Samuel not to rely on her, and he developed a controlling pattern of behavior. Here's a description of their interaction in the Strange Situation:

> Samuel appeared to be a precocious, but subdued little boy. Despite his attempts to dominate his mother when she was in the room, he was distraught during the second separation. The linchpin moment occurred

when Marie returned. Samuel was standing near the stranger, sobbing. He looked toward Marie as she reentered with her arms outstretched. She picked him up and took him to a chair. She uttered reassuring words, patting him, and wiping his tears, but her face showed her agonized uncertainty, and her touch had a frantic quality. Overall, her comfort seemed to be ineffective in helping him to settle his feelings. Within 30 seconds, she took him to the floor, and began to encourage him to look at the toys, defensively trying to get him onto the top half of the Circle [i.e., exploring], even though he was directly cueing her that he was on the bottom [i.e., seeking comfort]. He stopped sobbing, and then said he wanted his father, got up and walked away to the door. (Zanetti et al. 2011, p. 332)

This vignette is instructive in showing how a disorganized pattern of attachment can emerge without active maltreatment; indeed, the therapist highlighted the way in which Marie's response to Samuel's distress was well-intentioned—but ineffective. In reviewing this linchpin moment on videotape with Marie and the other parents in the group, the therapist helped Marie appreciate how she was encouraging exploration when Samuel needed comforting. In the course of this discussion, Marie came to appreciate that when Samuel became emotionally wound up, she responded in kind; she learned that the best strategy for comforting another person is "just to be with them...to let them know that you're there, and it's okay. To spend that time, to be *with* that person" (p. 335, emphasis in original). By the end of treatment, Marie showed more warmth in her interactions with Samuel and his aggressive behavior had diminished. When the Strange Situation was repeated, after the second separation Marie "was able to reassure Samuel when he ran after her, bringing him back into the room, and saying 'It'll be all right. Mummy wouldn't tell you if it wasn't'" (p. 338).

Conclusion

If you've diligently worked your way through the catalog of treatments in this chapter, your head might be swimming. Here is a positive spin on this situation: we have an embarrassment of riches in the field of psychotherapy. Yet, although treatment developers and researchers have ample reason to take pride in their many successes, we're hardly in a position to cheer. Not all patients benefit from the various treatments, and many drop out; moreover, those who do benefit may have residual symptoms and remaining problems in living. Furthermore, although we have a wide array of treatment options, not all the options are widely available, and the options are particularly limited in rural areas. Additionally, we have the ubiquitous problem of limited financial resources for health care.

As this entire chapter attests, even under the best of circumstances—access to the full array of treatment options—patients and therapists face the daunting problem of making choices among them with limited evidence to guide the choices. We have many effective treatments, but the differences among them in effectiveness generally are marginal. I remember Julian Rotter, one of my early graduate class teachers, lamenting in the late 1960s that we needed to figure out what kinds of patients are best suited to different kinds of treatment. Now, more than four decades later, the field still struggles to find a basis in research to determine what works for whom (Roth and Fonagy 2005).

In the next chapter, I present a counterweight to the problem of choosing among the dizzying array of treatment methods that are roughly equivalent in effectiveness: searching for the elements these treatments have in common that account for their effectiveness. In this search, consistent with the book's focus on attachment, I highlight the therapeutic relationship. As the present chapter attests, the honorific label "evidence-based treatment" has been awarded to treatment methods that have been subjected to experimental research (e.g., experimentally comparing the outcome of the particular treatment method with a control group, such as being placed on a waiting list). Yet this "evidence-based" label is somewhat arbitrary. As reviewed in the next chapter, extensive evidence supports the benefits of a therapeutic relationship. This fact should be no surprise, given the research on attachment reviewed in the first chapter of this book.

Key Points

◆ Virtually all effective treatments for PTSD entail controlled exposure to frightening stimuli—external and internal. Prolonged exposure is the best-researched and ostensibly simplest treatment approach, typically conducted in a dozen sessions. Yet the process by which fear and anxiety are diminished is not a simple one.

◆ The complexity of the process bears underscoring: exposure therapy improves anxiety tolerance as well as building new associations to anxiety-provoking stimuli; it entails exploring and understanding a wide range of emotions beyond fear; it promotes the development of a coherent narrative of traumatic experience; and it takes place in the context of a safe relationship—that is, an attachment context.

◆ Attachment trauma goes far beyond PTSD to impair emotion regulation in close relationships; hence, treatments developed for BPD are of cardinal importance in treating attachment trauma. Although DBT is the best researched and deservedly most widely known, other treatment approaches also have been demonstrated to be effective. All these are long-term treatments. Although the theoretical language differs, all these approaches address problems with emotion regulation in key relationships, and, in so doing, all promote greater awareness of emotions and conflicts in relationships. As I've not refrained from noting, TFP has demonstrated improvements in attachment security, and MBT has shown the most enduring effects in long-term follow-up research.

♦ The diagnosis of BPD, multifaceted as it may be, doesn't capture the full complexity of problems associated with attachment trauma. Complex traumatic stress disorders comprise a broad domain of diagnoses and problems for which complex treatment approaches have been developed, typically involving treatment in stages (attaining safety and stabilization, processing trauma, and enhancing functioning and quality of life). These long-term treatments are complex, and they cannot be highly prescriptive; hence, they are not easily researched, although research is under way and we have reason for encouragement.

♦ Individual psychotherapy has been the mainstay of psychosocial treatment for the full range of psychiatric disorders and has been most extensively researched in relation to trauma as well as other mental health problems. Ample research supports the value of group therapy for trauma, but little research-based guidance is available to recommend specific types of groups or to decide who might benefit most from groups. Of great concern is the relative paucity of research on couples and family therapy for trauma, given the prima facie benefit of efforts to promote mentalizing and secure attachment directly in the relationships where they matter most.

♦ It has been obvious for at least a half century that mental health problems are best addressed through prevention. The attachment literature is highly encouraging in this regard, showing promise for early interventions that promote parent-child interactions conducive to security; some of these interventions begin as early as pregnancy and include explicit attention to mentalizing. Indeed, this research demonstrates experimentally the potential benefits of mentalizing in attachment relationships, the justification for plain old therapy.

CHAPTER 5

Plain Old Therapy

My first experience as a psychotherapist was formative. I was an undergraduate psychology major in my last semester, headed for graduate school in clinical psychology. I had taken some graduate courses in clinical psychology. So it wasn't entirely outrageous over four decades ago—although it would never be done these days—for my senior advisor to propose that I see a patient in the Psychology Clinic. This plan was feasible only because I was to conduct a highly structured and well-researched treatment—systematic desensitization—for a patient with a very circumscribed problem: a public speaking phobia. He had taken a job that required speaking to groups, so he needed help. The procedure is straightforward: the therapist instructs the patient in relaxation techniques; after mastering relaxation, the patient is guided through a graded series of imaginal exposures (e.g., from speaking to a small and informal gathering of friends all the way up to giving a formal speech to a large audience of critical experts). The patient learns to maintain a state of relaxation while imagining otherwise anxiety-provoking situations. Albeit all in imagination, this experience generalizes to the real situation—as does imaginal exposure for posttraumatic stress disorder (PTSD).

Initially, my novice status notwithstanding, all went well. I taught my patient the relaxation techniques, and he successfully ascended his hierarchy of feared situations while maintaining a state of relaxation. But something insidious also was happening. At the beginning of the sessions, he wanted merely to talk to me about his problems. Moreover, over the course of the therapy, he wanted to talk more and desensitize less. Alas, he wanted psychotherapy, and I hadn't been trained to do it. With supervision from my advisor, I was able to help the patient reasonably well. Fortunately, apart from his phobia, the patient's mental health was sound.

Long after this initiation, I labored under the illusion that there was a structured procedure for psychotherapy; I merely didn't know it but was hopeful I could learn. I went to graduate school and earned my Ph.D. I took an academic position but continued doing psychotherapy and seeking supervision as well as providing it to graduate students. Not enough! I undertook postdoctoral training and, after completing the training, I had 5 years of additional psychotherapy supervision. I never managed to achieve this elusive goal of conducting psychotherapy as a structured procedure. Now I recognize the utter folly of my quest. Unknowingly, I began my career as a psychotherapist by practicing an evidence-based treatment according to the standards of the time. Only in recent years—after four decades of experience—have I fully appreciated the reasons for my plight when my patient merely wanted to talk with me. I've never found the manual, and I've stopped looking.

Limitations of Evidence-Based Therapies

The psychotherapy field's fecundity, merely glimpsed in the preceding chapter ("Evidence-Based Treatments"), has created a major problem, now widely acknowledged: no therapist can master all these evidence-based therapies. As long as a few decades ago, more than 250 therapies were current (Herink 1980). Psychotherapy researchers have aspired to sift the wheat from the chaff by winnowing therapies down to those that are empirically supported through randomized controlled trials, and this guided my review in the last chapter. But the winnowing effect of this effort has been marginal, as empirically supported treatments (ESTs) continue to proliferate. Considering that a decade ago, 145 ESTs were identified (Chambless and Ollendick 2001), one can only imagine the plight of the beleaguered therapist who aspires to treat a wide range of patients while employing ESTs: "unless there is functional equivalence among different manualized renditions of the same treatment, the practitioner who wants to apply ESTs to his or her practice is faced with the daunting problem of learning 150+ specific manualized treatments" (Malik et al. 2003, p. 151).

Over a decade ago, a skeptical patient in one of my trauma-education groups needled me about all our therapies. At the end of the group, she came up and silently handed me a slip of paper with the following statement that she attributed to Anton Chekhov's *The Cherry Orchard:* "If many remedies are prescribed for an illness, you may be certain that the illness has no cure." I discovered this was a paraphrase from the source, which, in one translation, reads:

> You know, when people suggest all sorts of cures for some disease or other, it means it is incurable. I keep thinking, racking my brains, and I come up with plenty of solutions, plenty of remedies, and basically, that means none—not one. (Chekhov 1904/1998, pp. 25–26)

Plainly, if we had a completely effective treatment, we'd be using it instead of continuing to develop all these alternatives. We must be honest: we can help, but we cannot cure.

The evidence-based therapies flourish in academic centers that recruit patients with *relatively* pure forms of specific disorders, although truly pure forms are nearly impossible to find in practice. But most psychotherapists—and I include myself in this group—treat patients with a wide variety of disorders, albeit limited by the range of our experience and expertise. As contrasted with those in academic centers, most therapists in the field are the counterpart to the general practitioner in general medicine—not specialists. Our colleague Jeremy Holmes represents us well: "I define my practice, both in the public and private sectors, as 'general psychotherapy' analogous in medicine to 'general practice': i.e., an open access, non-highly specialised, all-comers form of work" (Holmes 2010, p. xiv).

In defense of plain old therapy, I enjoy quoting the ironic point made by Peter Fonagy and his colleague Anthony Roth after their masterful review of the research literature on evidence-based therapies: "although there is an increasing requirement for practice to be based on evidence, we are not aware of systematic evidence demonstrating the benefit of this process" (Roth and Fonagy 2005, p. 502). Having devoted substantial portions of their careers to researching and obtaining it, Roth and Fonagy aren't discounting the value of evidence; rather, they emphasize the need to go beyond evidence in relying also on clinical judgment. They give due respect to the art of implementing evidence-based procedures, especially in the context of complex and severe psychopathology. I am not arguing against the need for evidence, but I take a broad view of the evidence that we therapists need to justify our practice.

As I envision it, two somewhat parallel streams of thought have been developing over the past several decades regarding psychotherapy. One stream, exemplified by the previous chapter, is the development of disorder-specific, evidence-based therapies. I hope that my review conveys my respect for this stream and gives a glimpse of what we general practitioners have to learn from it. Moreover, when patients need these disorder-specific treatments, we generalists must refer them to specialists. Yet, as my review also attests, as we move in complexity from PTSD to borderline personality disorder (BPD) and then complex traumatic stress disorders, the specificity in the disorders and their treatments necessarily decreases.

The second, equally venerable stream of psychotherapy research has focused on what is common among the various brands. A half century ago, Jerome Frank made this bold assertion: "Much, if not all, of the effectiveness of different forms of psychotherapy may be due to those features that all have in common rather than to those that distinguish them from each other" (Frank 1961, p. 104). Frank's claim now has been supported by decades of research, especially research on the patient-therapist relationship, which I highlight in this chapter. We're fortunate to have this research, not least because the two streams of thought about psychotherapy have put clinicians at odds with researchers. John Norcross and Michael Lambert (2011) introduced their systematic review of psychotherapy research as follows: "The culture wars in psychotherapy dramatically pit the treatment method against the therapy relationship. Do treatments cure disorders or do relationships heal people?" (p. 3). Here's their contrast in stark form: "Most practice guidelines and evidence-based practice compilations depict disembodied psychotherapists performing procedures on DSM disorders. This stands in marked contrast to the clinician's experience of psychotherapy as an intensely interpersonal and deeply emotional experience" (p. 7).

I have predicated this book on my conviction that we psychotherapists must be informed providers and, equally, our patients must be informed consumers. Moreover, we providers bear a significant responsibility for informing our consumers. On the basis of social forces shaping mental health care practices, therapists are liable to be better informed about various evidence-based brands of therapy than the common factors they share. I suspect that this is even truer of patients, who may have heard of cognitive-behavioral therapy (CBT) or Dialectical Behavior Therapy (DBT) but are unlikely to know of the pervasive similarities in outcomes or what these treatments have in common.

A Definition of Plain Old Therapy

Lacking a manual, plain old therapy isn't readily defined, which left me feeling at sea as an undergraduate when I was striving to continue desensitizing the patient who instead wanted to talk with me. I've proposed plain old therapy in protest against the proliferation of narrowly defined therapies with all their acronyms, but this tack identifies plain old therapy in opposition—by what it is not. Being relatively unstructured, plain old therapy has an inherent lack of specificity, and its concrete practice will reflect substantially the individuality of the therapist. I think the mark of a true psychotherapist is conviction in the sheer value of understanding and being understood, a conviction that's not easily achieved. I don't dispute the obvious value of problem solving; yet clarifying the problems comes first, and the main goal of psychotherapy isn't to solve specific problems but rather to help patients become better problem solvers. That's where improved mentalizing in attachment relationships comes in; this capacity emerges from the repeated process of understanding and feeling understood.

I'm being intentionally provocative in using the term *plain old therapy;* the term *talk therapy* is fine with me. Although I'm now far more comfortable with a lack of clear structure than when I was inadvertently thrown into conducting psychotherapy as an undergraduate, I've never given up my need to know what I'm doing.

I had an amusing interaction with a patient who resisted my efforts to find a focus for the therapy; she said she just wanted to talk and "vent." Hence, she experienced my questioning as something akin to an interrogation. In an effort to turn the tables, she asked if she could interview me. Willing to see where this role reversal would lead, I consented. She inquired about my educational background and then proposed a challenging question: What was most emotionally difficult for me about graduate school? The answer came to me immediately; I replied that learning to do psychotherapy was the hardest part, because there wasn't a straightforward procedure for it. Delighted with my response, she exclaimed, "I see you haven't given up your need for structure!" Having given me a taste of my own medicine, she was then more open to proceeding with a discussion of her own development.

I'll need the rest of this chapter to give some definition to plain old therapy as I aspire to practice it and encourage others to do likewise. By way of orientation, I propose that practitioners of generic psychotherapy—regardless of their thinking about what they're doing—are mentalizing and engaging their patients in the process of mentalizing while endeavoring to provide their patients with a safe relationship that bears the hallmarks of secure attachment. Moreover, to the extent that the therapy addresses problems in close relationships—including ways of relating to oneself—the content of the therapy process pertains to attachment.

Thus, in campaigning for my version of plain old therapy, I am merely explicating what I believe to be implicit in well-conducted generic psychotherapy. I think therapists intuitively attend to attachment relationships and strive to provide a secure therapy relationship. Moreover, therapists naturally have been mentalizing and helping their patients do so long before the advent of Mentalization-Based Treatment (MBT). But clarity helps; when I know what I'm doing, I can do it better. That's my justification for reviewing theory and research on attachment and mentalizing. I also think that educating patients about attachment and mentalizing helps them make better use of plain old therapy.

The source of greatest potential confusion involves the subtle distinction between plain old therapy and MBT. This confusion stems largely from the fact that MBT was developed as an evidence-based treatment for BPD; yet we also have proposed that mentalizing is common to psychotherapies more generally and, moreover, that mentalizing is applicable to a wider range of psychiatric disorders (Allen et al. 2008; Bateman and Fonagy 2012a). As I conceive it, plain old therapy is a generic version of MBT with a specific focus on problems in attachment relationships that occur in the full range of psychiatric disorders. Conducting psychotherapy and educating patients about treatment at The Menninger Clinic for decades provided the impetus for me to generalize the MBT approach to plain old therapy: I feel a need to maintain some conceptual coherence in an increasingly eclectic environment of diverse clinical practices and to help patients understand the essence of treatment in this complex and potentially bewildering environment (Allen et al. 2012; Groat and Allen 2011). Of course, the challenges in this local environment mirror the broader field of clinical practice, where I find conceptual coherence dismally lacking.

Here is another source of potential confusion in my presentation: I'm advocating plain old therapy as a way of treating attachment trauma while also implying that this approach is a good way to conduct psychotherapy more generally. Given my broad view of trauma as resulting from persistently feeling alone in emotional pain, I believe this version of plain old therapy has wide applicability. But I also acknowledge my skewed perspective on this point, because I have worked primarily with hospitalized patients struggling with severe and chronic problems, a population in which varying degrees of attachment trauma are pervasive.

As I envision it, plain old therapy provides just the right amount of structure. In addition to focusing on mentalizing and attachment, I like to collaborate with patients in developing a written formulation of the problems we're addressing, which affords a modicum of structure (and which the patient who interviewed me steadfastly resisted). And I think this moderately structured approach is helpful for us general practitioners who aspire to work flexibly and creatively with a wide range of patients and who find value in many different theoretical approaches, ranging from psychodynamic to interpersonal and humanistic to cognitive-behavioral.

Those who become embroiled in wars are liable to stereotype and caricature their opponents, and I am no exception. I join Patrick Luyten and colleagues (2008) in advocating a *person-centered* developmental approach to psychotherapy as contrasted with a *disorder-centered* approach, which characterizes many specialized evidence-based treatments. Yet we shouldn't turn broad distinctions into rigid dichotomies. Imagine asking a diverse group of therapists, from behaviorists practicing manualized treatments to psychoanalysts, "How many of you regard yourself as focusing more on the individual person than the psychiatric disorder?" I'd wager that all hands would go up. Thus, it would be downright offensive to imply that those who practice disorder-specific treatments aren't also person centered in conducting therapy. Nor should we generalists be characterized as ignoring evidence. On the contrary, we also have a place at the evidence-based table; yet to merit this place, we cannot rest content with the status quo but must continually refine our practice on the basis of contemporary theory and research. Moreover, I have no doubt of the superior efficacy of specialized treatments for circumscribed problems and disorders; we shouldn't be treating obsessive-compulsive disorder with plain old therapy when the patient would benefit from exposure and response prevention. But we always will need generalists alongside specialists—better as collaborators than adversaries. Furthermore, given the importance of commonalities among therapies and the centrality of the patient-therapist relationship in particular, I think specialists must be competent in the practice of plain old therapy on which their more prescriptive methods necessarily are superimposed. I learned this lesson the hard way in working with the first patient of my career. From this broad perspective, Table 5–1 summarizes my justification for reviving plain old therapy.

With this orientation, the rest of the chapter elaborates what I consider to be the basis of plain old therapy. First, I review research on some of the main common factors, as inspired by Frank's (1961) trenchant observation that patients benefit more from what therapies have in common than from the ways in which they differ from one another. Second, I expand on what I consider to be the essential elements of plain old therapy, enhancing attachment and mentalizing. I conclude by acknowledging that we have yet much to learn about how psychotherapy works. I believe that refining plain old therapy with knowledge to be gained from ongoing research on attachment and mentalizing puts us generalists on a productive path toward increasingly better practice.

Contributors to Psychotherapy Outcomes

Larry Beutler and Louis Castonguay (2006) introduced their monumental review of decades of psychotherapy research on a wistful note: "It is hard to find a treatment that works better than another treatment and all

---
TABLE 5–1.   Why we need plain old therapy

- Many psychotherapists are generalists who treat patients with a wide range of problems and disorders.
- Therapists cannot master a large number of specialized treatments.
- Many patients do not present with narrowly defined problems or single disorders but rather with complex combinations of problems and disorders.
- Therapists must learn to capitalize on factors that are common to the effectiveness of diverse treatment approaches and to optimal qualities of the patient-therapist relationship in particular.
- Specialized procedures must be superimposed on competence in plain old therapy.

---

seem to be better than doing nothing" (p. 5). This comment sets the tone for their history of the two streams of research, represented by two task forces: one reviewing empirically supported treatments and the other focused on relationship factors. A continuing stalemate led Beutler and Castonguay to form a third task force charged with integrating the results of the two previous task forces!

I reviewed treatment methods in the last chapter, and in this chapter I emphasize relationship factors. I first describe patient and therapist characteristics that influence treatment outcomes. I then cover two relationship domains consistently related to treatment outcomes: the therapist's manner of relating to the patient and the therapeutic alliance. To provide an overview, I've enumerated these major contributors to psychotherapy outcomes in Table 5–2. Throughout this section, I rely heavily on Beutler and Castonguay's (2006) monumental contribution, buttressed by Norcross's (2011) recent update of research on relationship factors, the product of yet another task force.

Patient's Characteristics

What we have long known to be true of psychotherapy, as of general medicine, is that the main determinant of the treatment outcome is the severity of the patient's illness (Norcross and Lambert 2011). By *severity*, I refer to the seriousness of the symptoms and impairment in functioning; the duration of the problems; the level of distress; and the sheer multiplicity of problems (e.g., in DSM terms, the number of different disorders). For example, substance abuse and personality disorders complicate the treatment of anxiety and depression. Further complicating treatment is environmental stress, which includes financial and occupational problems, living in poverty, and lack of social support.

TABLE 5–2.   Potential contributors to psychotherapy outcomes

- Patient's characteristics—most notably, severity of illness
- Therapist's characteristics—for example, expertise and flexibility
- Therapist's manner of relating to the patient—including empathy, positive regard, and authenticity
- Therapeutic alliance—including a trusting relationship as well as collaborative work and capacity to repair ruptures
- Treatment methods and procedures
- Extratherapy factors—for example, social support, stress, life events, and self-guided change

---

Here we face a catch-22: I argue that the therapeutic relationship is a main avenue of healing in all therapies, yet, as I've discussed, attachment trauma leads to problems such as distrust and alienation that make it difficult for patients to benefit from a therapeutic relationship. This catch-22 is demoralizing to traumatized patients who are keenly aware of their challenges in trusting therapists and benefiting from treatment. An important point to keep in mind is that the vast majority of research studies have been conducted on short-term treatments, which are inherently easier to study. All the research points to the relative benefits of long-term treatment for persons with more severe disorders, and long-term treatments are effective.

Therapist's Characteristics

We seem far more inclined to study therapies than therapists, despite indications that differences among therapists in treatment outcomes outweigh differences among treatment methods (Roth and Fonagy 2005). Accordingly, there is a relative dearth of research on therapist characteristics that predict outcomes of therapy (Castonguay and Beutler 2006). Gender has garnered some attention; although a handful of studies have shown a small advantage for female therapists, there's too little consensus to draw conclusions about whether female therapists are more effective than males, whether female patients benefit more than males, or whether there is any advantage to same-sex matching of therapists and patients. Of course, patients' preferences are extremely important and must be honored, such as when a woman who has been sexually abused or assaulted by a man feels safer working with a woman than a man.

There is surprisingly scant evidence demonstrating that better outcomes are associated with greater therapist experience or with therapist experience in treating specific disorders. As Roth and Fonagy (2005) conclude, experience is less important than expertise and competence. An important aspect of expertise is *flexibility*—that is, knowing when to deviate from the standard delivery of a particular treatment method. Pertinent to the domain of attachment trauma, flexibility is most needed in treating patients with complex and difficult problems, especially problems in relationships. Therapist characteristics have been singled out as being particularly important in the treatment of personality disorders. Here's the list of qualifications: comfort with long-term, emotionally intense relationships; patience; tolerance of feelings regarding the patient and treatment process; open-mindedness, flexibility, and creativity; and specialized training (Critchfield and Benjamin 2006, p. 255). Undergraduates need not apply.

Sidney Blatt's (2008) overview of an ambitious study of the treatment of depression highlights the contrast between methods and therapists. Sponsored by the National Institute of Mental Health, the Treatment of Depression Collaborative Research Program was, in Blatt's view, "probably the most extensive and comprehensive data set ever established in psychotherapy research" (pp. 224–225). Four brief treatment methods were compared: CBT, interpersonal psychotherapy, antidepressant medication with clinical management (i.e., a supportive and encouraging relationship), and placebo with clinical management. By now you should not be surprised that no overall differences were found in effectiveness, as measured by improvement at termination or at 18-month follow-up, among the three active treatments, although medication led to more rapid decreases of symptoms than the two psychotherapies. Although there were no differences among *therapies*, there were substantial differences among *therapists* in outcomes, regardless of the methods the therapists employed—including medication management. The effective therapists had a more psychological than biological orientation, appreciated the need for patients to have more sessions to derive benefit from treatment, and were able to work with a wide variety of patients. Blatt's conclusion will now be familiar: "Therapeutic outcome is significantly influenced by the interpersonal dimensions of the treatment process... rather than by the techniques and tactics described in treatment manuals" (p. 233).

Therapist's Manner of Relating to the Patient

Carl Rogers began developing Client-Centered Therapy in the 1940s. He incorporated the quality of the client-therapist relationship into the theory of therapy in the most thoroughgoing way imaginable. Specifically, Rogers (1951, 1957/1992) proposed that the therapist's *attitude* toward the client carried far more weight than any particular technique. He high-lighted three broad facets of the therapist's attitude that are essential to the development of an effective therapeutic relationship: empathy, posi-tive regard, and congruence.

Of these three, *empathy*—a key facet of mentalizing—is the linchpin:

> It is the counselor's function to assume, in so far as he is able, the internal frame of reference of the client, to perceive the world as the client sees it, to perceive the client himself as he is seen by himself, to lay aside all per-ceptions from the external frame of reference while doing so, and to com-municate something of this empathic understanding to the client. (Rogers 1951, p. 29)

For empathy to be effective, the therapist must not only feel it but also ex-press it, and the patient must perceive it (Elliott et al. 2011). In Dan Sie-gel's (1999) felicitous phrase, the patient must "feel felt" (p. 89).

Complementing empathy is *positive regard* for the patient, a broad concept that encompasses acceptance, affirmation, caring, nonpossessive warmth, and valuing of the patient as an individual. As Rogers's writing makes plain, positive regard balances relatedness and autonomy as well as the core values of love and respect. Notably, respect includes the convic-tion that no one can be more knowledgeable regarding the patient than the patient himself or herself; in this regard, the patient is the expert.

Lastly, Rogers advocated *congruence* in the therapist, also character-ized as genuineness and authenticity. Congruence entails being at ease and behaving naturally, as contrasted with enacting a constrained profes-sional role. Such congruence requires that therapists be self-aware as well as transparent—that is, willing to share their self-awareness in an open and honest manner. Congruence also enables the therapist to acknowl-edge mistakes and empathic failures and to explore the reasons for them in a nondefensive fashion.

These three therapist relationship capacities are widely recognized as core common factors in effective therapy, and each is supported by research (Castonguay et al. 2006). Of the three, empathy has been re-searched most extensively; its therapeutic benefits have been demon-strated in a combined sample of 3,599 patients in 57 separate studies (Elliott et al. 2011). Substantial research support also has been amassed for the benefits of positive regard (Farber and Doolin 2011) and congru-ence (Kolden et al. 2011). Hence, as Tracy Smith and colleagues (2006) concluded regarding this half-century-old Rogerian tradition, "One would think that long before...the present Task Force reports on the power of relationship had appeared, Client-Centered would have been listed as an empirically supported therapy approach" (p. 231).

In my mind, Rogers represents the plainest and oldest version of plain old therapy. Accordingly, I find much in the principles of Client-Centered Therapy to be compatible with a mentalizing approach (Allen et al. 2008). Plainly, empathy and congruence require that therapists be mentalizing with respect to their clients and themselves. We, too, put a premium on the therapist's attitude, which we construe as the mentalizing stance of nonjudgmental inquisitiveness (Allen et al. 2008; Bateman and Fonagy 2006a). Moreover, from the attachment perspective, Rogers anticipated John Bowlby's (1988) view of the therapist's role as providing a secure base for exploration, which includes painful feelings and meanings that otherwise are defended against:

> In the emotional warmth of the relationship with the therapist, the client begins to experience a feeling of safety as he finds that whatever attitude he expresses is understood in almost the same way that he perceives it, and is accepted. He then is able to explore, for example, a vague feeling of guiltiness which he has experienced. In this safe relationship he can perceive for the first time the hostile meaning and purpose of certain aspects of his behavior, and can understand why he has felt guilty about it, and why it has been necessary to deny to awareness the meaning of this behavior. (Rogers 1951, p. 41)

My admiration for Rogers's thought and contributions should be obvious. He not only shaped thinking about the therapeutic relationship but also pioneered psychotherapy research. Boldly, he focused on therapists' interpersonal skills as crucial to the outcome. But I have two reservations. First, Rogers construed a positive psychotherapy relationship as not only necessary but also *sufficient* for improvement (Smith et al. 2006). From Marsha Linehan's (1993a) perspective, given his focus on empathy, Rogers can be seen as emphasizing one side of the needed dialectic: that is, putting a premium on validation while downplaying help for change. A focus on mentalizing, similarly dialectical, requires a balance of empathizing with the patient's perspective while also challenging the patient by presenting alternative perspectives (Bateman and Fonagy 2006a); the capacity to appreciate varying perspectives lies at the heart of mentalizing. To put it simply, we therapists need to establish a good relationship for the purpose of *doing work*, providing a safe haven as well as a secure base for exploration, learning, and growth—change. Doing this work requires a problem focus, which will be informed only in part by psychiatric diagnosis.

My second reservation: in his theory of therapy, Rogers focused primarily on changes in the self. He proposed, not unreasonably, that the therapist's positive regard would serve as a platform for the patient's improved self-regard and, moreover, that this improved self-functioning would lead to improved relationships: "the person who completes therapy is more relaxed in being himself, more sure of himself, more realistic in his relations with others, and develops notably better interpersonal relationships" (Rogers 1951, p. 520). Rather than assuming that improved relationships will ensue from greater self-acceptance, mentalizing assiduously balances a focus on self, others, and relationships. In our educational groups, we often hear patients assert that you must love yourself before loving others. From the vantage point of early development, this proposition has the direction of causation backwards: self-love stems from being loved. More broadly, as described in the first chapter, the sense of self develops from being mentalized in relationships, and this development continues throughout life.

Therapeutic Alliance

Of all the patient-therapist relationship factors, the therapeutic alliance has been most extensively studied, with research from over 14,000 cases attesting to its positive impact (Horvath et al. 2011). Moreover, the strong relationship between the alliance and the treatment outcome holds regardless of the treatment method—psychodynamic, interpersonal, cognitive-behavioral, or substance-abuse focused.

The alliance is a highly complex concept that cannot be separated entirely from the demands of the treatment method or other aspects of the patient-therapist relationship (Roth and Fonagy 2005). Attesting to its breadth, the alliance "encompasses a positive affective bond, consensus about goals and means to achieve the goals, a sense of partnership and shared commitment and engagement, and acceptance of complementary roles and responsibilities" (Stiles and Wolfe 2006, p. 157). Broadly, there are two key facets to the alliance: a *trusting relationship* and a feeling of *working together* toward common goals. With regard to the second of these facets of alliance, my colleagues and I (Allen et al. 1984) have emphasized the importance of patients' *collaboration* in therapy—that is, active engagement in the treatment process and making optimal use of the therapy as a resource for constructive change. Such collaboration also includes respecting patients' preferences for type of therapist, treatment method, and treatment processes; not surprisingly, honoring patients' preferences decreases dropout rates and improves treatment outcomes (Swift et al. 2011). Notably, although we distinguish the trusting relationship from collaboration, these two facets are highly related in practice: it's hard to work cooperatively with someone without having a good relationship. Moreover, receiving competent help and benefiting from treatment will strengthen the relationship.

As already noted, we face a catch-22: problems in relationships consistent with a history of attachment trauma are liable to interfere with establishing a trusting and collaborative relationship, thus impinging on the development of a positive alliance and thereby limiting the benefit of treatment. Such problems have been observed most conspicuously in the treatment of patients with personality disorders (Smith et al. 2006). Such interfering problems include a history of poor family relationships, problems in current relationships, defensiveness, hopelessness, lack of interest in psychological understanding (mentalizing), negativism, and hostility, as well as perfectionism. All these problems are familiar in the context of attachment trauma. This perspective on the alliance illustrates a more general point: the patient's and therapist's contributions to the therapeutic relationship are inextricable. Although Rogers focused on the therapist's empathy, positive regard, and congruence, all these therapist qualities are influenced by the patient's manner of relating. We therapists have a harder time feeling empathy and acceptance for patients who are avoidant, detached, or hostile than we do with those who are collaboratively engaged. Moreover, like our patients, we therapists must feel safe and trusting in order to be transparent—that is, to be at ease and open in sharing our thoughts and feelings.

In the context of therapy with patients with BPD, we have found it misleading to think that we start by establishing a positive alliance and then proceed on a smooth course to a positive outcome. On the contrary, we found the quality of the alliance waxes and wanes across therapy, and even within single therapy sessions (Horwitz et al. 1996). When we think of attachment trauma, it may be more reasonable to think of a stable positive alliance as being a *result* of effective therapy rather than a precondition for it. Consistent with this view, much attention has been given to the value of *repairing ruptures* in the alliance (Safran et al. 2011). Such ruptures may occur in relation to either facet of the alliance. The feeling of trust may be breached, for example, by a therapist's wounding remark or failure to respond to a phone call. Collaboration may be undermined by disagreement about the goals or methods of therapy. To repair such ruptures, the patient must be willing to express negative feelings, an act that, paradoxically, requires a high level of trust. Concomitantly, the therapist must be nondefensive and empathic, for example, by acknowledging insensitivity and mistakes and validating the patient's reactions. Such validation sets the stage for exploring misinterpretations on the patient's part that can exacerbate responses to ordinary human failings. For example, if I were to make an ill-considered comment that was inadvertently insulting, I would acknowledge my error and apologize for it and then explore the patient's misinterpretation that I had desired to drive her out of therapy.

As I view it, secure attachment rests not only on a history of dependable sensitivity but also on a feeling of confidence that conflicts can be addressed and resolved. No relationship, from infancy onward, is characterized by continuous attunement; the norm is to fluctuate among engagement, disengagement, and reengagement. As my co-leader Denise Kagan was fond of saying in our educational group on attachment, the test of a relationship is its capacity to weather the storms. The following is an example of a relatively minor rupture in the alliance, noteworthy because it occurred within a matter of minutes in the first session.

Case Example

I had reviewed the psychiatric evaluation before I met Sarah, a young woman who had been admitted to the hospital for treatment of increasing depression and anxiety. By the time she started therapy, Sarah had begun responding to treatment, and she was pleasant and engaged. I let her know I had a general idea about her history but that we would need to figure out how to work together, and I'd like to hear directly from her what she'd like to work on. She talked about how crippling her depression had been and that she didn't see any reason for it. I agreed, letting her know that when I reviewed her history, I found her symptoms to be downright puzzling, given how well she had been functioning previously. She also was perplexed, but she said that she had a family history of depression and that she was sure it was "genetic." While acknowledging my view that biological factors are important, I let her know my "prejudice" that there also must be a psychological basis to her problems that we could explore together. To my surprise, she found this comment irksome and said, "You're twisting my mind!" I experienced her reaction as surprisingly paranoid, but didn't say so; paranoia was out of character with her general demeanor. Although I wasn't aware of it at the time, I suspect that my direct contradiction of her view had a hard edge to it, given my aversion to exclusive focus on biological factors. I responded by remarking with some surprise, "We've just gotten started and already we're at odds!"

Reinstating collaboration, Sarah then asked if I had a "theory" about her symptoms, and I confessed that I did have a hunch—namely, that a major separation from her family had something to do with them, notwithstanding that she seemed to have managed the separation extremely well at the time. We then explored her experience during the separation, and I quickly developed an appreciation for her talents, success, and general gumption. She resonated with my admiration and talked about her accomplishments with a feeling of pride. We were back on track and ended the session on this positive note. Thus, after merely noting the rupture, I made an end run around it, motivated simply by my interest in getting to know her better as a person.

In several subsequent sessions, we were able to make sense of substantial contributors to the severe exacerbation of attachment insecurity, which had erupted in a way that Sarah was unable to fathom at the time.

Albeit speculating, we also agreed on significant temperamental (genetic) factors that contributed to her vulnerability.

Attachment in Psychotherapy

Only relatively late in his career did John Bowlby (1988) articulate his view of the implications of attachment theory and research for psychotherapy in his eloquent book *A Secure Base*. I discovered the relevance of attachment theory to trauma through that book; I was astounded to realize that Bowlby so clearly articulated just what my traumatized patients most lacked and most needed—a secure base in attachment. Bowlby provided an attachment framework for psychotherapy in this oft-quoted passage in which he proposed that the therapist's first task is

> to provide the patient with a secure base from which he can explore the various unhappy and painful aspects of his life, past and present, many of which he finds it difficult or perhaps impossible to think about and reconsider without a trusted companion to provide support, encouragement, sympathy, and, on occasion, guidance. (p. 138)

My favorite pithy summary of Bowlby's view of psychotherapy emerged in an educational group on trauma. In the context of talking about the intrusive symptoms of PTSD, I remarked, "The mind can be a scary place." A young woman in the group quipped, "Yes, and you wouldn't want to go in there alone!" This is Bowlby's point, most succinctly put, and the best description of trauma therapy I've ever heard. Bowlby's thesis and the perspicacious patient's pithy version of it illustrate Holmes's view that attachment theory "provides a common-sense model of the therapist-client relationship," which he spells out as follows: "The architecture of the therapeutic relationship is that of a person in distress, seeking a safe haven and in search of a secure base, and a caregiver with the capacity to offer security, soothing, and exploratory companionship" (Holmes 2009, p. 493).

As I have outlined in this book, attachment theory began as a developmental model that eventually was extended to adult relationships. Only more recently, following Bowlby's lead, have clinicians been applying attachment theory and research to the conduct of psychotherapy. We clinicians don't have anything approaching a recognized school of therapy based on attachment theory. As I interpret it, Arietta Slade (2008b) articulated the current consensus:

> My perspective here is that attachment theory and research have the potential to *enrich* (rather than dictate) a therapist's understanding of par-

ticular patients. Attachment theory does not dictate a particular form of treatment; rather, understanding the nature and dynamics of attachment and of mentalization informs rather than defines intervention and clinical thinking. (p. 763, emphasis in original)

Consistent with Slade's view, Joseph Obegi and Ety Berant (2009b) declare, "There is no school of therapy for adults called 'attachment therapy'" (p. 2). Yet they're pushing the envelope in distinguishing two types of therapy derived from attachment theory. The first type, *attachment-informed psychotherapy*, is "a therapy that uses attachment theory and research as adjudicative sources of knowledge and that influences how presenting problems are conceptualized, assessed, and treated" (p. 3), but it uses this knowledge in the context of treating patients with established therapies. The second type, *attachment-based psychotherapy*, uses attachment theory to conceptualize the individual's development and problems, incorporates attachment theory into the structure of the psychotherapy, and attempts to demonstrate its effectiveness with outcome studies.

With the transition from attachment-informed to attachment-based psychotherapy, I can see the potential for yet another brand name, complete with another acronym, ABP. Averse to brands and acronyms, I don't think this is the way to go. As Slade (2008b) puts it, attachment theory informs and enriches our conduct of psychotherapy, whatever method we might employ—including plain old therapy. Whether the therapist attends to it or not, attachment will play a key role as a common factor in psychotherapy, because psychotherapy inherently evokes attachment needs and patterns: the patient in distress needs help. Once attachment needs are evoked, patients will rely on secure or insecure strategies to meet them as best they can.

There is a lot of ground to cover in this section. I start with more discussion of the point that attachment almost inevitably will come into the therapy relationship. I then describe how the specific patterns of secure and insecure attachment tend to play out in psychotherapy. This background sets the stage for considering how the therapist's attachment style and behavior influence the therapy outcome. I summarize two areas of emerging research: the extent to which patients' characteristic attachment patterns influence therapy outcome, and the extent to which psychotherapy improves attachment security. I follow this discussion of the interpersonal impact of attachment with a discussion of the impact of psychotherapy on developing an internal secure base—that is, a secure attachment relationship with oneself. To conclude, I discuss the extent to which changes in attachment within psychotherapy generalize to other relationships. Table 5–3 summarizes the main points I'll be making.

TABLE 5–3. Roles of attachment in psychotherapy

- Ideally, psychotherapy has the hallmarks of secure attachment, including providing a safe haven and secure base.
- Psychotherapy is limited in meeting attachment needs by virtue of its essential professional boundaries.
- All the patterns of secure and insecure attachment potentially are manifested in the patient-therapist relationship.
- Patients are likely to repeat their pattern of attachment with parents in their relationship with their therapist.
- Patients who are securely attached develop more positive alliances and benefit more readily from psychotherapy.
- Patients who are insecurely attached are more likely to seek psychotherapy.
- Psychotherapy has the potential to improve attachment security.
- Psychotherapists who are secure in attachment are more able to relate flexibly to patients with different patterns of insecurity so as to help them move in the direction of greater security.
- Psychotherapy can be helpful in promoting a secure relationship with oneself—that is, an internal secure base.

Psychotherapy as Attachment Relationship

I've already affirmed that psychotherapy is an attachment relationship, but this statement oversimplifies things. Mario Mikulincer and Phil Shaver (2007a) neatly summarized the way in which psychotherapy is likely to become an attachment relationship:

> When the therapeutic relationship develops as intended by the therapist, he or she becomes a genuine attachment figure for the client (i.e., a reliable and relied-upon provider of security and support). Clients typically enter therapy in a state of frustration, anxiety, or demoralization that naturally activates their attachment system and causes them to yearn for support and relief. Attachment needs are easy to direct toward therapists, because therapists, at least when a client believes in their healing powers, are perceived as "stronger and wiser" caregivers, possessing the hallmarks of good attachment figures. Therapists are expected to know better than their clients how to deal with the clients' problems, and they occupy the dominant and caregiving role in the relationship. Therefore, the therapist can easily become a target of the client's proximity seeking and projection of unmet needs for a safe haven and secure base. (p. 411)

Consistent with this proposal, research on patients' experience of therapy (Eagle and Wolitzky 2009) has demonstrated that patients rely on their therapists as a safe haven and secure base; they have concerns about their therapist's availability; and they may respond with protest to separations occasioned by illness or vacations (e.g., by detachment, irrita-bility, or missed appointments). Yet clinicians also recognize the substantial differences between psychotherapy and other attachment relationships, the prototype being the mother-child relationship. As Bowlby (1988) put it, "In providing his patient with a secure base from which to explore and express his thoughts and feelings the therapist's role is *analogous* to that of a mother who provides her child with a secure base from which to explore the world" (p. 140, emphasis added).

Many differences between therapy and parent-child relationships have been delineated, in part related to the unique features of psycho-therapy (Florsheim and McArthur 2009). Psychotherapy is a professional relationship, most notably, a service for which the patient pays. Maintain-ing professional boundaries is crucial to the effectiveness of psychother-apy. Such boundaries entail scheduled sessions in the therapist's office (sometimes including explicit agreements about telephone contact be-tween sessions) as well as limited self-disclosure on the part of the ther-apist. If the relationship morphs into a social relationship, a friendship, or—at the extreme—a sexual relationship, the relationship is no longer therapeutic but rather downright destructive. Moreover, the safe haven in most attachment relationships entails not only emotional attunement but also physical comforting; although there are individual differences among therapists in their use of touch, the emotional comforting and connection in psychotherapy fundamentally relies on *psychological* attunement—mentalizing.

Given these differences and limits, Holmes (2010) explicates a para-dox in the psychotherapy relationship as follows:

> The intensity of the therapeutic relationship is both "real"—the client may develop an intimacy with his therapist more intense than any previously experienced in adult life—and "unreal" in that it remains encapsulated within the ethical and physical confines of the contract and the consulting room. Ultimately the therapist is a *quasi-secure base* rather than the real thing. (p. 57, emphasis added)

Given this paradoxical nature of the relationship, perhaps most con-spicuously evident in paying for the service and in divorcing touch from emotional comforting, we must be mindful that the professional nature of the relationship accounts for its unique effectiveness. To put it starkly, we therapists would be far less capable of being consistently empathic if we were living with our patients. The professional boundaries of the re-lationship limit the attachment in ways conducive to therapeutic explo-ration. But I think we must be careful with language here—that is, with such terms as *analogous* and *quasi*. As Rogers (1951) made plain over a half century ago, the relationship must involve real caring, or it will be useless as an attachment relationship.

Attachment Patterns in the Psychotherapy Relationship

When Bowlby (1988) characterized the psychotherapy relationship as providing a secure base for exploration, he was articulating an ideal. Exaggerating to make the point, one could say that the patient who could readily use therapy as a secure base for exploration wouldn't *need* psychotherapy. In fact, the vast majority of psychotherapy patients are insecure (Slade 2008b). Particularly for a patient with a history of attachment trauma, it's a major achievement, not a given, for the patient to be able to experience a psychotherapy relationship as a safe haven and secure base (Eagle and Wolitzky 2009).

Given the pull for attachment in the patient-therapist relationship, we can anticipate that predominant attachment patterns will be reexperienced and reenacted in that relationship. Broadly speaking, this is merely one instance of ubiquitous *transference* in relationships—that is, the repeating of past patterns in current relationships. To take the prototype, patterns of relating to parents can be repeated in the relationship with the therapist. Diana Diamond and colleagues (2003) confirmed this repetition in a small case series, employing the Patient-Therapist Adult Attachment Interview to assess patients' attachments to their therapists. These researchers compared attachments to therapists with attachments to parents as assessed by the standard Adult Attachment Interview. They found a high degree of concordance: attachments to therapists were highly similar to attachments to parents.

We can see transference as the manifestation of interpersonal learning; more or less consciously, we all generalize from the past to the present. This inevitable generalization will be more or less adaptive, depending on the goodness of fit between the past and the present. If your boss or your therapist is indeed as critical and domineering as your father, wariness will be appropriate. In the first section of this book, I described the basic attachment prototypes: secure, avoidant, ambivalent, and disorganized. You will recognize them easily from the following descriptions of the manner in which patients with different attachment patterns are likely to engage in relationships with their therapist. Here, I merely summarize observations from clinical practice and research (Slade 2008b; Obegi and Berant 2009a).

Unsurprisingly, patients with secure attachment best fit Bowlby's (1988) ideal of using the therapist as a secure base for exploration. They are more likely to seek psychotherapy if they need it, and having done so, are likely to form a solid therapeutic alliance. Given their positive internal working models, they're likely to be trusting, viewing the therapist as dependable, sensitive, attentive, and supportive. Hence, they're relatively self-disclosing as well as able to tolerate disappointment, frustration, and anxiety in the relationship. Accordingly, they're able to reveal their negative feelings such that ruptures in the alliance can be explored and repaired. For patients with a proclivity for insecure attachment, and a history of attachment trauma in particular, this vision of psychotherapy is something to work toward, and it may be a very long time in coming. I won't forget my experience of working with a woman who had suffered severe trauma and who still struggled to trust me after 5 years of intensive therapy, during which time I had been reasonably dependable and trustworthy.

Patients who show avoidant-dismissing attachment are relatively unlikely to seek therapy, and when they do, they have difficulty establishing an alliance. On the relatedness-autonomy dimension, they are imbalanced in the direction of autonomy, denying attachment needs and striving to be self-reliant. Thus, they have difficulty forming an emotional bond as well as developing a collaborative relationship. They're disinclined to make themselves vulnerable by expressing needs for help, and they're likely to view the therapist as disapproving and rejecting; thus they're prone to feeling ashamed and humiliated. They're more likely to focus on others' shortcomings—including the therapist's—than their own. They're openly skeptical of therapy and tend to approach it as an impersonal business relationship, as if they were consulting an expert, with little sense of the therapist as a caring individual. Because of their difficulty expressing feelings, ruptures in the alliance are liable to remain underground and thus impervious to repair. Their therapists will have difficulty empathizing and are liable to feel as disengaged emotionally as the patient—indeed, emotionally shut out. When I asked trainees in a treatment seminar to provide a visual image to symbolize their relationship with a patient, one therapist came up with "a block of ice" to characterize his experience with an avoidant patient. Ironically, this is a hopeful metaphor: ice melts, and the patient was indeed warming up—very slowly.

Case Example

Thelma sought hospital treatment in her 40s to interrupt a spiraling pattern of impulsive, self-destructive behavior that included what she called a "sex addiction" as well as drug abuse and self-cutting. She said she'd never had a healthy romantic relationship and that she was more comfortable with "meaningless sex." She had a history of being sexually molested by a teenager when she was a child, and she was raped in college and again in later adulthood. She described her mother as a "rageaholic," and she learned to depend on her father, as she'd continued to do throughout her adult life. Yet she described her father as being "emotionless," and she depended on him for practical problem solving rather than emotional comfort.

Thelma stated flatly at the beginning of therapy that she didn't want to depend on anyone, and she didn't want anyone to depend on her. She talked about what I felt to be alarming and serious problems with a cheerful demeanor that she developed deliberately to keep people at a distance. But she also revealed a cold and detached side of herself; she was critical and contemptuous to the point of being "cruel," proclaiming that she was "the ice queen."

Given Thelma's emotional distance, she was extremely hard to engage in psychotherapy. She talked about her problems openly, but she was so detached emotionally that the psychotherapy seemed to have no meaning or influence on her. She made an effort to connect by bringing in some artwork and poetry that expressed profoundly painful emotions and implied a yearning for comfort and connection, but she couldn't express her pain directly. When she was frightened as a child by her mother's rages, she hid in her room. When she was distressed in the hospital, she did the same—retreating to her room. She left treatment early when she had a disagreement with her treatment team about participating in the addictions program; she protested that she didn't like the 12-step focus on a "higher power," because she was her own higher power. She eventually transferred to another program that she thought would give her "more space."

In contrast to those who are avoidant, patients who are ambivalent-preoccupied are likely to seek therapy and to become emotionally engaged quickly, with a seemingly positive alliance. They're emotionally intense and expressive, highly self-disclosing. On the relatedness-autonomy dimension, they're imbalanced in the direction of relatedness to the point of excessive dependency; they fear self-assertion and autonomy, which portends a feeling of being alone. Accordingly, the positive alliance is vulnerable to ruptures; the therapist's inevitable failings confirm the patient's expectations that the therapist will not be dependable. The early positive alliance can be an illusion; disillusionment is in the offing. Although the patient easily expresses distress and a need for help, the help may be hard to take in. One of my early teachers, psychoanalyst Stuart Averill, commented that a patient had a strong "sender" and a weak "receiver." On the one hand, given the inherent limitations of a professional relationship, the therapist's caring may be experienced as frustratingly inadequate—as one patient expressed it, akin to putting a thimble of water into the ocean. On the other hand, the patient may resist the therapist's encouragement to change inasmuch as movement toward autonomy can be threatening because it heralds terminating the treatment and losing the tenuous connection with the therapist.

Case Example

Ursula sought hospital treatment in her early 20s after extensive outpatient psychotherapy failed to prevent recurrent suicidal crises. She described herself as "needy" and "codependent," and she attributed these characteristics to being a "sad, neglected kid" throughout her childhood. Her mother had chronic medical problems that included severe pain; she said her mother would be bedridden for days at a time, often "moaning and wailing" in a way that was excruciating to hear. She said her father was "bipolar" and extremely unpredictable, ranging from loving and funloving to irritable and punitive to depressed and withdrawn—sometimes sitting alone in his recliner for hours "staring into space like a zombie."

Ursula said she moved quickly into romantic relationships, starting in junior high school. She said she didn't bother making serious friendships with girls because these never met her needs for love. She "glommed onto" boyfriends and became "intoxicated" with love. She said the intoxication temporarily assuaged her "self-loathing." She tried to ensure that her boyfriends would stay with her by "showering them with love" and attempting to meet all their needs. To the extent that her boyfriends reciprocated, their efforts were relatively futile, as Ursula's unrelenting self-loathing ultimately returned to the fore. She described herself as being like a "colicky baby" and "immune to consolation." She'd come to recognize in previous therapy how her behavior was smothering and controlling; she became extremely possessive and jealous, and as her boyfriends withdrew, she lashed out in anger. The ruptured relationships inevitably left her feeling let down and neglected.

When she was in high school, one of Ursula's friends committed suicide. The funeral made a big impression on Ursula: she was struck not only by the outpouring of sorrow and care but also by the expressions of regret that others hadn't been sufficiently caring and loving when her friend needed it most. With this model in her background, Ursula increasingly came to rely on suicidality as a means of eliciting care from her parents and preventing her boyfriends from leaving her. She repeated this pattern in outpatient psychotherapy and in the hospital. Her suicidality was extremely confusing to clinicians, who alternately felt she was "playing games" and were alarmed for her safety. Ursula shared this confusion; she acknowledged that she sometimes used suicide as a "distress signal" but that as she "rehearsed" suicide through increasingly dangerous attempts, she became more genuinely suicidal. Thus, increasingly quickly, she could slide from "sounding the alarm" to wanting to die.

Ursula's suicidality became a focus of treatment. I conveyed that she was sabotaging treatment, because clinicians felt "tormented" and "terrorized" by her suicidal behavior, which had put an end to her outpatient treatment and jeopardized her hospital treatment. Ursula was unaware of any conscious intention to torment others, even though she was keenly aware of her frustration and resentment. Yet, with help in mentalizing, she was able to appreciate that regardless of her intentions, others *felt* tormented and thus resentful. As I put it, even though her suicidal behavior might glue others to her through fear, eventually the relationships would "tear apart" as others became "fed up." Indeed, her romantic relationships and previous treatments had done so, and her current treatment also was on the brink of tearing apart.

Replayed in her hospital treatment relationships with staff members and fellow patients, the self-sabotaging nature of her behavior became glaringly obvious to Ursula with the help of psychotherapy. Her "immunity to consolation" also began to give way as she was able to talk about her painful history of relationships in her family and in romantic relationships. This shift enabled others to be connected to her through concern rather than fear. Ursula also came to appreciate how she could empathize with her peers and provide some consolation to them, and thus she felt more valued and developed some self-regard; she said she was moving from "self-loathing" to "self-dislike" with a bit of "self-appreciation." After a long struggle, she was able to discharge from the hospital with better prospects for using continuing treatment without undermining it.

As it is in the Adult Attachment Interview, disorganized attachment in psychotherapy is intermingled with organized patterns (Slade 2008b). In parallel with their lapses in the interview, patients with a history of attachment trauma, particularly when they're struggling with intrusive memories of trauma and dissociative disturbance, are liable to experience marked disruptions in the therapy relationship. I remember vividly a patient who was seeing me as her abusive deceased father—not as *reminding* her of her father or *as if I were* her father but rather as *being* her father in the moment. Not uncommonly, when traumatic experience and painful emotions are evoked, patients with disorganized attachment may lapse into dissociative states to the extent that they feel profoundly detached or, at the extreme, "gone."

Giovanni Liotti (2011) points out that like the initially traumatizing attachment relationship, the therapy relationship can present the patient with the insoluble dilemma of fright without solution: fear of the therapist evokes attachment needs, but the closeness that would assuage these needs is frightening. Unlike the ambivalent patient who manages to maintain relatedness at the expense of autonomy, or the avoidant patient who manages to sustain autonomy at the expense of relatedness, the disorganized-fearful patient is relatively incapable of sustaining either relatedness or autonomy. Unable to maintain a balance, the patient potentially oscillates between frightening and engulfing closeness and withdrawal that portends utter aloneness.

Case Example

Vic, a young adult who had not been able to leave his family's orbit, was hospitalized when his family could no longer tolerate his reckless behavior and temper outbursts. His stonewalling their efforts to help, for example, when he locked himself in his room for long periods, especially frustrated his parents. They described this pattern of "impossible" behavior as virtually lifelong, and they described the family as being "in shambles," which they said often had been the case throughout Vic's life.

In psychotherapy, Vic starkly manifested the pattern of fright without solution, and I confess that I was unable to find any stable solution to helping him out of it. In the first session, Vic stated that he was "fine." He said he'd solved all his problems on his own, he had nothing to work on in therapy and, indeed, he had "nothing to say." He acknowledged that "being fine in a nuthouse" was a contradiction. He said that no one but his friends could understand him and the doctors merely "came down" on him, pushed him around, and experimented on him as if he were "an animal in a maze." Notwithstanding his declaration that he had nothing to say, he talked a blue streak. When I pointed out this contradiction, he said that he wanted to "dominate" the conversation so that I would have no opportunity to talk and "beat him up." Nonetheless, Vic's anguish was palpable. Although he couldn't focus on any single problem, he made it clear that he'd battled unsuccessfully with addiction to narcotics, felt guilty about the enormous strain he'd put on his parents, and suffered an extremely painful breakup in a romantic relationship that he'd hoped might lead to marriage. He said he felt "adrift" and was afraid he'd never amount to anything. Accordingly, even though we had absolutely no basis for a therapeutic alliance, I said at the end of the session that he seemed "very troubled," such that it made sense for us to continue to meet. He agreed.

Over the course of more than a dozen sessions, at which point Vic abruptly quit hospital treatment, we continued in this stalemate. Vic generally continued to flood the sessions, briefly alluding to obviously traumatic experiences in his relationships but denying any desire for help despite the fact that he was frequently tearful or agitated. He rebuffed my efforts to explore painful matters and said he simply needed to "blow off steam." Indeed, he said blowing off steam was helpful because otherwise his head would "burst."

Frequently, I was bewildered by flat contradictions. For example, Vic said that his father was trying to make him feel insecure by making sure that he was secure, and he expressed frustration with a friend who tried to help him calm down when he was "freaked out" because he was "perfectly comfortable" and needed no help. Any attempt to clarify contradictions only added to his defensiveness. To the extent that he acknowledged difficulty with his mental functioning, he attributed it to psychiatrists' "botched" use of medications.

I continued the therapy on the principle that actions speak louder than words. Vic consistently stated that he had no need for therapy and nothing to work on, yet he attended his appointments regularly, talked about many problems, and expressed painful emotions. Over time, we were able to achieve some narrative coherence in portions of sessions. Vic wasn't completely unsympathetic to my struggles. In one session, in response to my statement that it's hard for me as a therapist not to have problems to work on, Vic asked me what would make *me* feel "more comfortable." I responded, "If you came in saying you had a problem, such as a relationship problem." Vic then proceeded to talk about his frustration that he hadn't been able to "open up" to his girlfriend and that he'd felt scared to do so, even though he couldn't think of any reasons for his fear. He understood that she was frustrated with him; in fact, when she broke up with him, she told him she felt "helpless" because she knew he was hurting but he "shut her out."

Even though he was continually at odds with treatment, Vic ultimately was able in psychotherapy to acknowledge straightforwardly a "character flaw" that he recognized influenced his relationship with his girlfriend and played out in treatment. He said that he felt ashamed and weak that he'd never been able to talk with anyone about his personal problems and that he couldn't help "shutting down" when he felt a need to confide. He knew that others were aware of how "upset" he was, but they had no way to understand because he shut them out, being unable to tolerate "being in the spotlight." I let him know that I had this experience throughout the therapy: I could see how "anguished" he was, and my natural inclination was to try to understand, but I had a hard time doing so. Plainly, this problem was the bane of his treatment; I found it somewhat hopeful that we were able at least to articulate it.

In describing these attachment patterns as they are enacted in therapy, I have relied on prototypes—perhaps stereotypes, if not caricatures. We therapists need to be mindful that these patterns are evident in degrees (e.g., more or less ambivalent or avoidant); are potentially fluid (e.g., in movement from ambivalence to avoidance, or in a collapse from avoidance to a fearful, disorganized pattern); and are intermingled (e.g., as when avoidance masks a profound and ambivalent hunger for solace, as Ursula's experience exemplifies). Moreover, as discussed next, the patient's attachment behavior will interact with the therapist's attachment proclivities. The attachment pattern always is a joint production—a relationship or *partnership*, as Bowlby (1982) characterized it.

Psychotherapist's Contribution to Attachment

It takes two to create an attachment relationship. Although comparatively little research is available on the contribution of therapists' attachment patterns to the psychotherapy process, the literature to date presents a relatively consistent picture (Obegi and Berant 2009a).

The benefits of a therapist's attachment security are obvious: the secure therapist is likely to function well in a caregiving role, as does the secure parent. This role entails being available, dependable, and emotionally responsive (i.e., mentalizing). Attachment security also is associated with better capacities for emotion regulation, such that the securely attached therapist will be better equipped to accept emotional distress and to address conflicts in the patient-therapist relationship as well as to explore and repair ruptures in the therapeutic alliance. Accordingly, secure attachment in therapists has been associated with more positive therapeutic alliances (Levy et al. 2011) and better treatment outcomes (Beutler and Blatt 2006).

Most psychotherapy patients have insecure attachments, and the therapist's job is to move insecure patients in the direction of greater security. The two fundamental directions of insecurity are too much autonomy and distance (i.e., avoidance) and too much relatedness and dependency (i.e., ambivalence). Hence, the job of the therapist is to move patients from the extremes (distance or closeness) toward the middle—that is, toward a better balance between relatedness and autonomy. Securely attached therapists are better able to do this balancing by virtue of their flexibility—that is, their tolerance for closeness as well as distance.

Therapists naturally tend to complement their patients' attachment styles; that is, they can be relatively cognitive with avoidant patients and relatively emotional with ambivalent patients. Secure therapists, however, also have the capacity to counter their insecure patients' attachment proclivities by moving toward more emotional engagement with avoidant patients and toward more emotional containment with their ambivalent patients. In other words, they're able to do as Arietta Slade (Slade 2008b) counsels: "I've suggested…that there is value in gently challenging an individual's predominant defensive style. This means…using more feeling-based or empathic responses for dismissing patients, and more intellectual or structuring responses for preoccupied patients" (p. 774). Alternatively, therapists might consider tailoring the method to the patient's attachment pattern, as Beutler and Blatt (2006) propose:

> While preoccupied patients pull for emotional-experiential interventions, they appear to benefit from a more cognitive-behavioral strategy that helps them modulate overwhelming feelings…. Likewise, avoidant patients pull for rational-cognitive interventions, but appear to benefit from strategies that facilitate emotional engagement. (p. 35)

Such flexibility—complementing while gently countering patients' insecure attachment patterns—will be more challenging for the insecure therapist. As Brent Mallinckrodt and colleagues (2009) noted, "The optimal therapeutic distance tends to produce tension and discomfort in avoidant clients, whereas it tends to produce frustration for anxious clients" (p. 243). Insecure therapists will have difficulty tolerating the discomfort associated with maintaining this optimal distance. Avoidant therapists are liable merely to complement avoidant patients' attachment behavior, engaging in a relatively intellectualized therapy process and thereby perpetuating the avoidant pattern. Also, avoidant therapists are liable to feel frustrated with their ambivalent patients' wishes for more emotional engagement and closeness, potentially responding with anxiety, hostility, and distancing. In contrast, ambivalent therapists are liable to be highly emotionally responsive, complementing their ambivalent patients' emotional style and failing to assist them with emotion regulation. They're also liable to feel frustrated with their avoidant patients' wish for emotional distance. Moreover, ambivalent therapists are liable to have difficulty dealing effectively with ruptures in the alliance, given their sensitivity to abandonment and rejection.

In educating patients about psychotherapy, I often refer to the "H-factor"—that is, therapists are human. Unquestionably, as this brief discussion attests, therapists must be relatively secure to do their work effectively. But therapists' insecurities inevitably will come into play, contributing to withdrawal and excessive distance or emotional entanglements. It makes no sense for therapists to avoid such imbalances assiduously; they're inevitable in all attachment relationships. Therapists, however, are obligated to be aware of such departures from security and to do their best to rectify them—that is, to engage in repairing these ruptures. Therapists must be mindful and mentalize. Quite often, therapists need help, and secure attachment in therapists will be associated with a willingness to seek such help—be it in personal therapy or supervision with senior colleagues or peers.

Relation Between Attachment Patterns and Therapy Outcomes

As discussed earlier in the chapter, better therapeutic alliances predict better treatment outcomes, and securely attached patients are more likely to develop a positive alliance. Hence, the logical inference would be that securely attached patients are likely to improve more than insecurely attached patients in psychotherapy. Although the research literature is limited, it supports this supposition.

In general, securely attached patients are functioning at higher levels both at admission to treatment and at termination (Berant and Obegi 2009). Ken Levy and colleagues (2011) combined results from 14 studies and used a dimensional assessment of attachment, relating degrees of attachment anxiety and avoidance to extent of improvement with psychotherapy. As expected, secure attachment was associated with greater improvement; notably, of the two dimensions of insecurity, anxiety but not avoidance was associated with poorer improvement.

Although they might have more difficulty benefiting from it, patients with insecure attachment are most likely to need psychotherapy insofar as problems in attachment relationships are a major reason for seeking psychotherapy. Not surprisingly, patients who are insecurely attached are likely to need longer treatment (Berant and Obegi 2009), and they benefit from it. For example, Fonagy and colleagues (1996) found that compared to patients with other attachment classifications, a far higher proportion of avoidant patients improved in long-term psychodynamic treatment. Similarly, Blatt (2004) showed that patients with self-critical depression (which is associated with avoidant-dismissing attachment) benefit from longer-term psychotherapy. Overcoming avoidance is an inherently slow process, but it is possible if patients can remain engaged in treatment.

Relation Between Psychotherapy and Improved Attachment Security

One key benefit from psychotherapy for patients with a pattern of insecure attachment is improved security. As I described in Chapter 1 (see the section Stability and Change), attachment patterns show a mixture of continuity and change over the course of development. Establishing trusting and enduring relationships is one potential source of change, and psychotherapy provides one opportunity to do so.

Although the number of studies examining change in attachment security over the course of psychotherapy is small, the results are consistent: the proportion of patients classified as secure increases, and the proportion classified as insecure decreases (Berant and Obegi 2009). For example, researchers have employed the Adult Attachment Interview to assess attachment status before and after a course of psychotherapy. Fonagy and colleagues (1995) reported that whereas none of their patients showed secure attachment at the beginning of treatment, 40% were classified as secure at the end of receiving psychodynamic psychotherapy in an inpatient setting.

Similarly, as reported in the preceding chapter, Levy and colleagues (2006) reported a significant increase in the number of patients with BPD showing secure attachment after a year of Transference-Focused Psychotherapy (but not with Dialectical Behavior Therapy or supportive psychotherapy). Notably, in the transference-focused group, narrative coherence in the Adult Attachment Interview also increased, and narrative coherence is a marker for attachment security. We would hope for this result in a psychotherapy process aimed at exploring attachment relationships and conversing about them in an emotionally rich and authentic way. Notably, Levy and colleagues found that Transference-Focused Psychotherapy led to a modest decrease in the number of patients classified as unresolved with respect to trauma and loss, but this finding was not statistically significant. In contrast, in a study of treatment outcomes for women with a history of child abuse who were diagnosed with PTSD, Stovall-McClough et al. (2008) found a significant decrease in unresolved status over the course of treatment.

Although research on attachment security as an outcome of treatment is in its early stages, the findings are generally encouraging. Yet the extent to which greater security presumably achieved in the patient-therapist relationship generalizes to relationships with key attachment figures, such as romantic partners and family members, remains uncertain. Bowlby (1988) proposed that "the focus of psychotherapy must always be on the interactions of patient and therapist in the here and now, and that the only reason for encouraging the patient at times to explore his past is for the light it throws on his current ways of feeling and dealing with life" (p. 141).

Plainly, individual psychotherapy provides a vehicle to examine attachment patterns in three domains: childhood relationships with parents, the patient-therapist relationship, and current attachment relationships outside the therapy. Yet there is much to be said also for working directly with patients and their partners to improve their responsiveness to each other for the sake of greater attachment security. We should keep in mind that since we humans evolved, our natural attachment relationships have provided trauma therapy, and they continue to be our main source of solace. When it functions well, individual psychotherapy can facilitate making better use of these relationships. Yet Sue Johnson (Johnson and Courtois 2009) has been a strong proponent of bolstering the healing capacity of these relationships more directly in couples and family therapy so that we need not rely solely on generalization from individual psychotherapy. Mentalization-Based Family Therapy (Asen and Fonagy 2012) has evolved to fill this need. But there is another potential value of individual psychotherapy in healing from trauma that we should not overlook: improving one's relationship with oneself.

Cultivation of Internal Secure Base

When I read some years ago the idea that self-love entails *bonding* with oneself (Swanton 2003), it occurred to me that one could think of secure attachment as a model for relating to oneself (Allen 2005). In other words, you could respond to your emotional distress by mentalizing and being mindful—that is, being attentive to your feelings, accepting of them, and curious about the basis of them. With this attitude, you could comfort yourself, just as you might comfort others or receive comfort from them. Unfortunately, insecure attachment also provides a model for relating to yourself: you can ignore your feelings, or you can criticize yourself for your feelings. At worst, you can relate to yourself in a neglecting or abusive way. To get a line on the security of your attachment with yourself, you merely need to pay attention to what you say to yourself when you're feeling anxious, sad, angry, guilty, or ashamed. Periodically throughout this book, I have made a point of contrasting experiential avoidance with experiential acceptance; you could think of experiential avoidance as based on an insecure relationship with yourself and experiential acceptance as requiring a secure attachment relationship with yourself.

Mikulincer and Shaver (2004) proposed that activating mental representations of secure attachment relationships—remembering, imagining, or thinking about them—evokes a feeling of security that provides a buffer from stress. Accordingly, a feeling of security is based on internalizing attachment relationships: "A well-treated child incorporates the protecting, soothing, approving, encouraging, and coaching functions originally performed by a security-enhancing attachment figure into his or her own mental processes" (Mikulincer and Shaver 2007a, p. 152). Thus, securely attached persons are able to "mobilize caring qualities within themselves" (p. 162); in so doing, they activate internal working models of being loved and valued in a way that provides relief from distress.

Mikulincer and Shaver (2007b) found several ways to put secure internal working models to work by what they call *security priming*, analogous to priming a pump. Such priming activates attachment representations—for example, by encouraging individuals to think, talk, or write about secure attachment experiences. The wide-ranging experimental effects of security priming are remarkable, including improvement in mood, mitigation of distress related to reminders of trauma, improved feelings of self-worth, and enhancement of caregiving as evident in increased compassion and altruistic helping. Among these remarkable findings, security priming enables persons who are characteristically avoidant or anxious-ambivalent to function temporarily in ways characteristic of those who are more securely attached. In effect, security priming tones down insecurity temporarily.

To my amazement, security priming has these beneficial effects even when the priming is done *subliminally*—that is, without conscious awareness. Such subliminal priming is accomplished by projecting a stimulus on a screen for an extremely brief period (e.g., about one-fiftieth of a second) so that it doesn't register consciously. Many such subliminal stimuli have been employed: a Picasso drawing of a mother cradling an infant; the names of persons with whom the participant is secure; or the words "caring," "love," "secure," or "affection." Such security priming has been shown to lead to less defensive responses for avoidant participants and less maladaptive coping for ambivalent participants; that is, each group of insecure participants responded more like secure participants after security had been primed (Cassidy et al. 2009).

Holmes (2001) uses the term *internal secure base* to refer to a person's capacity to mobilize secure internal working models to provide a feeling of security when distressed. Psychotherapy has the potential to provide an external secure base, with the proviso that the relationship has the positive therapeutic qualities described earlier in this chapter. Psychotherapy also has the potential to enhance security in other relationships that provide an external secure base. Yet psychotherapy also has the potential to strengthen the patient's internal secure base through internalization—taking in the empathic qualities of the relationship. This opportunity is especially valuable in the context of attachment trauma, wherein the patient hasn't had experiences of psychological attunement conducive to developing and internalizing secure working models. Sadly, attachment trauma is conducive to *insecurity priming*, activating internal models conducive to neglectful and abusive ways of relating to oneself.

We spend a lot of time in psychotherapy discussing present and past relationship problems—insecure attachments. Perhaps we should be spending more time bringing to mind experiences of secure attachments. I've latched onto Mikulincer's (Shaver and Mikulincer 2011) concept *islands of security*. Invariably, patients with a history of attachment trauma have experienced islands of security—with siblings, members of their extended family, teachers, coaches, or members of the clergy. We therapists need to spend time revisiting these islands so the relatively secure relationship experiences come more easily to mind. I recall working with a woman who had grown up in a violent household, feeling continually frightened without solace. Yet I had been struck by her warmth and caring, and I asked her how she had developed these characteristics. She recalled childhood visits to her loving grandmother, which she had not thought about for a long while. The joy she expressed in recalling this experience was palpable, and appreciating fully what she had internalized from this relationship made a significant difference in her sense of herself as well as her feeling of psychological security.

Limitations of Attachment

I've been thoroughgoing in the use of attachment theory, but there is far more to life than attachment. Attachment theory is founded on the premise that attachment is only one among many behavioral systems (Cassidy 2008): people explore, develop skills and talents, socialize, affiliate with groups, enjoy sex, and provide care. So there's much more to talk about in psychotherapy than attachment. Yet Mikulincer and Shaver (2007b) remind us that "attachment theory makes security the *developmental foundation* for optimal functioning of other behavioral systems, such as exploration, caregiving, affiliation, and sex," and they go on to add, "No one imagines that good sex, saintly virtues, complex play, or friendship can emerge first and then make room for security later on" (p. 205, emphasis added). Accordingly, they state, "This is why we consider safety and security to be primary, but it does not mean that safety and security are everything" (p. 205).

Fonagy and colleagues (2008) also acknowledged the limitations of attachment theory as follows: "Attachment theory cannot and does not aspire to specify the full richness of the subjective contents that preoccupy the ordinary mind, let alone the mind in distress. This is the ambition of psychoanalysis" (p. 802). I share their view that psychoanalytic theory and practice has provided us psychotherapists with the most thoroughgoing psychological understanding of individuals and their relationships. Yet we also have much else to learn from other theoretical approaches, as I hope this book attests. And I'll reiterate that psychology, psychiatry, and psychotherapy are all new; we also have much to learn about ourselves from philosophy, literature, and art—and most of all, from living life fully. All these contributions to our knowledge—and our individual humanity—play into our capacity to mentalize in psychotherapy, our next agenda.

Mentalizing in Psychotherapy

My colleagues, Peter Fonagy and Anthony Bateman, and I made a bold claim in proposing that mentalizing "is *the most fundamental common factor* among psychotherapeutic treatments" (Allen et al. 2008, p. 1, emphasis in original). This claim might seem megalomaniacal if we hadn't tempered it by our previous acknowledgment that our focus on mentalizing is "the *least novel* therapeutic approach imaginable" (Allen and Fonagy 2006, p. ix, emphasis added). The terminology might be new, but the basic idea is not. I can't imagine psychotherapy of any brand that does not involve attention to mental states—thoughts, feelings, and the like. In my view, arguing that psychotherapy revolves around mentalizing would be relatively banal if it were not for developmental research that has established the foundation of mentalizing in attachment relationships. Moreover, to claim that psychotherapy rests on mentalizing isn't to say that we psychotherapists mentalize consistently or skillfully. John Oldham (2008), chief of staff at The Menninger Clinic, made this point: "Mentalizing, even if not always explicit in our language, is implicit in many forms of psychotherapy and is an invaluable conceptual beacon to guide us in our work. Allen and colleagues, of course, have already said this, when we suggest: 'You're already doing it. And indeed we are, *if we're doing our job.*'" (p. 346, emphasis added). We have learned from attachment theory not only what promotes mentalizing but also what prevents us as therapists and our patients from "doing our job": the foremost obstacle is attachment trauma.

Although mentalizing came into prominence in the treatment of BPD, it is being applied in an increasingly wide range of contexts (Bateman and Fonagy 2012a), consistent with our view of mentalizing as a common factor that cuts across different schools and brands of therapy. Accordingly, I've come to view a focus on mentalizing as a *style* of plain old therapy, and I begin this section by illustrating the style as I aspire to practice it, with varying degrees of success. I go on to illustrate the process of mentalizing trauma in psychotherapy, and I summarize research on the impact of psychotherapy on mentalizing. I conclude the section by acknowledging that attachment relationships, fundamental as they may be, aren't the only route to mentalizing.

Mentalizing as a Style of Plain Old Therapy

There is nothing unique about a mentalizing approach to psychotherapy such that if you were observing a session using this approach, you could say, "That must be Mentalization-Based Treatment—MBT!" There are no eye movements, no thought records, no mindfulness practice, no couch. In its generic implementation, it's plain old therapy. Although Bateman and Fonagy (2006a) have published a treatment manual, it isn't highly constraining but rather consists of relatively broad principles and suggestions for the conduct of psychotherapy. They convey well their style of practice in their recent handbook (Bateman and Fonagy 2012b), and I'll illustrate my efforts to implement it in plain old therapy. Though not a unique approach, mentalizing is a somewhat distinctive style of practice that many therapists find appealing.

I believe that many therapists practice something akin to this style of plain old therapy without having heard the word *mentalizing.* Occasionally, I work with patients who express concern that after they leave the clinic, they won't be able to find an outpatient therapist who practices mentalizing therapy. I reassure them that good therapists mentalize without calling it that, and they need to find a therapist who understands and works well with them. Yet I also believe that bearing the concept of mentalizing in mind, as well as understanding its foundations in attachment relationships, helps us therapists practice in this style more consistently and thus more effectively. Furthermore, helping patients to understand mentalizing and attachment assists them to collaborate with us in this style of therapy.

As I strive to practice it, the mentalizing style of psychotherapy feels very natural in being conversational, informal, commonsensical, and engaged. The approach is highly collaborative in the sense that the patient and the therapist are in the same boat: both are engaged in a mentalizing process, and their capacity to mentalize together will depend on their ability to manage emotions (i.e., thinking while feeling and feeling while thinking), which will be rooted in their attachment histories as well as their feeling of safety and security in their relationship at any given moment. Mentalizing is a two-way street: if my experience is any guide, patients help their therapists mentalize as well as get help in mentalizing from their therapists. I don't mean to imply that there's no difference in roles; there are many differences, not least of which is that the therapist has training and expertise in the process as well as ultimate responsibility for maintaining the professional nature of the relationship. I believe that we therapists—whatever brand of therapy we practice—have an *obligation* to mentalize.

Our patients have no such obligation. Thus, it's our job to engage them in the mentalizing process, providing whatever assistance we can. Yet, while not ignoring the professional or technical nature of the relationship, I am keenly aware much of the time that individual therapy boils down to two people in a room trying to make sense of themselves and each other. I am not aware that all I have learned about mentalizing has made me a better mentalizer, but it has made me somewhat more aware of my difficulties and failures so that I can get back on the rails after I've gone off (e.g., by saying to a patient, "We seem to be out of sync, and I think I've misunderstood something…").

Because we all know how to do it, mentalizing sounds easier than it is. Even when I'm deliberately aspiring to do it, I can go wrong.

Case Example

I had a session with a hospitalized patient, Will, who was so profoundly depressed that he barely talked, and he didn't look at me; he spent most of the session with his head down, looking at the rug. I felt completely incapable of helping him. One reason for his depressive plummet was that his psychiatrist was out on leave and his best friend in the hospital had left to attend a funeral. Will also resented other patients who were being more "needy" and thus drawing the staff's attention. Will felt neglected and alone. I was concerned about him and, given his psychiatrist's absence, the only useful thing I did was to offer him an additional session the next day. By that time, his mood had improved and he was somewhat more engaged and able to look at me some.

Knowing that Will's depressive swings had damaged his relationships, I initiated a discussion about our difficulty interacting in the previous session. Specifically, I explored his inability to look at me, which made interacting especially problematic. He said that when he's acutely depressed, he doesn't look at people (e.g., his mother or his wife) because he believes that they will be critical of him or will feel distressed by his plight. He can't stand seeing them in pain—then he feels guilty and even more depressed.

Encouraging mentalizing, I asked Will what he thought he would have seen in my face in the previous session, had he looked. Will responded that he hadn't thought about it, so I requested, "Think about it now." He said the depressive part of him might have thought I would view him as being "a mess" or "dramatic," but the more reasonable part of him might have seen me as trying to help. He also said he was grateful that I gave him "a break" by not demanding that he interact more with me.

Aspiring to share my mind with Will, I told him that *he would have seen me* as puzzled about how to help. I also let him know that struggling to help him gave me a glimpse of how hard it is for others to relate to him when he's depressed as well as how hard it is for him to interact when he's in that state. Here's my mentalizing slip: I don't know what he would have seen had he looked at my face. I can only state what I felt, as best as I understood it.

The heart and soul of this treatment approach is maintaining a *mentalizing stance*, which, for therapists, entails being curious, inquisitive, and open-minded about what's going on in the patient's mind and relationships, including the relationship with the therapist. Therefore, therapists also must remain curious about their own thoughts, feelings, and motivations in the relationship. Therapists who maintain this stance may thus inspire their patients to join in this stance: as in development, mentalizing begets mentalizing. Therapists and patients will lose this mentalizing stance for the same reasons—feeling distrusting, or frightened, or angry, or ashamed and, more generally, feeling defensive and thus being closed off or in a self-justifying mode rather than being inquisitive and open-minded.

Anthony Bateman once said to me that the hallmark of a mentalizing approach is the therapist's making "I" statements—thinking out loud with the patient. I find that this approach gives me a great deal of freedom to state what's on my mind without having to make any claims about holding the truth or having the correct understanding. Often, I'm quite active early in the process, even in the first session: "I know we've just gotten started, but let me tell you what I'm thinking so I can see if I'm on the right track...." I sometimes work with patients who don't expect their therapist to talk, in which case I need to intervene: "Pardon me for interrupting, but I've found that I need to be able to talk in order to be of help...." Understanding comes not only through listening but also through interacting.

In this mentalizing process, I am not making expert declarations about the patient's mind—much less the patient's unconscious—but rather offering my thinking and feelings for our mutual consideration: "I'm thinking that I might have insulted you." "I'm wondering if you might be feeling proud of yourself but not wanting to show off too much." "I'd been thinking that you felt intimidated by him, but now I see you were being cautious about provoking him." "I confess that I've lost track of what we're working on." "I'm feeling like we're butting heads [as I put my fists against each other]." "I feel sad, hearing what you went through." "I think you're right; I *was* feeling critical of you, now that I think of it, because I was thinking, 'He shouldn't be putting up with that.'" I'm eager to be corrected when I'm off track, and I encourage patients to speak up when they think I've misunderstood them. I find it embarrassing to be completely off base, but I can tolerate it.

I like this mentalizing style of plain old therapy for its *transparency*: I strive to share my mind with patients just as I wish them to share their mind with me. I am particularly fond of this statement by Bateman and Fonagy (2006a): "The patient has to find himself in the mind of the therapist and, equally, the therapist has to understand himself in the mind of the patient if the two together are to develop a mentalizing process. Both have to experience a mind being changed by a mind" (p. 93). I make it a point to let patients know when they have changed my mind or when I have come to see them differently after getting to know them better. I told a patient, for example, that I'd seen him initially as being like "steel" and very "controlling" and that I came to appreciate that he is very "tender" in his feelings and also able to go along with others' wishes or needs. He said his tenderness was a side he rarely showed. Such shifts are not all positive; I have also let patients know that I've come to appreciate how "ruthless" they can be.

Do I say everything I think and feel? By no means! As in any relationship, I bite my tongue sometimes and aspire to be tactful and respectful, aiming to be helpful. But I don't strive to control my facial expressions, posture, or voice—those natural expressions are ways of sharing my mind and feelings for the patient's consideration. To emphasize a point, I have even, on occasion, gotten out of my chair and made a gesture of banging my head on the wall or bent down and lifted the corner of the rug to look for what I think we just swept under it. Although I have no interest in being treated badly by patients, I do encourage them to speak their mind without concern about being tactful. When they feel sheepish about swearing, I let them know I was in the Navy so they need not worry. I am averse to automatically answering patients' questions with a question, while aware of the importance of the "question behind the question." Within reason, I like to answer the question and *then* ask about the reasons for the question.

To repeat, I think it's important for therapists to be "natural" in their work. I don't feel as if I'm being a "therapist," but I do feel that I'm *working*, and the work is generally hard. I don't think there's a right way for everyone to practice plain old therapy, because what feels natural to me won't feel natural to another therapist. Although I'm not enthusiastic about highly structured, manualized therapies (such as the systematic desensitization on which I cut my teeth), I'm not comfortable with a freewheeling therapy that has no direction. To my chagrin, I can't always achieve a consistent focus; sometimes, the therapy meanders and the patient nonetheless seems to benefit. Yet, seeking direction, I ask patients early in therapy to complete a brief worksheet (Table 5–4), which I developed with the input of my cognitive-behavioral colleague Tom Ellis.

I often find it helpful to provide the patient with a written formulation of the problems as I understand them, and I invite patients to let me know what I might have gotten wrong or left out. Sometimes, I pull up the formulation on the computer and edit it until we agree. For example, I worked with a patient to understand the complex experience that went into his suicide attempt. With the aid of a suicide note provided by his father, it became clear to me and the patient that his attempt was in part an expression of anger; in case anyone might be left in doubt about the culprits, he'd named two individuals who'd let him down. Yet, in reading the formulation, when he got to the point where I stated that his attempt was an "angry act," he balked and said, "I disagree with this part." I was surprised, because we had agreed on this point in the previous session. But I realized that what I had written could be interpreted to mean that his suicide was *deliberately intended* to strike back at those who had failed him. I amended the formulation to clarify this matter, and then he was entirely in accord with it.

It is a truism that any therapy needs to be tailored to the needs and capacities of the patient. Not every patient and therapist can work together, and the first task always is to make that determination. Some patients may need a specialized approach that I cannot offer, and I'm also a firm believer that the "chemistry" must be right—or at least reasonably good. Gender often is significant—for example, as I've noted, some women

TABLE 5–4.   Focus for psychotherapy worksheet

Instructions: I find that we can accomplish more in the relatively brief timeframe
for individual psychotherapy at The Menninger Clinic if we can agree on a central
focus for therapy, that is, a formulation of the main problems we are working on. I
also find that coming up with a focus of the main problems is not necessarily easy.
This is an example of a task that requires "mentalizing," by which we mean being
aware of your own thoughts and feelings as well as the thoughts and feelings of
others. Thus, mentalizing includes not only empathy for others but also empathy for
yourself. Because the problems that typically bring people to treatment include not
only difficulties within the individual but also conflicts in key relationships, we rely
on mentalizing of both self and others to clarify these problems and to work on
them. As a starting point for our work in finding a focus, I would appreciate your
answering several questions.

- What are the main problems that you would like help with?
- What would you like to change about yourself?
- What has kept you stuck or prevented you from making progress?
- Is there some problem or conflict you have not been facing or dealing with?
- If you achieved your goals in therapy, what would you be doing differently?
- What gives you hope?

who have been sexually abused by men understandably feel more comfortable working with a woman. Gender was a prominent issue for a man
who was considering switching from working with a woman to working
with me, because with her, he was having difficulty bringing up sexual issues that were critical to his treatment. He was in a quandary and wanted
to base his decision about switching on the "chemistry," and I agreed with
the reasonableness of his criterion. After a couple of sessions, he said he
preferred working with her because the "chemistry" was better, yet he
thought it was the right thing to do to work with me instead, because he
would be more able to address the crucial issues. I agreed with the pru-
dence of his decision, and the chemistry improved over time.

For some patients, mentalizing in psychotherapy comes naturally, and
we're off and running. Others—for example, those who are profoundly
depressed or extremely anxious—find it extremely difficult to engage in a
mentalizing process. They need more encouragement, education, and direct guidance than anything else. In such instances, I'm not averse to giving advice if I have it. When the patient can engage in mentalizing, I make
an effort to balance focus on mentalizing self and others: if the patient is
too self-focused, I inquire about the patient's understanding of others'

mental states; if the patient is too focused on others, I direct attention back to the self. I also engage the patient in mentalizing regarding our relationship and interactions, so as to help the patient directly appreciate differences in perspectives; I like to explicate the difference between what the *patient* thinks I'm thinking and feeling and what *I* think I'm thinking and feeling.

Case Example

Joe was mired in depressive rumination and feeling totally hopeless about his life. He declared, "I know I'm the worst patient you've ever had and you hate working with me." I replied that I didn't *hate* working with him and wondered if he was responding to my feeling *frustrated* in working with him. I explained that my frustration related to my difficulty helping him to detach from his ruminations and to see his situation as anything but hopeless. We discussed the parallel between my frustration and his wife's frustration, which was all too evident to him.

Joe expressed worry that his wife would leave him and that I would give up on him. I replied that I am accustomed to being frustrated and that I'm very persistent; being frustrated doesn't mean I'm going to give up. I asked if he thought his wife couldn't tolerate her frustration with him. He said, on the contrary, that she's "incredibly patient" and, indeed, "stubborn" in her belief that he can overcome his depression in time. He was able to see, at least momentarily, that his conviction that both of us would give up on him was part and parcel of his depressive ruminations—belief, not fact. I asked him about the basis for her belief that he would eventually recover, and he said that he's been stuck in this "obsessive" and "hopeless" pattern before, and he's gotten out of it. Then we went on to discuss how he had done so.

Broadly, such interactions entail working with transference in the sense of using our relationship to promote mentalizing. I think clinicians who employ plain old therapy without incorporating transference in this broad sense are bypassing a golden opportunity to practice mentalizing in relationships. As discussed earlier in this chapter, mentalizing is essential in repairing ruptures in the therapeutic alliance. However, the main point of mentalizing regarding the patient-therapist relationship is assisting the patient to develop the inclination and skill to mentalize more effectively in *other* relationships—attachment relationships most prominently. It was important for Joe to consider that I wasn't about to give up on him, but it was far more important for him to recognize that his wife wasn't about to leave him.

I recognize, however, that talking directly about our relationship (e.g., the patient's feelings about me) can be quite threatening. It's not something people do in ordinary conversation, and it may feel intrusive or downright rude to patients who are unfamiliar with doing it. Moreover, patients are liable to perceive therapists who focus excessively on the patient-therapist relationship as being self-centered: "It's not all about *you*, you know!" I try not to overdo the focus on the therapy relationship or to overestimate its importance, but I find it easier to help the patient work on something I can see with my own eyes rather than using secondhand knowledge. I might say, "I feel like we're getting locked in a debate. Is this similar to the problem you talked about having when you try to get your point across to your wife?"

I hope these discursive comments serve to clarify the difference between a style of therapy and a set of procedures or techniques. To a large degree, each patient and therapist need to figure out how to work together. As with building and maintaining any significant relationship, there's much art to it; we begin learning this art early in life and we refine it over a lifetime. We learn by example, and I have provided a few here. Table 5–5 offers tips for therapists regarding the ways in which they might promote—or unwittingly undermine—mentalizing. Patients also might use these tips to gauge the extent to which their therapist is practicing in a mentalizing style.

I've protested the idea that a good relationship is sufficient for a good treatment outcome by posing this question: What are we doing while we're relating? I don't want to convey that we merely promote mentalizing without addressing the question, What are we mentalizing *about*? We relate, and we work. Thus, we must define the work. We therapists must engage our patients in a mentalizing conversation to arrive at an explicit formulation of the problems that provide a focus for therapy. Here's a formulation I wrote for a patient who was struggling to overcome avoidance in his attachment relationships:

> I thought it might be helpful to you for me to summarize my thinking about the main issues for psychotherapy. Given the fact that we've worked together for such a short time, I'm taking the liberty of speculating, with the hope that some of my thoughts will be useful to you.
>
> You're correct in believing that I am concerned with "trauma," which, in my view, revolves around experiences of feeling alone in emotional pain. Your account of seeing your father collapse before dying of a heart attack when you were 9 years old illustrates: your mother "fell apart" and all the attention of the rest of the family was focused on her in the months thereafter, leaving you feeling "invisible." As you put it, she was center stage and you were left in the wings. Thus, you were left pretty much alone with your grief and the horror of what you experienced.
>
> And we've barely touched many other stressful experiences, including being uprooted from your home and friends when your mother moved to remarry; your stepfather's harsh discipline and cruel punishment; your

TABLE 5–5. Tips for therapists on influencing mentalizing

Promoting mentalizing

- Maintaining an inquisitive, curious, not-knowing stance
- Offering interventions that are simple and to the point
- Promoting a level of emotional engagement that is neither too hot nor too cold
- Providing a secure-base experience that facilitates the patient's exploration of mental states—their own and yours
- Maintaining a balance between engaging patients in exploring mental states of self and of others
- Engaging in a mirroring process in which your emotional responsiveness reflects the patient's mental state and feelings back to the patient
- Engaging in judicious self-disclosure about your interactions with the patient
- Validating the patient's experience before offering alternative perspectives
- Engaging the patient in viewing interactions and self-experience from multiple perspectives
- Letting the patient know what you are thinking so as to permit the patient to correct your distorted mentalizing
- Acknowledging when you do not know what to say or do and enlisting the patient's help in moving the process forward
- Acknowledging your own mentalizing failures and endeavoring to understand misunderstandings
- Acknowledging mistakes and actively exploring your contribution to the patient's adverse reactions
- Challenging patients' unwarranted assumptions about your attitudes, feelings, or beliefs
- Working with the patient-therapist relationship so as to help patients understand how their mind is working in the room at the moment

Undermining mentalizing

- Striving to be clever, brilliant, and insightful
- Offering complicated, lengthy interventions
- Presenting your ideas about the patient to the patient with a sense of certainty
- Attributing mental states to the patient based on your theoretical preconceptions
- Engaging in "psychobabble"
- Allowing prolonged silences
- Attributing the patient's experience of a relationship to a general pattern rather than exploring the experience and its basis in more detail
- Responding to the patient with intense reactive (nonmentalized) emotion

Source. Adapted from Allen JG, Fonagy P, Bateman AW (eds): *Mentalizing in Clinical Practice.* Washington, DC, American Psychiatric Publishing, 2008, pp. 166–167. Used with permission.

brother's hiking accident and disabling injuries; running away from home and living on the streets for some periods; being assaulted by a gang; and attempting suicide and then being terrified that you were going to die.

You were rightly proud of being able to "pull it together" in developing a solid relationship with Jill and in making good progress in a promising career. Unfortunately, "it all came apart" when Jill started complaining about your being "addicted to work," and you discovered she was unfaithful. Your feeling that your new supervisor didn't appreciate your talent and your hard work compounded this betrayal. Thus, you became disillusioned with all you'd worked for, and you started to think that suicide was "the best way out."

You now see that perhaps beginning with your father's death, you adopted a coping strategy of "building walls." You recognize that you've walled off emotional pain, for example, by shutting off thoughts and feelings connected with traumatic experiences. You're afraid of the grief and explosive anger behind this internal wall in your mind. You've buttressed the wall with alcohol, but I wonder if alcohol also hasn't started crumbling the wall—you've said you're more likely to "fly off the handle" when you've been drinking. You also have an external wall in the sense of not letting others know about the emotions you feel. This wall, unfortunately, has perpetuated the experience of being alone in emotional pain, and I think it's likely that the lonely isolation behind the wall has contributed to your depression.

For a long time, you believed that your walls were a source of strength and essential to your achievements. You're now beginning to see that the walls are blocking the help you need. Helpfully, you're reaching out. You've recognized your need for security, and you've been able to rely on prayer and a feeling of closeness to God, which provides some comfort. I think you've also made significant headway in allowing yourself to become attached to Melanie, despite your apprehension about trusting another woman. But making the connection and allowing yourself to receive affection goes against the grain. And your desire to refrain from burdening Melanie with your needs could backfire: she's letting you know that she feels frustrated and helpless when you don't confide in her, especially when she's afraid about the severity of your depression. From what you say, she's not at all keen on the walls.

Particularly in light of the walls you've erected, I think you've made remarkably good use of psychotherapy. You see a need for the walls to come down, but we both agree that we can't just smash through them. I like your image of "slowly chipping away." You've shown trust in letting me know a lot about you in this short time, and you've given me some glimpses of your sadness as well as your warmth. You've allowed me to spend some time on your side of the wall. I think you've made a wise decision in seeking treatment in a setting that will give you many opportunities to chip away at the wall, not just with us staff members but also with your fellow patients. I was encouraged by your telling me that you opened up in group therapy and felt safe in doing so. And I like your idea that you and Melanie can use help from your social worker in talking about the difficulty you've had in confiding in her.

Mentalizing Trauma

I don't see mentalizing trauma in plain old therapy as being fundamentally different from doing so in any other confiding relationship. Mentalizing trauma can be profoundly difficult, but the basic principle is simple: I aim to help patients think, feel, and talk about the experience so as to be able to have the experience in mind without being overwhelmed by it. I don't aim to "desensitize" the patient to the experience but rather to help patients remember it as painful but not unbearably so; when the pain is bearable, they won't need to resort to desperate efforts to avoid it. And I try to help patients make whatever sense of the experience can be made, generally with the aim of developing a less self-critical and more forgiving and compassionate attitude toward what they have endured.

This mentalizing approach differs from a "cathartic" approach that some patients seek and that I consider counterproductive. In my view, there's nothing to be gained and much potentially to be lost in extensive, detailed exploration of traumatic experience for its own sake. My approach is focused on the present: I concentrate on ways in which the past is influencing the present (or, more commonly, ways in which avoidance of the past is influencing the present). To state the obvious—which can be overlooked—the goal of trauma treatment is living better in the present and future. Excessive immersion in trauma, particularly when the patient lacks secure attachments and the capacity to manage emotional distress, can undermine the aspiration to live well. There may be a grain of truth in the old saw that you need to *feel* worse before you can feel better; however, if your *functioning* deteriorates in the process, something is going wrong.

The following examples illustrate my approach to treating trauma with plain old therapy.

Case Examples

Yolanda entered the hospital after escalating substance abuse that included intermingling of heroin and cocaine. She was referred by her hospital psychiatrist for "trauma therapy" to talk about her experience of being molested repeatedly by an uncle in early childhood. She had avoided thinking about the abuse for most of her life, and she now blamed herself for not talking about it when it happened. She had made a concerted effort to carry on as if everything were normal. She talked about the abuse for the first time with a college roommate after her roommate revealed a history of being molested. Then she began to talk about the abuse with her outpatient therapist, but doing so escalated her substance abuse, and she was referred for hospital treatment.

Although the sexual abuse had a significant impact on her past and present, it was merely one facet of an extensively traumatic past. Yolanda witnessed parental violence throughout childhood, and she also was bullied in school. She complained of being misunderstood and criticized by her mother and said she felt more secure with her father, but when she entered high school and began using drugs, she became more defiant and she became embroiled in continual battles with him. She also "got sucked into" a physically abusive and humiliating long-term relationship with her boyfriend. She said she stayed in the relationship because she was "terrified of being alone," especially at night. Furthermore, in conjunction with cocaine use, she was raped at a party, which escalated the conflict with her boyfriend when he learned about it a few days later. Coupled with the ongoing abuse in her romantic relationship, the rape further escalated her drug use.

Yolanda initially found psychotherapy to be difficult. She started by stating that she knew she needed to talk about the sexual abuse, but she didn't remember much of it—only isolated incidents akin to snippets of scenes in a movie. She said these isolated images bothered her, mainly because she felt "grossed out" and "disgusted" with herself. I made a point of stating that I was not inclined to encourage her to remember more but rather to be able to talk about images in her mind that troubled her. Despite agreeing to this plan, she avoided coming to therapy sessions, and when she did, she presented various excuses and denied that missing sessions related to her anxiety. Eventually, however, she was able to talk about her anxiety about our work together and we proceeded as initially planned, which turned out to be less distressing to her than she'd anticipated.

We agreed to focus not only on the sexual abuse but also on the impact of the extensive additional trauma. Once she overcame her initial apprehension, Yolanda used the therapy very productively. Albeit with considerable distress, she was able to talk forthrightly about some patchy memories that were disturbing and disgusting to her. She then talked spontaneously and freely about the impact of various traumas on her functioning. Over the course of the therapy, her intrusive memories of the sexual abuse became less frequent and less distressing. She saw how her anxiety about being alone had essentially made her "a slave" to her boyfriend. An extended period of sobriety contributed profoundly to her confidence in managing her emotions.

The containment provided by the hospital enabled Yolanda to use psychotherapy in a way that was not formerly possible—previous therapy was entirely crisis oriented, "putting out one fire after another." Yolanda was no longer anxious about talking about trauma in therapy, and she was ready at the point of discharge to use further psychotherapy in conjunction with intensive substance abuse treatment to examine her problematic relationships with men. Moreover, her sobriety put her in a position to begin repairing her relationship with her father, which had been a mainstay of support earlier in her life.

Andrea was hospitalized after a suicide attempt by carbon monoxide poisoning. She was discovered and rescued by a neighbor by happenstance, and she was initially angry to be alive. But she decided to work on getting rid of her "childhood baggage," which she believed to be contributing to problems in her marriage that triggered her suicide attempt.

Andrea grew up in a violent household, with recurrent fights between her mother and father, both of whom fought violently with her older brother as well. Her brother hanged himself in his early 20s. Andrea said she was "freaked out" when she thought of the violence, and she blamed her parents for her brother's death. At one point in a therapy session, Andrea noticed a photo lying on my desk that was dark and shadowy; she merely got a glimpse of it, and she panicked. She asked me to put it away, and I did. Naturally, I inquired about her reaction to the photo, but she was unable to discuss it. We worked on helping her calm down, which she was able to do.

Andrea brought up her reaction to the photo in the subsequent session; I asked if she could talk about what it evoked, and she was able to do so. She remembered a particularly painful episode of violence between her parents that occurred in the nighttime. She described her father's brutal and humiliating attack on her mother. What she found most distressing, however, was not the violence but rather the fact that she was alone in the dark and her parents were totally oblivious to her. She was furious, more generally, about their ignoring the impact of all the fighting on her and its contribution to her brother's suicide. Not incidentally, her suicide attempt was triggered by her husband's dismissing attitude about the impact of his "foul moods" on her.

Andrea worked hard in treatment to discuss the "baggage" and, with the help of her social worker, she was able to talk to her husband about her feelings in a way that led to her feeling heard by him. She said she was in a better position to "make peace" with him as well as to set the baggage aside. She saw clearly that her husband's moods were "merely aggravating" in contrast to her parents' fights, which were "horrifying."

Toward the end of the therapy, Andrea spontaneously asked to see the photo that had put her into a panic, which I had kept in a drawer ever since. The photo had functioned like a Rorschach inkblot, a projective test; it was a landscape with a scene of dark clouds in which she'd glimpsed a menacing figure. When she looked at it again, she saw the beauty in it, and she remarked on "the power of different perspectives."

Ben sought treatment after escalating marital violence led him and his wife to feel alarmed about the potential for grave harm to both of them. The antecedents of the violence were transparent; each had grown up in a violent household, and this shared history was one reason for their initial attraction to each other. Ben said he was told countless times to "stuff it" when he complained to his parents about anything; he was grateful to find a "soul mate" who was eager to listen to him. Ostensibly, they were drawn to each other with the conviction that having this history, their marriage would be different. Sadly, as it turned out, their marriage became more violent than either of their parents' marriages had been.

Ben was "a wreck" when he entered treatment, partly because he no longer had access to alcohol to "obliterate" memories of violence. He was angry about the restrictions of the hospital, got into arguments with the staff, and felt "undone" when he was in earshot of others' conflicts and raised voices. He couldn't stand the noise, including the TV. He sought refuge in his room and resented efforts to help him engage with others.

Ben entered treatment "drowning" in trauma. He couldn't stop thinking and talking about it. Immediately in the psychotherapy, he provided a helpful metaphor: he said he opens the lid to the trunk in the attic and, having done so, he can't stop rummaging through all the contents. I suggested that we needed to help him close the lid, and he agreed. I also alerted him to the possibility that asking him to close the lid could lead him to feel like I was encouraging him to "stuff it." He agreed that we should be mindful of this danger but said he mainly wanted to stop drowning.

We used the metaphor of the trunk in the attic throughout therapy, striving to strike a balance between opening the lid and closing it. When Ben started becoming flooded with memories, I pointed out that he'd started "rummaging in the trunk," which was a cue to focus our attention elsewhere—not always easily achieved. Over time, Ben was able to be selective in examining the contents of the trunk—for example, stating how a phone call with his wife reminded him of an incident with his parents but not getting caught up in a flood of memories and out-of-control fury. He was able increasingly to open and close the lid spontaneously. I was impressed by his ability to talk angrily without feeling like he was drowning. Moreover, his anger gradually was tempered by his acknowledgment of fear as well as his painful sadness. For example, he remembered treasured periods of respite during which he and his parents would visit his maternal grandparents; he felt intimidated by his grandmother, but he loved his grandfather and talked tearfully about how much he always looked forward to being hugged by his grandfather after they'd spent time together. Leaving his grandparents' house after a visit was one of his most poignantly painful memories of childhood.

Ben and his wife acknowledged that their violent attachment was like "toxic superglue," and they agreed upon a separation as a pathway to divorce. They realized that they could interact only in "limited doses," and Ben realized that a major contributor to keeping his head above water rather than drowning was the limited contact with his wife. He also came to see that the strategy of trying to "obliterate" his traumatic memories with alcohol backfired; with his health restored, especially his sleep, he felt a level of "mental clarity" that he hadn't experienced for years. Moreover, confiding in his peers—especially a male age-mate who had a similar experience—rekindled his appreciation of the importance of friendships, which he'd neglected as he unwittingly had become increasingly "trapped" in his marriage. Renewing a long-standing friendship was crucial in helping him feel less alone as he anticipated the separation from his wife.

Reading these examples, you might wonder, "What's new about this approach?" If there's something new in it, I can't discern it. As Bowlby (1988) would have agreed, the mind can be a scary place, and you wouldn't want to go in there alone. I've used these examples not only to illustrate plain old therapy but also to highlight the benefits—extremely rare in current mental health care—of conducting therapy to enhance mentalizing in the context of a psychotherapeutic hospital milieu (Vermote et al. 2012). The hospital provides containment and safety as well as an opportunity to cultivate confiding and greater security in peer relationships. In addition, the multimodal treatment approach includes couples and family work to address problems in key attachment relationships and promote mentalizing in the family system more broadly.

Research on Mentalizing in Psychotherapy

Based on residential and outpatient treatment programs, Bateman and Fonagy (2008, 2009) have established a solid evidence base for MBT for BPD. Yet relatively little direct research is available showing that psychotherapy improves mentalizing. Thus, to a large degree, I am extrapolating from developmental research in my conviction that psychotherapy can harness the potential for secure attachment to promote mentalizing and vice versa.

Ironically, some research support for the conviction about psychotherapy's potential to enhance mentalizing comes from other treatment approaches. As I summarized in Chapter 4, Transference-Focused Psychotherapy for BPD has been shown to improve mentalizing capacity as well as narrative coherence in the Adult Attachment Interview (Levy et al. 2006). Sheree Toth and colleagues (2008) also assessed changes in mentalizing by mothers suffering from depression who were engaged in a yearlong course of toddler-parent psychotherapy. Their treatment intervention was designed to enhance mothers' awareness of the emotional impact of their interactions with their child as well as to help mothers appreciate the effects of their earlier relationships on these interactions. As intended, the intervention improved mentalizing: compared with mothers in the control groups, a significantly greater proportion of mothers in the depressed-intervention group moved from a low level to a high level of mentalizing. At the same time, toddlers in the intervention group also improved in attachment security. The authors found no direct evidence, however, that the changes in toddler security could be attributed to improvement in maternal mentalizing. They speculated that a direct relationship might emerge if changes in mentalizing regarding the mother-toddler relationship were assessed, rather than mentalizing in relation to the mothers' childhood attachments (i.e., in the Adult Attachment Interview).

Rudy Vermote and colleagues (2010) took up the challenge of assessing changes in mentalizing over the course of a yearlong psychodynamically oriented hospital-based treatment program modeled after Bateman and Fonagy's (2006a) approach. Contrary to prediction, the researchers found no overall improvement in mentalizing, and no relation was found between mentalizing changes and treatment outcome. A more refined examination of the results revealed more subtle patterns of change (Vermote et al. 2011)—that is, two clusters of patients. A *stable* cluster showed gradual and steady improvement in mentalizing capacity over the course of treatment, whereas a *fluctuating* cluster showed increases and decreases in mentalizing over the course of treatment, likely related to disruptions in the alliance. For example, mentalizing could be adversely affected by getting into emotion-laden conflicts in the middle of treatment or by anxiety related to facing impending separation toward the end of treatment.

Measures of mentalizing capacity and attachment security in the Adult Attachment Interview imply that we're dealing with stable traits of individuals: some individuals are better mentalizers than others, and some individuals are securely attached, whereas others are insecure. Yet we know that, even at 1 year of age, an infant can be securely attached to one parent and insecurely attached to the other. Hence, I take seriously the concept of internal *working models* of attachment relationships—that is, *models* (plural), as in *multiple models*. We don't apply the same model to all relationships (or if we do, we're in trouble). We employ relationship-specific models (Bretherton and Munholland 2008). Diana Diamond and colleagues (2003) have taken a similar view of mentalizing as being relationship specific. Like attachment, mentalizing in psychotherapy is a *dyadic* process: something the patient and therapist do—or fail to do—*together*. Accordingly, as Diamond and colleagues' research showed, a therapist might mentalize more effectively with one patient than another. Furthermore, given its relationship-specific and dynamic nature (P. Luyten, P. Fonagy, L. C. Mayes, R. Vermote, B. Lowyck, A. Bateman, and M. Target, unpublished manuscript, September 21, 2011), mentalizing capacity will vary not only from one relationship to another but also *within* a given relationship from time to time. Thus, you might mentalize more easily when interacting with your mother than with your father, but you might have more difficulty mentalizing with your mother when you feel she's being intrusive and controlling. Therefore, there can be *islands of insecurity* within a given relationship, and mentalizing will be more difficult when you're stranded on one of these islands.

Research on the dyadic nature of mentalizing underscores the fact that mentalizing isn't a one-way street in any relationship, including the therapy relationship. I don't believe that therapists help patients mentalize and not vice versa. I know better from extensive personal experience: frequently enough, my patients help me mentalize when I'm off base, and

I count on them to do so. Telling me I've misunderstood is a common example. Also, patients can assist in repairing ruptures in the alliance.

Case Example

I recall with some chagrin a therapy session during which I was at odds with a patient. I was trying to get Kevin to explore what I thought was his sabotaging of progress, whereas he felt he was working hard against many obstacles to carry his treatment forward. I was preoccupied with Kevin's safety after he left the hospital, and I felt his "negativity" was blocking my efforts to help him make concrete plans to prevent further episodes of dangerous self-cutting. Likely projecting my own feelings onto him, I was feeling frustrated but asked him if *he* was feeling irritated.

Kevin replied that he wasn't irritated and explained that he felt I was off course; he wanted to understand where I was coming from. He explained that he was merely trying to explain his thinking to me, and he wanted to understand my thinking. When I voiced my concern about his safety, he said he also felt alarmed. He went on to help me understand the sheer difficulty he was having making adequate plans as well as his efforts to do so that I hadn't realized. Accordingly, he was inviting *me* to mentalize, and ultimately we got back in sync. This interaction exemplifies patient-assisted collaboration, which illustrates the mentalizing partnership as well as the role of mentalizing in understanding misunderstandings.

As stated earlier, I like viewing therapy from the perspective of attachment and mentalizing because doing so puts us therapists and our patients in the same boat, despite the differences in our roles: "Both parties bring themselves—their origins, cultures, personalities, psychopathology, expectations, biases, defenses, and strengths—to the human relationship" (Norcross and Wampold 2011, p. 429). No matter how we theorize about psychotherapy, according to Holmes (2010), "in the end the therapist and patient are on their own with their relationship and the human qualities they bring to it" (p. xii).

Mentalizing Beyond Attachment Relationships

I have emphasized the link between mentalizing and secure attachment, but I shouldn't overstate it. As Fonagy and colleagues (2008) cautioned, "It would be *absurd* to suggest (from either a scientific or a common-sense perspective) that secure attachment is the only relationship influence on the development of mentalization" (p. 797, emphasis added). We must learn to mentalize when we are being manipulated, bullied, or mistreated, as well as when we're competing and at risk for being outwitted. We learn to mentalize not only with parents but also with kin and peers, romantic partners and strangers, friends and foes, therapists and patients.

Nonetheless, as Fonagy and colleagues conclude, attachment relationships are "the *primary* teaching context within which the understanding of minds in self and others occurs" (p. 802, emphasis added). As I understand it, the reason for this claim is simple: these are our most intimate and enduring relationships and, given a modicum of security, those in which each member is likely to be most fully known to the other. Furthermore, as I hope will now be obvious, being known by others and being self-aware are inextricable, beginning in infancy.

Psychotherapy is my main concern here, and mentalizing is fundamental to psychotherapy. As the foregoing implies, however, psychotherapy is not our only source of help in mentalizing. That is a good thing: psychotherapy is a recent cultural phenomenon, only a century old, and other relationships have served the human community well for all that time—indeed, well enough for consciousness and mentalizing to evolve in the first place (Hrdy 2009). Yet trauma in attachment relationships can undermine the individual's capacity to make use of these ordinary confiding relationships, and we've developed a profession of psychotherapy to fill in this gap.

The Need for Plain Old Therapy

My answer to the question "Do we really need plain old therapy?" hardly requires explicating, but current trends in the delivery of mental health care bring the question to the fore. Alan Kazdin and Stacey Blasé (2011) pose forcefully a contemporary version of a decades-long argument that traditional psychotherapy in all its versions—individual, group, and family—is grossly inadequate to meet the needs for care. Not only is the distribution of services grossly uneven geographically, but also the pervasive limitations of resources become more glaring in the context of global economic woes.

Thus, not without justification, Kazdin and Blasé argue that a far broader array of nonpsychotherapeutic interventions must be developed and disseminated, even if the magnitude of their effectiveness is more limited. These authors' advocacy of greater emphasis on prevention is not new; the potential benefits of early intervention also are evident in the attachment literature. Yet, as my commitment to plain old therapy would imply, I am jarred by their advocacy of impersonal interventions abetted by technology and the ever-increasing devotion to computers and the Internet in particular. Telephone therapy is not new, and enhancing it with video seems eminently sensible; this expansion of service delivery can greatly enhance the likelihood of developing therapeutic relationships. How much is lost (or gained?) in video versus face-to-face interactions is an empirical question. But, as Kazdin and Blasé review, we now have an expanding array of computer-based interventions and smartphone applications that can be used, for example, to monitor mood and promote coping skills.

I cannot fault Kazdin and Blasé's fundamental point that we therapists need to expand the reach of services and that any form of help we can provide—even if it's modest in its effectiveness—is all to the good. Moreover, as these authors state, new technologies can serve well as adjuncts to psychotherapy. But, as much as I love my iPad, I find the prospect of ubiquitous iPad therapy chilling. Sole reliance on impersonal technology goes against the grain of all we've learned from a half century of research on attachment relationships and the therapeutic value of good patient-therapist relationships. Although we don't seem to be able to live without them, computers don't mentalize. For that, we need parents, friends, romantic relationships, and—especially when things have gone drastically wrong in attachment relationships—psychotherapists.

How Plain Old Therapy Works

Kazdin (2007) put the issue simply: "We know well that therapy 'works,' i.e., is responsible for change, but we have little knowledge of why or how it works" (p. 2). It has not been unreasonable to develop different methods of therapy and to see if some work better than others. Yet, as Kazdin points out, "It is remarkable that after decades of psychotherapy research, we cannot provide an evidence-based explanation for how or why even our most well studied interventions produce change" (p. 23). Thus, Kazdin asserts that we must identify *mechanisms of change* in psychotherapy, "the basis for the effect, i.e., the processes or events that are responsible for the change; the reasons why change occurred or how the change came about" (p. 3). If we could figure out what accounts for the benefits of therapy, we could tailor our interventions to the mechanisms rather than continuing to proliferate and experiment with techniques and manuals. As Roth and Fonagy (2005) stated, "The promise of identifying key, mutative psychological processes is especially attractive given its potential to bring order to the current proliferation of therapeutic approaches, and to identify what is, or is not, both effective and common across orientations" (p. 508). Moreover, Roth and Fonagy as well as Kazdin advocate that we should aspire to link these mechanisms of change to the developmental processes that led to the disturbances that we endeavor to ameliorate—attachment trauma in the present instance.

I haven't concealed my bias that we should highlight the therapeutic relationship and the therapeutic alliance as the broad territory in which we search for mechanisms of change, and there's considerable evidence to support this approach (Norcross 2011). And I have aspired to anchor the alliance and relationship in developmental research by focusing on mentalizing in the context of attachment. By Kazdin's (2007) exacting standards, it would be jumping the gun to nominate mentalizing and secure attachment as mechanisms of change. Rather, given the solid grounding in developmental research, I believe this is promising territory for the further exploration of mechanisms of change—especially with respect to the treatment of attachment trauma. As reviewed earlier in this chapter, research on attachment and mentalizing in psychotherapy is in its early stages. As Kazdin argued compellingly, we're a long way from identifying mechanisms of change and doing so will require extensive programmatic research. Meanwhile, I believe the focus on mentalizing in attachment relationships keeps us headed in the right direction.

As a proponent of talk therapy, I employ one all-purpose technique: conversation. Of course, this isn't ordinary conversation. Thus, mentalizing explicitly, I have my mind on the content of the conversation. But the therapeutic attachment relationship is built as much—or perhaps far more—on the nonverbal interaction than on the content of the conversation. One of Fonagy and colleagues' (Fonagy and Target 1997) main contributions has been to privilege *skill* over *insight:* insights come and go, but it's your inclination to mentalize and your aptitude for it on a moment-to-moment basis—remaining in the mentalizing stance—that forms the basis of healthy relationships. And healthy relationships include your relationship with yourself: keeping your internal secure base alive in your mind requires mentalizing. Thus, there's much to learn *about* yourself and your relationships in psychotherapy, but the main value of psychotherapy is *learning by doing,* that is, mentalizing and becoming better at it— in other relationships. Moreover, internal working models are revised not primarily by reflection but mainly in *action.* When you take a chance and confide in someone regarding a shameful experience, you learn to become more trusting. As with other skills, with practice, the application of the skill becomes more automatic; you do it without having to think about it. Then, when something goes awry—as in misunderstandings and miscommunication—you go back to mentalizing explicitly to sort it out.

Thus, psychotherapy is a continuous process of mentalizing implicitly in a way that moves toward more freedom in relationships—greater spontaneity and openness to experience stemming from an accepting relationship and increasing self-acceptance. Rogers (1951) proposed that such a relationship can be healing in itself. But we cannot take this assumption for granted. To be of full benefit, what the patient learns explicitly and implicitly in psychotherapy must provide a bridge to mentalizing and increased security in *other* attachment relationships. When I've used this metaphor in patient education groups, I've been told that it's hard enough to get on the bridge but even harder to get off. But we must use the therapy to enhance functioning in current relationships. Mentalizing and attachment security in therapy relationships must become the route to change in other relationships. We should recognize the limitations of individual psychotherapy in this respect. Paul Wachtel (2008) cautioned,

> I have noticed with some frequency a pattern that has troubled me. The person describes how wonderful his therapist is, while it seems to me, from all I hear or know about the person, that he is still *living his life* in the same painful and self-defeating way. From what I can discern, the relationship to the therapist *has* improved. There is a vitality, aliveness, and genuine connection in the room that perhaps was not there when they began. Consequently, the therapist too has probably felt that good work was being done. But the patient's life outside the sessions isn't nearly as different. He continues to live in a way that is painful or constricted. The therapist becomes a wonderful oasis, but the patient still lives in the desert. (p. 267, emphasis in original)

Individual psychotherapy can help by addressing problems in current relationships, but the skills need to be applied in other relationships—hence the benefits of group, couples, and family therapy.

Skill in Being Human

Where does this orientation to mentalizing leave the therapist? In focusing on skill over knowledge, psychotherapy is closer to piano lessons than history lessons. But there's no sheet music or score to follow in a mentalizing approach to therapy. Improvised music, such as jazz, is a better analogy. Practicing plain old therapy and being a consumer of it requires a high tolerance for ambiguity. I agree wholeheartedly with Wachtel's (2008) firm conviction that "there is no single right way to conduct psychotherapy" (p. 303), just as there's no single right way to behave in a marriage or any other relationship. We therapists have our theories to guide us, but the ties between theory and practice are loose. Wachtel puts it wonderfully, acknowledging that his book on therapeutic practice "reflects not just my theory but who I am as a person. This is *my* way of working with people. It bears a significant relationship to what my theory is, but it is partly simply me" (pp. 266–267, emphasis in original). As described in the introduction to this chapter, my unintended introduction to plain old therapy as an undergraduate student left me longing for a procedure. But, despite my yearning for structure, I haven't been able to give up plain old therapy, never having become enamored of the popular alternatives: empirically supported and manualized therapies of the cognitive-behavioral variety. I was in no position as an undergraduate to come to terms with the fact that doing psychotherapy was in large part simply being me.

I have learned to tolerate ambiguity, and generally I've been able to help my patients do so. I have adopted the view of psychotherapy as an art (Allen 2008), although Holmes (2010) has argued persuasively that the term *craft* is preferable to *art*. In his view, craft draws from art and science while being distinguishable from both. A craft cannot be learned from books; it requires apprenticeship; it is noncompetitive; it requires belonging to a community or guild with rites of passage; and it implies finesse or skill. A craft cannot be reduced to a standardized procedure. Analogizing psychotherapists to master gardeners or chefs, Holmes put it this way: "It is up to everyone to cultivate their garden or kitchen to the best of their ability and resources. Similarly, each psychotherapist-patient relationship has its own unique quality deserving of honour" (p. x). As Wachtel says, there's no single right way to do it. Although I may not have conveyed it in my caricatures, the same is true of manualized therapies, which call for improvisation and creativity in their application (Newman et al. 2006). We need procedures and scientific methods, but we need to use them artfully. As I discovered in my first exposure to conducting psychotherapy, evidence-based treatments must be grounded in plain old therapy. As I stated earlier in this chapter (see A Definition of Plain Old Therapy), to varying degrees, specialized techniques must be *superimposed* on plain old therapy—ordinary therapeutic conversation. For this reason, I believe that developing greater skill in mentalizing and becoming more knowledgeable about attachment is valuable for *all* therapists and patients.

What skill goes into the craft of psychotherapy? As I've construed it, mentalizing is the therapist's core skill. Like their patients, therapists will mentalize most skillfully when secure in their attachment. But we've seen that attachment is relationship specific, and, if my own experience is any guide, mentalizing skillfully requires a feeling of security with the patient. I can't mentalize freely when I'm feeling wary, on edge, or self-conscious—any more than I can play the piano well under those conditions. How does the therapist enable the patient to mentalize more skillfully? In psychotherapy as in development: by mentalizing. To repeat, the process must be one of learning by doing. From whence comes the therapist's skill? From development, beginning in childhood and refined over the course of a lifetime.

This view brings me to a humbling inference: if the key to our distinctness as a human species is our mentalizing capacity as it evolved in communal caregiving (Hrdy 2009), our ability to conduct effective psychotherapy rests on our *skill in being human*. At this most fundamental level, we psychotherapists bring nothing special to our work, either as professionals or as individuals. Our effectiveness rests ultimately on our common humanity. Thus, in the treatment of attachment trauma, *we must use our humanity to heal from the effects of our inhumanity*. If it comes down to our skill in being human, the essence of therapy cannot be manualized, any more than parenting or marriage can be. Admittedly, as the extensive psychotherapy research literature and abundance of self-help books attest, that fact has not deterred psychologists from aspiring to manualize our relationships. I prefer plain old therapy.

A final comment is in order, lest you wonder: If effective psychotherapy rests on our skill in being human, why do therapists need professional training and experience? Plainly, for all our remaining ignorance, we've learned a great deal from research about the helpfulness of psychotherapy and the essential qualities of professional relationships. There is much we need to know. Professional knowledge helps us mentalize patients' experience. As I hope the first chapter of this book attests, knowledge gained through attachment research enables us to mentalize traumatic experience—that is, to mentalize what it is that renders stressful experience traumatic. Moreover, without professional knowledge, we have great difficulty mentalizing behavior that is influenced by psychiatric disorders. Indeed, difficulty mentalizing without such knowledge contributes substantially to conflicts between patients and their bewildered family members and friends—hence the need for public education. Ironically, we find it most difficult to mentalize nonmentalizing as it occurs in posttraumatic flashbacks, dissociative states, suicidal behavior, nonsuicidal self-injury, paranoia, depressive convictions of being evil, sadistic behavior, and the like. I have included the chapters on trauma-related disorders in part as an aid to mentalizing. Finally, as I hope this chapter attests, we have much to learn about how therapy works so as to conduct it most skillfully, and we have much yet to discover. Hence, skill in being human is necessary but not sufficient to conduct psychotherapy skillfully; however, if it's not superimposed on skill in being human, professional knowledge will be of little value to therapists and their patients. The final chapter of this book ("Existential-Spiritual Perspectives") addresses the most profound challenges in healing from attachment trauma, those which put our therapeutic skill in being human to the ultimate test.

Key Points

- The field of psychotherapy research has privileged specialized treatments, but we need to pay equal attention to refining psychotherapy as practiced ubiquitously by generalists. Attachment trauma commonly leads to complex disorders that cannot be addressed with narrowly focused approaches. Plain old therapy capitalizes on commonalities among effective therapies for diverse problems; the quality of the patient-therapist relationship is central to these commonalities. Moreover, the conduct of specialized treatments must be superimposed on skill in plain old therapy insofar as the therapeutic relationship is central to the success of all treatments.

- Attachment trauma impairs emotion-regulation capacities; improved attachment security is a cornerstone of emotion regulation. Different patterns of insecure attachment invariably are manifested in the patient-therapist relationship, and therapists' own attachment security plays an important role in their ability to relate flexibly to insecure patients so as to assist them in becoming more secure.

- A style of plain old therapy conducive to treating attachment trauma employs basic principles from Mentalization-Based Treatment. This treatment approach builds on attachment research indicating that mentalizing is conducive to attachment security and vice versa. By maintaining a mentalizing stance, therapists enable their patients to do likewise—in psychotherapy and in key attachment relationships.

- We know from extensive research over the past half century that psychotherapy works, but we have much to learn about why it works. Research on attachment and mentalizing points in a promising direction for future research on mechanisms of change. For example, exposure plays a central role in trauma treatment, but exposure doesn't take place in a vacuum, and it entails far more than desensitization. Mentalizing trauma in the context of a secure attachment relationship renders painful experience more meaningful and bearable, and this therapeutic process paves the way for greater mentalizing capacity and attachment security where it counts most: in other close relationships.

CHAPTER 6

Existential-Spiritual Perspectives

I base this chapter on the conviction that the existential-spiritual impact of trauma—especially in attachment relationships—deserves as much consideration as the psychiatric consequences we therapists are trained to treat. By "existential-spiritual" impact, I'm referring to such phenomena as disillusionment, loss of trust in people and the world, cynicism, bitterness, alienation, nihilism, hate, self-loathing, loss of faith, and a sense of futility or meaninglessness. As difficult as the trauma-related psychiatric problems may be, I believe that the existential-spiritual impact is even harder to address; we can be truly at sea. Here, without specialized treatment manuals, we must fall back on plain old therapy, relying on our skill in being human.

As I mentioned with regard to identity in Chapter 2, Ronnie Janoff-Bulman (1992) proposed that all people hold three fundamental assumptions: the world is benevolent, the world is meaningful, and the self is worthy. Traumatic experiences potentially shatter these assumptions, creating an existential crisis. From this existential perspective, focusing treatment on cognitive distortions is too superficial. As Chris Brewin (2003) pointed out:

> Although negative thoughts and beliefs are much in evidence after
> trauma, it is possible that they are often a reflection of some deeper, un-
> derlying process.... Experiences such as mental defeat, with its oblitera-
> tion of a sense of personal agency, seem to describe a more fundamental
> assault on what it is to *be* a person, rather than just what that person is
> made to think. (p. 67, emphasis in original)

Of course, persons with a history of attachment trauma in childhood
may not have the luxury of developing positive assumptions, and subsequent trauma may merely cement nihilistic expectations. Yet I believe that
disillusionment can take root early in life. Attachment theory supports the
view that we're prepared by evolution for a relatively benevolent caregiving environment and that—even if it happens at a preverbal level—attachment trauma violates expectations in some unfathomable sense.

As a psychologist, I confront these existential-spiritual concerns with
trepidation. I assume that the vast majority of psychotherapists, like me,
have no expertise in philosophy or theology. Yet, unless we're downright
blind to them, we cannot avoid confronting existential-spiritual concerns
when we work with persons who have been traumatized. We must do so,
however, with an attitude of profound humility as we test the limits of
our mentalizing capacity. Millennia of philosophical and theological inquiry have failed to resolve these concerns, and we psychotherapists
hardly can expect to do so for our patients. What we can do, if we're willing, is to help our traumatized patients think and talk about them.

Having hewed relatively closely to scientific research in the preceding
chapters, I might well seem to be going off the rails in this last one. Perhaps so. I write this chapter with full awareness that doing so is an act of
hubris. I have no authority on these matters. I identify with philosopher
Thomas Nagel's (1985) disclaimer at the beginning of his book *The View
From Nowhere:* "I do not feel equal to the problems treated in this book.
They seem to me to require an order of intelligence wholly different from
mine" (p. 12). I'm fond of quoting the ancient Stoic philosopher Epictetus as a model for all my endeavors: "To do anything well you must have
the humility to *bumble* around a bit, to follow your nose, to get lost, to
goof. Have the courage to try an undertaking and possibly do it poorly.
Unremarkable lives are marked by the fear of not looking capable when
trying something new" (Lebell 1995, p. 87, emphasis added). I also find
this a good motto for conducting psychotherapy, no matter how experienced the psychotherapist. Comfortable with bumbling, I don't aspire to
provide any firm answers in this chapter. Rather, in the spirit of the mentalizing stance, I merely draw attention to the value of inquisitiveness
about these matters. Existential-spiritual concerns, above all, put us
firmly into the "not-knowing" standpoint we advocate in mentalizing.

My only justification for bumbling through this territory without any authority is the luxury of relying on the work of many true authorities from whose writings I'll quote liberally. You might treat this multitude of quotations as a gallery of ideas; I serve the role of curator, surrounding them with some explanatory text. Not entirely going off the rails, I maintain a thread of continuity with the previous chapters by keeping attachment and mentalizing in mind and by continuing to make use of research when it is available. Rushing in where angels fear to tread, I devote this chapter to three main topics: the problem of evil, attachment to God and spiritual connection, and cultivating hope. Broad as these topics are, they hardly exhaust the vast domain of existential concerns. But I grapple frequently with each of these three matters in treating traumatized patients, so I have given them a lot of thought.

The Problem of Evil

Case Example

Clarissa entered the hospital in a state of suicidal despair, feeling betrayed by her husband, who had decided to file for divorce after declaring that he was fed up with her depression. She found his decision to be profoundly unjust, as she had put all her energy into caring for him and their two children, including putting up with his alcohol abuse for years.

Clarissa believed that she was "born depressed." She could remember only unrelenting joylessness in her home throughout her childhood. She described her mother as a "religious fanatic" for whom any infraction or failing was a "sin." She characterized her father as an "evil, drunken sadist." While her older brother was allowed to "run wild," she was restricted to the house, required to help her "crazy perfectionist" mother who was "obsessed with dirt" take care of the house. In addition, she was required to care for her ailing maternal grandfather, whom she described as a "cantankerous ingrate." Clarissa didn't bend easily to her mother's domination; she described being subjected to "drunken tirades" and being "beaten senseless" by her father when she couldn't contain her fury and cursed at her mother. When Clarissa developed an interest in boys in adolescence, her mother redoubled her efforts to maintain rigid control. When her mother found a picture of a boy in Clarissa's night table, she called Clarissa a "dirty whore" and told her that God would see that she "burns in hell" for her sins.

Clarissa recalled one "saving grace" in her childhood: she had pet rabbits whom she loved, cared for, cuddled, and confided in. Her father repeatedly threatened her with getting rid of her rabbits if she didn't mend her ways, and he occasionally locked them in the barn to make his point. She remembered the single most traumatic event in her life: her father punished her for an act of rebellion by putting the rabbit cage in the back of his truck, declaring that he was going to drown the rabbits in the river.

The rabbits reappeared two days later, but the damage had been done: Clarissa remembered that event as an act of "pure evil" that she thought broke her faith in some irreparable way.

Clarissa said the only way she maintained a "shred of sanity" was by going to school—a haven of benevolence and safety compared to her home. She was diligent in her work and thrived on her teachers' respect for her talents. She was well liked by her peers but reluctant to develop deep friendships, knowing that any relationships would be confined to school, because she'd never bring anyone home or be allowed to visit their homes. She developed a confiding relationship with a girl whose home life was "equally hellish" but felt bereft when the girl moved away.

In therapy, Clarissa made no bones about her hatred for her parents, whom she "detested" and regarded as "vile." Fortunately, her experience at school made her aware that she need not live a life of torment and deprivation. She said she made her "escape" to college. Not surprisingly, after living under her mother's "iron-fisted rule," she made the most of her freedom. Sadly, her "partying" led to trouble: after a few months, she became pregnant and arranged for an abortion. She concealed the pregnancy from her parents, but she couldn't conceal it from her mother in her mind. Her mother's prophecy came back to haunt her: she felt like a "dirty whore," convinced she was "evil" and sure to be "damned."

Through remarkable determination after the abortion, Clarissa managed to get her "act together," partly with the help of a trusted friend who got her engaged with a tolerant church. Clarissa came to envision an alternative to the "monster God" she'd feared in her childhood, and she was convinced that God would "come through" for her in the end. But she couldn't leave the legacy of her childhood behind. She married, had children, and worked part time to keep the household afloat. But she never felt good enough. She was horrified by her occasional outbursts of frustration with her two young sons, notwithstanding that these outbursts were nothing compared to the cruelty she'd endured. She also berated herself for not being the loving mother she'd envisioned; she said she lacked "enthusiasm" for her life, often forcing herself to keep going in a "duty-bound" way. As she became more depressed, she came to feel that she was a burden to her husband. She was disheartened and resentful that she'd been unable to overcome the psychological legacy of her childhood, despite what seemed to me to be her heroic efforts to do so—including extensive psychotherapy and trying many different medications. In therapy, she said with great shame that she'd given up on God, just as he'd given up on her. As she'd become more depressed, she said she was "consumed by hate" for the lasting damage her parents had done to her. She felt she'd been "duped" into believing that someone would care for her and stick with her; neither her husband nor God had done so.

I address the problem of evil in this chapter not only because patients like Clarissa contend with it explicitly but also because centuries of philosophical and theological concern with evil underscore the sheer gravity of trauma. I don't mean to lose sight of the fact that trauma comes in degrees, and my focus on evil highlights the extremes. But we therapists do face the extremes in our work—as Clarissa's experience attests—and we have much to learn about the full range of trauma from the extremes, not least the need to find meaning. In the past few decades, the word *trauma* has become so common in the lexicon and in the professional literature that we've become habituated to it. We act as if we can "treat" trauma as if it were like any other illness. I think not. For the extreme of attachment trauma such as Clarissa experienced, I think this melioristic therapeutic attitude is too complacent. Employing the venerable framework of evil forces us to take the word *trauma* seriously: one doesn't necessarily "get over it" or "reach closure." Somehow, with varying degrees of success, one learns to live with it.

I must state at the outset that notwithstanding the historical connotations of the term *evil*, in using the term I'm not referring to anything supernatural; on the contrary, evil is all too natural. I am mindful that *evil* is an inflammatory and potentially dangerous word that can lead us to demonize and dehumanize others; ironically, such demonizing contributes to acts of evil. And I'm keenly aware that using the term *evil* is extremely heavy-handed. Many traumatized patients, in my experience, use the term not only to characterize those who have harmed them but also as the ultimate form of self-condemnation. As will be evident in the following discussion, I'm not entirely averse to placing blame when it seems due, but I'm far more inclined to seek understanding.

I start this section by justifying my concern with evil, based on its intrinsic relation to trauma. Then I give some definition to evil and its various forms. I also consider ways we have of trying to come to terms with evil and to make sense of it, from both religious and secular perspectives. Lastly, I address the dauntingly complicated problem of forgiveness.

Evil, Diabolical Evil, and Spiritual Trauma

In reading Susan Neiman's (2002) profound book *Evil in Modern Thought*, I quickly realized that evil is evil by virtue of the trauma it inflicts. Neiman makes the point that evil inflicts innocent and meaningless suffering: "Every time we make the judgment *this ought not to have happened*, we're stepping onto a path that leads straight to the problem of evil" (p. 5, emphasis in original). If my experience is at all representative, we psychotherapists must help our traumatized patients grapple with the effort to understand how what ought not to have happened, happened. How often I hear, "How could he have done that?" "How could she have done that?" "How could they have done that?" I think—and sometimes say—we're trying to make sense of the senseless. Neiman notes, "The pursuit of understanding leads to the judgment that the world exists to drive us mad" (p. 144).

In her book *The Atrocity Paradigm*, Claudia Card (2002) defined *evils* as "foreseeable intolerable harms produced by culpable wrongdoing," and she added, "the nature and severity of the harms, rather than perpetrators' psychological states, distinguish evils from ordinary wrongs" (p. 3). Thus we're at the extreme end of a continuum of possible harms: "Evils tend to ruin lives, or significant parts of lives. It's not surprising if victims never recover or are never quite able to move on, although sometimes people do recover and move on" (pp. 3–4). Card focuses on *atrocities*—large-scale evils—and she gives a discouragingly long list that includes attachment trauma: "genocide, slavery, torture, rape as a weapon of war, the saturation bombing of cities, biological and chemical warfare unleashing lethal viruses and gases, and the domestic terrorism of prolonged battery, stalking, and child abuse" (p. 8).

Card goes on to construe *diabolical evil* as "knowingly and culpably seeking others' moral corruption, putting them into situations where in order to survive they must, by their own choices, risk their own moral deterioration or moral death" (pp. 211–212). Such diabolical evil is an extreme form of what Antonia Bifulco and colleagues (2002) categorize as psychological abuse, which includes corruption of children—sadly if shockingly common in engaging them in sexual and criminal activities as well as substance abuse.

We all have been made excruciatingly aware of sexual abuse of children by Catholic priests, a form of attachment trauma that qualifies as psychological abuse and fits Card's concept of diabolical evil (i.e., corruption). Ken Pargament (2007) aptly characterized such abuse as "a desecration of the survivor's soul" (p. 95). In this context, Thomas Doyle (2003) highlighted the underappreciated dimension of *spiritual trauma*. Doyle linked the traumatic impact of sexual abuse by priests to the context of *clericalism*, the power and the influence of clergy stemming from their close relationship to God: "a cleric should be considered a man chosen and set apart from the midst of people, and blessed in a very special way with heavenly gifts—a sharer in divine power, and, to put it briefly, another Christ" (p. 219). Accordingly, clerics command the highest respect and obedience.

What Doyle calls *religious duress* stems from the priest's authority, which is not only inculcated in the child by the church but also reinforced by the parents. When the child has become emotionally attached to the priest as a haven of security, the sexual abuse places the child in an unbearable conflict that goes beyond other forms of attachment trauma: God is in the psychological field of the abuse. The church implicitly sanctions the priest's behavior but also has taught that sex is sinful: "The Catholic Church has consistently taught that illicit sex is a most grave offence, and now one of the 'teachers' leads an impressionable victim into that very realm of sin" (Doyle 2003, p. 226). Quoting Patrick Carnes, Doyle frames abuse by clergy squarely in the domain of existential-spiritual trauma:

> Betrayal by the spirit means that the person who betrays the victims also plays a critical role in the resources the victim has for defining meaning. The victim's spiritual path is blocked. The fundamental question all victims have to answer to themselves is: "Why do bad things happen to good people?" It is a far more troubling question when the cause of the problem is supposed to be the resource for the answer. (Carnes 1997, pp. 68–69; quoted in Doyle 2003, p. 225)

Compounding the offense, to the extent that the abuse is shrouded in secrecy, the church takes the role of the neglectful parent—for example, the mother who fails to protect the child from the father's abuse. Protecting the church's public image and neglecting the psychological and spiritual trauma constitutes what Doyle construed as the church's worst fault: failing to provide needed care to the traumatized children and their families.

We are certainly in the field of diabolical evil when the child is corrupted by a relationship that the church has condemned as sinful. But it doesn't necessarily end there. I worked with a patient who suffered additional psychological torment when the priest who'd just abused him insisted afterward that he confess his sins because he'd committed such "unnatural acts." I worked with another man whose priest convinced him that his parents would die and go to hell if he revealed the sexual abuse. This context exemplifies my focus on being psychologically alone in trauma. And we should be mindful that adults also are vulnerable to sexual exploitation by virtue of the profound power of clericalism in conjunction with the authority of God. This too constitutes a particularly pernicious form of attachment trauma that puts the adult in the middle of an irresolvable moral conflict.

Comprehending Evil Through Religion: Theodicy

As if mere evil were not enough, we have *extreme* evils: atrocities and diabolical evil. Religion has been one resource for coming to grips with evil, but it provides no easy answers: "The pervasiveness of evil appears to be the most widely held objection to theism in both the Western and Eastern philosophy of religion" (Taliaferro 1998, p. 299). Neiman (2002) tersely summed up the challenge: "The problem of evil occurs when you try to maintain three propositions that don't fit together. 1. Evil exists. 2. God is benevolent. 3. God is omnipotent" (p. 119). Theodicy is a branch of theology that strives to reconcile the pervasiveness of evil with the existence of an omnipotent, omniscient, and wholly good God (Peterson 1997). This reconciliation requires that God is just and that evil is not gratuitous but rather exists for the sake of a greater good, such as thoroughgoing human freedom:

> If God is to bestow upon man a kind of freedom which is not just artificial but really significant, He must allow man a wide scope of choices and actions. Indeed, the kind of freedom which is basic to the accomplishment of great and noble actions is the kind of freedom which also allows the most atrocious deeds. In creating man and giving him free will, God thereby created an astonishing range of possibilities for both the creation and the destruction of value. (Taliaferro 1998, p. 306)

Fyodor Dostoevsky's protest against such theodicy bears full hearing. In *The Brothers Karamazov*, Ivan confronts evil:

> There was a little girl of five who was hated by her father and mother, "most worthy and respectable people, of good education and breeding." You see…it's a peculiar characteristic of many people, this love of torturing children, and children only. To all other types of humanity these torturers behave mildly and benevolently, like cultivated and humane Europeans; but they're very fond of tormenting children, even fond of children themselves in that sense. It's just their defencelessness that tempts the tormentor, just the angelic confidence of the child who has no refuge and no appeal, that sets his vile blood on fire. In every man, of course, a demon lies hidden—the demon of rage, the demon of lustful heat at the screams of the tortured victim, the demon of lawlessness let off the chain.… This poor child of five was subjected to every possible torture by those cultivated parents. They beat her, thrashed her, kicked her for no reason till her body was one bruise. Then, they went to greater refinements of cruelty—shut her up all night in the cold and frost in a privy, and because she didn't ask to be taken up at night (as though a child of five sleeping its angelic, sound sleep could be trained to wake and ask) they smeared her face and filled her mouth with excrement, and it was her mother, her mother did this. And that mother could sleep, hearing the poor child's groans! Can you understand why a little creature, who can't even understand what's done to her, should beat her little aching heart with her tiny fist in the dark and the cold, and weep her meek unresentful tears to dear, kind God to protect her? (Dostoevsky 1912/2005, pp. 223–224)

Ivan longed to understand "what it has all been for"; recognized that all religions are "built on this longing"; declared, "I'm a believer"; yet was caught short: "But then there are the children, and what am I to do about them?" (p. 226). Ivan's anguish could not be assuaged by theodicy:

> I renounce the higher harmony altogether. It's not worth the tears of that one tortured child who beat itself on the breast with its little fist and prayed in its stinking outhouse, with its unexpiated tears to "dear, kind God!" It's not worth it, because those tears are unatoned for. They must be atoned for, or there can be no harmony. But how? How are you going to atone for them? Is it possible? By their being avenged? But what do I care for avenging them? What do I care for a hell for oppressors? What good can hell do, since those children have already been tortured? (pp. 226–227)

Ivan passionately articulated the spiritual agonies that many traumatized persons suffer. Survivors are fortunate to have options: accepting theodicy, reconciling themselves to their inability to comprehend the mystery of God's ways, and finding meaning outside theology. I am partial to Neiman's (2002) expanded concept of theodicy that encompasses "any way of giving meaning to evil that helps us face despair" (p. 239). To reject theodicy in this broad sense "becomes the rejection of comprehension itself" (p. 325).

The Enlightenment provided us with a secular alternative to theodicy: at the risk of oversimplifying, we should stop blaming God, think for ourselves, and take responsibility for preventing evil. Thus, it's up to us: "The God of the scientists, one is tempted to suggest, created man in his own image and put him into the world with only one Commandment: Now try to figure out by yourself how all this was done and how it works" (Arendt 1971, p. 137). This brings us to psychology.

Comprehending Evil Through Science: Mindblindness

Card (2002) defined *evil* on the basis of the extent of harm done rather than focusing on the state of mind of the evildoer. Yet, in experiencing events as evil, as well as in striving to make whatever sense of evil we can, we cannot ignore the state of mind of the person who inflicts the damage. We cannot escape trying to mentalize—even though the extremity and seeming senselessness of the deeds may thwart our effort to do so. Card includes the culpability of the evildoer in the definition of evil, which encompasses negligence and recklessness as well as evil *intention*—namely, "a culpable intention to do someone intolerable harm" (p. 20).

It's a big leap from evil *acts*, which do great harm, to evil *persons*, who commit such harms. We must not slip unknowingly from one to the other. We have no more damning characterization than calling someone evil, and I've heard the term often enough in my work with trauma survivors—in relation to the self as well as others. More often, I hear words that point in the direction of evil: *mean, cruel, heartless,* and *sadistic*—terms that go hand in hand with psychological abuse. Roy Baumeister (1997) made the provocative points that "the perpetrators of evil are often ordinary, well-meaning human beings with their own motives, reasons, and rationalizations for what they're doing" (p. 38) and that "understanding evil begins with the realization that we ourselves are capable of doing many of these [evil] things" (p. 5). Accordingly, something we're not eager to hear, "otherwise decent people, much like you or me, can come to participate in evil acts" (p. 103).

Based on studies of rapists, violent policemen, and other violent offenders, Baumeister (1997) concluded that only roughly 5% of persons who commit such violent acts do so in pursuit of sadistic pleasure. Moreover, among these 5%, few start off as sadists; on the contrary, most initially are disgusted or horrified by the impact of their violence. Yet, over time, sadistic pleasure eventually can become an acquired taste, and an addictive one. Erich Fromm (1973) captured this transformation in construing malignant aggression as a character-rooted passion, pinpointing the core of sadism as "*the passion to have absolute and unrestricted control over a living being*, whether an animal, a child, a man, or a woman" (p. 322, emphasis in original).

If evil is rarely done with evil intent, how do we understand it? John Kekes (2005) conducted in-depth case studies highlighting several common motives: faith, ideology, ambition, honor, envy, and boredom. But I find it instructive to consider what is *missing*. I was jarred into taking this tack on evil by Hannah Arendt's (1963/1994) controversial writing on the Holocaust. She highlighted the sheer *banality* of evil as exemplified by Nazi war criminal Adolf Eichmann, a man

> whose only personal distinction was perhaps *extraordinary shallowness*. However monstrous the deeds were, the doer was neither monstrous nor demonic, and the only specific characteristic one could detect in his past as well as in his behavior during the trial and the preceding police examination was something entirely negative: it was not stupidity but a curious, quite authentic *inability to think*. (p. 159, emphasis added)

Echoing Baumeister (1997), Arendt (2003) observed that some war crimes "were not committed by outlaws, monsters, or raving sadists, but by the most respected members of respectable society" (p. 42). She proposed that the inability to think can be found in intelligent people, and that "wickedness is hardly its cause, if only because thoughtlessness as well as stupidity are much more frequent phenomena than wickedness. The trouble is precisely that no wicked heart, a relatively rare phenomenon, is necessary to cause great evil" (p. 164). As Arendt (1963/1994) noted, one psychiatrist who evaluated Eichmann declared him "more normal, at any rate, than I am after having examined him" (p. 25).

When I first read these passages, I immediately translated "inability to think" into the more precise formulation, inability to *mentalize*. I found Simon Baron-Cohen's (1995) term *mindblindness* to be most apt in characterizing the extreme mentalizing failure in such evildoing (Allen 2007). Baron-Cohen employed mindblindness to characterize the absence of mentalizing in autism. Intuitively, Arendt perceived mindblindness in Eichmann. Equally mindblind, Eichmann's lawyer referred to what had been done at Auschwitz as a "medical matter" (Arendt 2003, p. 43). Kekes (2005) described an astonishing level of mindblindness in Franz Stangl, commandant of Treblinka, whom Heinrich Himmler awarded an Iron Cross for his clockwork-like efficiency in carrying out the extermination:

> Who was this man, Stangl, in white [riding] clothes supervising the daily murder of thousands of people, enjoying his lunch of meat and potatoes with homegrown fresh vegetables, and having a quiet nap between herding naked men, women, and children into the gas chambers and disposing of their corpses? What manner of man would preside over this hell on earth and organize its smooth functioning? (p. 51)

In Stangl's own words:

> I rarely saw them as individuals. It was always a huge mass. I sometimes stood on the wall and saw them in the tube [the path to the gas chamber]. But—how can I explain it—they were naked, packed together, running, being driven by whips like…[the sentence trailed off]. When I was on a trip once, years later in Brazil, my train stopped next to a slaughterhouse. The cattle in the pens…this reminds me of Poland; that's just how the people looked, trustingly…. Those big eyes…which looked at me…not knowing that in no time at all they'd all be dead…. Cargo…They were cargo. (Kekes 2005, pp. 61–62)

In his book on evil, Baron-Cohen (2011) aspires to give a scientific account based on research on empathy, construed in a way that overlaps mentalizing. Extensive research reveals that, like our intelligence, our capacity for empathy can be measured in degrees. Baron-Cohen grades empathy on a seven-point scale ranging from zero (no empathy at all) to six (remarkable empathy). He proposes that evil stems from *empathy erosion*. He reviews extensive evidence for neurobiological contributors to lack of empathy, including genetic factors along with evidence of alterations in brain activity in multiple brain areas associated with empathizing (and mentalizing). He reviews many forms of zero degrees of empathy, ranging from different types of personality disorder to autism-spectrum disorders. Obviously, evildoing is not inherent in lack of empathy, but—as Arendt's and Kekes's descriptions attest—lack of empathy sets the stage for evildoing. That is, doing harm becomes possible by virtue of lack of attun-ement—at worst, obliviousness—to others' mental states.

Baron-Cohen (2011) concludes that empathy "is the *most valuable re-source* in our world" (p. 153, emphasis in original). He believes empathy is an underutilized resource and a universal solvent: "Any problem im-mersed in empathy becomes soluble" (p. 186). He takes a hopeful view: "no one—however evil we paint them to be—should be treated as 100% bad or as beyond responding to a humane approach" (p. 175). Baron-Cohen isn't naïve about the challenges of enhancing empathy in persons who are deficient in it. The more we can learn about the conjoint contri-butions of genetic and other neurobiological contributions to impaired empathy (or mentalizing) as they're intertwined with environmental ad-versities—including attachment trauma—the better position we'll be in to cultivate this most valuable resource.

Our mentalizing capacity enables us to see things from different per-spectives and to recognize the differences in perspectives among us. In discussing evil, I've been juggling moral and scientific perspectives. As stated earlier, my profession inclines me more to understanding than con-demning. The work of Arendt, Baumeister, and Baron-Cohen should humble us all in pointing to our natural and shared human capacity for doing harm when we are mindblind. Paul Pruyser (1974) pointed out that "theodicy is no longer an abstract business but a very personal quest" (p. 175). Countering our all-too-human penchant for externalizing blame and, at worst, demonizing, he continued,

> I do not know how one comes to an integrated and realistic view of good and evil, but observations of normal (or optimal) psychological develop-ment give some pointers about the way we integrate the benevolent and malevolent experiences in our lives. One step in this integration consists of trimming our important human objects gradually down to realistic size: fa-ther and mother are neither gods nor demons. They are sometimes benev-olent, sometimes malevolent; they love and they hate. They are only human. They are frail and faltering beings, mixtures of love and hate, as their parents and grandparents were before them. And so am I: I am neither a god nor a demon, neither all benevolence nor all malevolence. (p. 175)

This brings us to forgiveness.

Forgiveness

Trauma in attachment relationships by no means always rises to the ex-tremes of evil; evil is at the far end of a continuum of wrongdoing, and we have no way of drawing bright lines. Regardless of the extent of harm and the culpability of the harm doer, those who suffer trauma will struggle not only with finding meaning and restoring trust but also in figuring out how to relate to the person by whom they were traumatized. Forgiveness is a pathway to repairing relationships, but it's a potentially tortuous journey.

I recall vividly an educational group in which I was talking about constructive and destructive anger as well as various shades of anger: feeling annoyed, irritated, frustrated, pissed off, angry, livid, furious, and enraged. A patient spoke up and pointed out correctly that I had left out "outrage." This was indeed a glaring omission in the context of trauma, which rightly evokes moral indignation. Glibly counseling traumatized persons, "You just need to forgive," overlooks justified moral indignation. I don't intend to convey that forgiving is undesirable; there's good evidence to support its benefits (Plante 2009). I merely contend that forgiving is not easy, and it must be a matter of personal choice. We must approach forgiveness thoughtfully. Some survivors choose never to forgive; others say they could not heal until they were able to forgive. Research reveals no simple relation between forgiveness and recovery from trauma (Connor et al. 2003).

We are accustomed to thinking of forgiveness as a virtue and resentment as a vice. The destructiveness of resentment is undeniable. Resentment is conducive to vengefulness and aggression, whereas forgiveness is conducive to reconciliation and peaceful relationships. Smoldering resentment is one way of being traumatized; it can poison relationships and your own well-being. So it might seem surprising that moral philosopher Jeffrie Murphy (2003) urged that we not be too quick to let go of resentment in favor of forgiveness. In his provocatively titled book *Getting Even: Forgiveness and Its Limits*, Murphy counsels that, as a response to wrongdoing, resentment can maintain self-respect, promote self-protection, and reinforce respect for the moral order. He proposes that forgiving too readily is tantamount to acquiescing to wrongdoing—an extreme example being the battered spouse who returns to the batterer and, in so doing, fails to respect and protect herself. As the patient who spoke up in the educational group made us all aware, we must leave room for outrage and moral indignation.

In a similar vein, philosopher George Sher (2006) published a book with the provocative title *In Praise of Blame*. Sher takes us mental health professionals to task for our antipathy toward blame and for glibly promoting a nonjudgmental stance. Sher views blame as intrinsic to morality; that is, if we embrace morality, we accept our natural reaction of feeling wrongdoing to be blameworthy. Of course, we differ from one another in our propensity to blame and in the intensity of our reactions and our judgments about blameworthiness, which are based on mentalizing (or nonmentalizing).

We excuse harmful behavior when, as Sher (2006) puts it, the wrong-doer "either could not recognize or could not respond effectively to the moral reasons for not doing what he did" (p. 118). We cannot help making these excusing judgments, yet they're profoundly difficult to make. Baron-Cohen (2011) amassed evidence for neurobiological contributions to empathy failures, and these neurobiological contributions potentially are intertwined with the intergenerational transmission of attachment trauma, as I discussed in the first chapter of this book. As I mentioned earlier, I am almost invariably disposed to move from blaming to understanding, but I'm also aware that we cannot and should not give up our natural inclinations to make moral judgments and the feelings that go along with them.

We must think in terms of degrees. Sher (2006) distinguishes our feelings of blame from what we do about them—for example, whether we communicate them. In addition to making room for excuses—also a matter of degree—he recognizes the value of improving our relationships by lowering the condemnatory volume. He concludes his book with a point that pertains to us mental health professionals:

> It is one thing to say that living a fully moral life requires blaming those who ignore or flout morality's demands, but quite another to say that it requires the kind of toxic anger that makes future harmony more difficult to achieve. That we would be better off if we were to weaken the connection between blame and rancor may be the kernel of truth in the anti-blame ideology, but that we would be better off if we abandoned blame itself is the larger falsehood in which that kernel is embedded. (p. 138)

Many traumatized patients take the position that they will forgive but not forget. Consistent with this view, my mentor Len Horwitz (2005) made the case that forgiveness entails letting go of obsessive rumination about the injury as well as giving up the wish for retribution. This is a prescription for mental health as well as for improved relationships.

I think of forgiveness not as a one-time act but as a long-term project. Card (2002) proposed that forgiveness is not an all-or-nothing proposition but rather a complex process with several facets: renouncing hostility out of compassionate concern for the offender; acceptance of the offender's contrition; forgoing opportunities to punish; and renewing the relationship (i.e., reconciliation). This complex structure is consistent with the idea of *partial* forgiveness. Moreover, I believe that forgiveness isn't a once-and-for-all matter but rather can come and go. As events over the lifetime reevoke memories of trauma, feelings of resentment are likely to resurface. Finally, writing in the context of extreme wrongdoing—evil—Card advocates a cautious approach toward forgiveness and takes seriously the idea that some actions may be unforgivable.

We mental health professionals champion our patients' self-forgiveness, perhaps even more than forgiveness of those who have wronged and harmed them. Self-forgiveness is important given the pervasiveness of unwarranted self-blame in the context of trauma. Although self-blame can be a strategy to maintain an illusion of control, it is pernicious in contributing to feelings of guilt and shame, and it perpetuates posttraumatic stress disorder (Foa et al. 1999). Here again, we must make room for complexity. Like forgiving others, forgiving yourself is a complex achievement; as Card (2002) points out, it requires that you renounce hostility toward yourself and adopt a compassionate attitude toward yourself. Murphy (2003) states, however, that we should take self-forgiveness no more lightly than the act of forgiving others, or self-forgiveness would be meaningless. Like forgiveness of others, self-forgiveness may be partial; we all must live with some legacy of guilt feelings for harm we've done. But we must maintain a crucial distinction between actual guilt and guilt *feelings;* in traumatized persons with whom I've worked, the latter generally greatly outweigh the former. And we must be on guard for the danger of moral perfectionism and aspirations for moral purity that can wreak emotional havoc (Nussbaum 2001, p. 234). I point out patients' "moral perfectionism" when I discern it—not infrequently. Whereas guilt feelings can be a useful source of moral motivation, intense suffering under the weight of guilt and shame can be tantamount to moral masochism, and it doesn't make us better persons; on the contrary, "ultimately, people need to be able to get on with the business of life, taking care of one another rather than condemning the self" (Tangney and Mashek 2004, p. 163).

Readers might find my bald lack of therapeutic neutrality downright shocking, but I have already acknowledged my view that psychotherapy is an inherently ethical endeavor as much as a professional and scientific endeavor (Allen 2008). Invariably, I judge—others and myself. But my main aspirations are therapeutic: to understand for the sake of improvement. Here, I must acknowledge what might seem like an utter contradiction. In the context of mindfulness and the mentalizing stance, improvement often requires adopting a nonjudgmental attitude toward experience. Similarly, scientific understanding entails an attitude of detachment. A nonjudgmental stance is necessary and helpful for much of the work we do, but it's an alternative to a moral stance, not a substitute for it. To hammer home a basic point, our mentalizing capacity is grounded in our ability to see our experience from multiple perspectives, including moral as well as religious and spiritual perspectives. Conducting psychotherapy with patients traumatized by wrongdoing is a messy business; no manual can render it neat and tidy.

Attachment to God and Spiritual Connection

By no means do all trauma survivors struggle with religious concerns or their relationship with God. Many are not religious and don't believe in God. Hence, for many patients, my concern with these matters will be irrelevant. But these matters are highly relevant for *all* of us psychotherapists, regardless of our personal beliefs; many of our traumatized patients struggle with their religion, and many experience profound conflicts in their relationship with God that mirror conflicts in other attachment relationships. We all must be mindful of the fact that patients generally are more inclined than therapists to discuss concerns about religion and spirituality.

Making my personal views explicit will help orient you to this section. While disclaiming authority and passing the buck to others whom I quote, I must acknowledge responsibility for the set of authorities I've chosen, which reflects my biases. I find the mentalizing approach appealing because I have a strong bias against certainty; while continually striving to know more, I *enjoy* not knowing. I write about God in this chapter because struggles with God are common among traumatized patients and attachment research informs us about these struggles as well as highlighting how religion is a potential resource for healing. My personal views are located well in the title of a book—*Between Belief and Unbelief*—by Paul Pruyser (1974), my mentor at The Menninger Clinic in Kansas. I was brought up in a religious home but lost interest in religion in adolescence, and for much of my adult life I believed that science will provide us with all we need to know about the world and our place in it. In more recent years, I've become disillusioned with this narrow view, yet I sometimes feel I need a crowbar to pry open my mind. The authorities I have chosen to quote exemplify that intellectual crowbar. I find that this position between belief and unbelief helps me as a therapist work with a wide range of patients. At my best, I'm simply interested in what they think and believe. Science minded as I obviously remain, I need to keep the crowbar in place. Doing so, I feel equally comfortable with atheists, doubters, believers, and those who remain utterly confused. The key to navigating this murky territory is respect; disdain for belief or unbelief undermines therapeutic exploration.

What I have learned about attachment and mentalizing has enabled me to work with traumatized patients' struggles with God in a way that I was unable to do previously. As we do with persons beginning in childhood, we also can form an attachment relationship with God. As we do with persons, we form this attachment through mentalizing. In so doing, we apply our internal working models of attachment—for better or for worse. For example, in conjunction with attachment trauma from childhood through adulthood, God may be viewed as a savior, a tormentor, or painfully neglectful. But I'm not content merely to make glib parallels; we must think clearly about this religious territory before we set foot in it, because we're treading on private and sacred ground.

I begin this section by elaborating the thesis that attachment relationships influence relationships with God. Next, I address what I consider to be a fundamental barrier to helping patients with traumatic attachments to God—namely, a history of professional disdain for reliance on religion, which is embedded in the broader cultural ethos of reverence for science that shapes our professional practice. This cultural context also influences our attitudes toward attachment, that is, our acceptance of our need to depend on others—including God—for emotional security. With this stage setting completed, I then summarize research that documents the potential for secure and insecure attachment to God. This research warrants our attention because, as in human relationships, attachment to God shows potential for stability and change; as in human relationships, movement from traumatic attachment to secure attachment carries significant benefit. I conclude this section by advocating a mentalizing stance toward God that I find professionally freeing in exploring this sacred and potentially treacherous ground.

For orientation, the main tenets of my argument are outlined in Table 6–1. After discussing attachments with God, I discuss spirituality as an alternative resource for healing, and I conclude this section by summarizing recent efforts to integrate religion and spirituality into psychotherapy. I entered this territory of religion and spirituality through the window of attachment trauma, yet the understanding I gained has turned out to be valuable in my work as a plain old therapist more generally. For that reason, I don't entirely confine these sections on religion and spirituality to the domain of trauma.

Gods and Persons

Karen Armstrong (1993) asserted, "All religion must begin with some anthropomorphism" (p. 48)—that is, attributing human characteristics to nonhuman entities. More specifically, "Judaism, Christianity and—to a lesser extent—Islam have all developed the idea of a personal God...who does everything that a human being does: he loves, judges, punishes, sees, hears, creates and destroys as we do" (p. 209). Taking a developmental perspective, Ana-Maria Rizzuto (1979) proposed that all children in the

---

TABLE 6–1.   Roles of attachment and mentalizing in
                 relating to God

- Relating to God requires imagination.
- God can be imbued with personal attributes—that is, mentalized.
- Trauma heightens dependence, potentially dependence on God.
- God becomes an attachment figure, and the attachment can be relatively secure or insecure.
- The quality of attachment to God can correspond to other attachments (e.g., to parents).
- A secure attachment to God can compensate for insecurity in other attachments.
- Secure attachment to God can contribute to an internal secure base.
- A mentalizing stance facilitates therapists' ability to explore patients' relationships with God.

Western world form an image of God, and this image relates to their experiences with parental figures. Of course, as Pruyser (1974) pointed out, God potentially offers far greater security: "The theistic family, which is conceived to have greater power, greater wisdom, greater love, and greater durability and constancy, does what the natural family fails to do for the individual" (p. 159).

Yet images of God are far more diverse than Pruyser's ideal, and our internal working models of attachment influence these images. Hence, our images of God are liable to be narrow and skewed, as Pargament (2007) captures in his enumeration of *small gods:* the Grand Old Man, out of touch with modern reality; the god of Absolute Perfection who insists on flawlessness from us; the Heavenly Bosom who provides limitless care; the Resident Policeman who keeps us in line; and the Distant Star god who leaves us cold. Those who have been traumatized might well wish for the Heavenly Bosom while feeling left out in the cold with the Distant Star god.

For believers, one profoundly traumatic consequence of attachment trauma is a feeling of alienation from God, which can contribute to the anguish of feeling alone in unbearable emotional pain. Like any human attachment figure, God can be experienced as abandoning, indifferent, emotionally neglectful, and oblivious to pain.

Case Example

Victoria grew up in a family ruled by her "hyperreligious" grandmother, whom Victoria said continually "threw God in my face" when she failed to comply with her grandmother's perfectionistic demands. She said she learned to "detest God" at an early age, equating God's standards with those of her grandmother. Moreover, her grandmother's refrain that "all troubles are God's will" infuriated her. When she left home for college, Victoria joined a liberal church and felt free to think for herself, developing an image of a compassionate God that enabled her to live more comfortably with her shortcomings.

Over time, however, Victoria suffered a series of betrayals and losses. She "fell head over heels in love" with a charming man in college, only to learn he was sleeping with other women—including her roommate. She gave up on love but not sex, and to her horror, she became pregnant. Her enduring religious beliefs prohibited abortion, but she was in no position to raise a child. She said the most traumatic event in her life was giving up the child for adoption. In her 30s, Victoria said, she "regained her senses," and she developed a satisfying teaching career. She made a concerted effort to find a satisfying romantic relationship but, inevitably, she broke off relationships, typically feeling some combination of being exploited and taken for granted. She also realized that she stayed somewhat distant emotionally, which she connected with enduring feelings of shame.

By the time she reached her early 40s, Victoria had become progressively depressed, and a tipping point was her involuntary transfer from a school and colleagues whom she valued to a new school where she felt "alone and adrift." The transfer was especially painful, because her school principal had been so "heartless" when she informed Victoria of the decision. She experienced "an old feeling of despair" and, for the first time, felt suicidal, at which point she sought hospitalization.

Victoria and I had many problems to address in psychotherapy, but her relationship with God was prominent among them. I was struck by Victoria's cynicism and bitterness. She said she'd come to feel profound resentment toward God; her grandmother's prophecy that "all troubles are God's will" came back to haunt her, and she felt tormented. Moreover, in the back of her mind, she realized that she'd developed the conviction that if she endured the troubles long enough, God would reward her. With some embarrassment, she said the reward would be a good love relationship. Feeling betrayed by God was pivotal in her suicidal state: she remembered a moment of acute frustration in the midst of prayer when she realized that her hopes were "absurd" and "futile," after which she thought about ending her life.

With her history of developing a feeling of connection with a compassionate God, Victoria recognized that she had "regressed" in the face of the loss of her security in her school. She was insightful: she could see how her grandmother's pernicious beliefs had come back to haunt her and how her experiences with men and her principal had colored her view of God. But these insights, in my view, weren't particularly significant in Victoria's regaining a more solid connection with God. Rather, as she overcame her feeling of alienation by developing connections with her fellow patients and staff members in the hospital, her mood improved and she developed more compassion for herself; these shifts helped open her mind about relationships, including her relationship with God. Then she was able to see how skewed her images of people and God had become.

Dependency

William James (1902/1994) put it plainly: "Here is the real core of the religious problem: Help! Help!" (p. 181). Sigmund Freud agreed, but he didn't conceal his disdain for this psychological strategy, which he equated with wishful and primitive thinking:

> We shall tell ourselves that it would be very nice if there were a God who created the world and was a benevolent Providence, and if there were a moral order in the universe and an after-life; but it's a very striking fact that all this is exactly as we're bound to wish it to be. And it would be more remarkable still if our wretched, ignorant and downtrodden ancestors had succeeded in solving all these difficult riddles of the universe. (Freud 1927/1964, pp. 52–53)

Hence, Freud considered the illusions of religion akin to obsessional neurosis and said of devout believers, "their acceptance of the universal neurosis spares them the task of constructing a personal one" (p. 72).

Freud's views of religion had a two-centuries-old precedent in Enlightenment thought: by relying on reason and science, we can cease depending on God and learn to take care of ourselves. Freud's predecessor, philosopher Ludwig Feuerbach (1873/2004), advocated, "Be courageous and consistent enough to give up God altogether, and to appeal only to pure, naked, godless nature as the last basis of your existence" (p. 48).

I think we can be seduced by the Enlightenment narrative into equating maturity with the courage to give up reliance on God, but we should recognize this seduction as such (Taylor 2007). This Enlightenment narrative commends autonomy over relatedness to anything transcendent. It encourages scientific exploration while cutting us off from any transcendent safe haven or secure base. We then might struggle to find ourselves at home in the universe—at worst, in traumatic attachment terms, afraid and alone. As I see it, as much as he prized human connections, Freud's position on religion is akin to the stance of avoidant attachment.

I think we need a better balance. As Pruyser (1974) made clear, belief and unbelief can be equally mature or immature. From the perspective of attachment theory, accepting dependency is the route to autonomy. Traumatic events render us helpless and heighten our sense of vulnerability and dependence; as Pargament (2011) argues, "Religion offers a response to the problem of *human insufficiency*" (p. 278, emphasis added). I agree with Rizzuto (1979) that imagination is the wellspring of all our connections, and as long as we need creative fantasy to contend with our longings for care, our fears, and our limitations, we will continue to have gods: "Nature and the world will continue to be personalized no matter how many 'progressive' efforts we make to computerize every corner of the universe. Freud's ideal man without illusions will have to wait for a new breed of human beings, perhaps a new civilization" (p. 54).

Research on Attachment Patterns in Relation to God

Pehr Granqvist and Lee Kirkpatrick (2008) make a strong claim: "No model of adult interpersonal relationships in general, or attachment relationships in particular, will be complete without explicit acknowledgement of the role of God and other imaginary figures in people's relationship networks" (p. 928). Extensive evidence justifies considering God to be a bona fide attachment figure (Kirkpatrick 2005). Many religious believers maintain a personal, interactive relationship with God; they experience the relationship as loving in maternal and paternal ways; they seek proximity to God, especially when they're distressed (most extensively through prayer but also by being in a house of worship); and they experience separation from God as painful (e.g., in loss of faith or feeling God forsaken). The relationship has all the hallmarks of a *safe haven* insofar as God is accessible and responsive in providing comfort in times of distress, most notably in the face of loss. In addition, the relationship provides a *secure base* in the sense of relative freedom from anxiety and a sense of strength, self-assurance, and competence. In my view, a relationship to God also can be viewed as potentially contributing importantly to the *internal secure base* that bolsters self-dependence and autonomy. No doubt there are significant differences between attachment to God and attachment to persons, not least that persons are directly observable. Moreover, God is an exalted attachment figure, profoundly stronger and wiser as well as continuously available to provide love and protection—in theistic terms, not only benevolent but also omnipresent, omniscient, and omnipotent.

For better or for worse, research demonstrates a straightforward *correspondence* such that internal working models based on human attachments are extended to one's relationship with God (Kirkpatrick 2005). Children who have positive relationships with their parents are more likely to have a positive relationship with God. The same is true in adulthood: securely attached individuals are more likely to identify with their parents' standards, and thus if their parents are religious, these secure individuals are likely to have a loving relationship with God. More specifically, a positive self-image is associated with an experience of God as loving, and a positive model of others is associated with a close personal relationship with God. In contrast, avoidant individuals are most likely to be agnostic or atheistic and to view God as distant and inaccessible.

The relationship with God, however, may not correspond to attachments with parents but rather may *compensate* for insecure attachments. As Kirkpatrick (2005) explains it, "The *lack* of adequate human attachments might be expected to motivate or enable belief in a God who is, in important ways, *unlike* one's human attachment figures" (p. 127, emphasis in original). Plainly, a history of attachment trauma contributes to vulnerability to this scenario. In the context of ambivalent attachment, for example, God may provide a stark contrast to unreliable parents, offering unconditional love so that the believer need not fear rejection or abandonment. To the extent that the relationship with God provides a feeling of security and enhances self-worth, this relationship might provide a stepping-stone to more secure human attachments. Yet the compensatory relationship with God, founded on insecure attachment, can suffer the fate of other ambivalent attachments. Victoria's experience in the midst of her depressive crisis attests to Kirkpatrick's point that "although anxious adults may be the most likely to turn to God as a surrogate attachment figure, they are also most likely to discover later that their relationship with God is not adequate to meet their attachment needs either" (pp. 141–142).

Mentalizing in Relation to God

James (1902/1994), a paragon of open-mindedness, issued a warning that we narrowly science-minded psychotherapists should take to heart: "nothing can be more stupid than to bar out phenomena from our notice, merely because we're incapable of taking part in anything like them ourselves" (p. 124). Nowhere is a mentalizing stance more essential in psychotherapy than in relation to religious concerns. As a therapist working with diverse patients, this stance enables me to explore evenhandedly the full range of beliefs, from unbelief to questioning to various forms of belief. The mentalizing approach has been enormously freeing. I never push a religious agenda, but I enjoy talking with patients about their experience with God whenever they bring it up, because I find this territory fascinating. Yet I also have ample experience with the same territory as being excruciatingly painful and confusing—as centuries of theological and philosophical literature on evil as well as research on the influence of insecure attachment on relatedness to God attest.

My mentalizing stance in exploring relationships with God is fostered by my belief that relationships with God are based on mentalizing. As our capacity to empathize illustrates, mentalizing requires imagination.

Karen Armstrong (1993) wrote that when she started out in the religious life, she would have been spared a great deal of anxiety had she heard that "in an important sense God was a product of the creative imagination" and that "I should deliberately create a sense of him for myself" (p. xx). A master mentalizer, Armstrong expanded her point about imagination:

> Today many people in the West would be dismayed if a leading theologian suggested that God was in some profound sense a product of the imagination. Yet it should be obvious that the imagination is the chief religious faculty. It has been defined by Jean-Paul Sartre as *the ability to think of what is not*. Human beings are the only animals who have the capacity to envisage something that is not present or something that does not yet exist but which is merely possible. The imagination has thus been the cause of our major achievements in science and technology as well as in art and religion. The idea of God, however it is defined, is perhaps the prime example of an absent reality which, despite its inbuilt problems, has continued to inspire men and women for thousands of years. The only way we can conceive of God, who remains imperceptible to the senses and to logical proof, is by means of symbols, which it is the chief function of the imaginative mind to interpret. (p. 233, emphasis in original)

In this vein, I like to think of God as a symbol for a mystery, consistent with Pruyser's (1987c) advocating "a religiously modest spirit that leads to the position of letting God be God and accepting one's creaturely limitations" (p. 6).

From this perspective, to feel loved—or hated or neglected or abandoned—by God requires imaginative mentalizing. So does praying. Accordingly, relating to God activates the same brain areas involved in mentalizing during social interactions (Schjoedt et al. 2009). Moreover, as the attachment research just reviewed attests, the way in which you mentalize God is influenced by the way in which you mentalize other relationships. Attachment trauma undermines mentalizing, and consequently you can be locked into rigid thinking. You can be convinced, for example, that God has condemned you to suffering—as if you could read the mind of God. Thus, in the face of loss and depression, Victoria regressed to a conviction that God willed her pain and abandoned her in it. Regaining mentalizing when she became more reflective in treatment, she was able to open her mind to other possibilities, as she had done earlier in her life after she left home.

Mario Mikulincer and colleagues (2004) summarize evidence that, compared with their avoidant and ambivalent counterparts, securely attached persons are likely to be more comfortable grappling with existential concerns and with viewing religion and spirituality as a *quest*. Thus, I wonder if a sense of security facilitates a mentalizing stance toward God:

a capacity to engage in imaginative thinking, an ability to suspend belief, tolerance for ambiguity and uncertainty, and an ability to reexamine and revise working models of God—just as mentalizing fosters openness to change in other attachment relationships. I also find mentalizing conducive to tolerance for diverse points of view more generally. For example, founded in attachment security, freedom to think without needing to be rooted in certainty is compatible with theism, atheism, and any middle ground between belief and unbelief.

As I see it, mentalizing puts us in the breach—not knowing while seeking knowledge. I worked with a young man who grew up in a highly religious family and who felt guilty and ashamed about his doubts about God, which stemmed from his intellectual inquisitiveness. After exploring his beliefs and feelings, I referred him for pastoral counseling, which he found reassuring. Meanwhile, I didn't refrain from conveying my opinion: I expressed my hope that he might come to enjoy his puzzlement rather than feeling guilty about it. I had done so in Armstrong's (2009) spirit: "Human beings seem framed to pose problems for themselves that they cannot solve, pit themselves against the dark world of uncreated reality, and find that living with such unknowing is a source of astonishment and delight" (p. 311). As it turned out, when my patient felt comfortable talking openly with his family, he discovered that they had no objection to his making up his own mind.

Spirituality

Case Example

I saw Eddie in psychotherapy after he developed posttraumatic stress disorder in his 50s. Eddie had been brutally dominated and subjected to violent harangues and beatings by his stepfather—a drill sergeant—throughout his childhood. He characterized himself as a "loner" who nevertheless married but maintained a somewhat distant relationship with his wife. He said he became "unglued" after he was assaulted violently by a gang and robbed when he got lost in an unfamiliar neighborhood and stopped his car to ask for directions. In the following weeks, he became increasingly plagued by horrifically violent images of assaults; out of the blue, he'd imagine being assaulted by others or assaulting them. He felt he was "going crazy," because sometimes his intrusive images were so vivid he actually felt as if a stranger on the street was assaulting him or vice versa.

Eddie said that he'd survived his childhood by immersing himself in nature. He'd seek safety in the woods in a park in the neighborhood, where he felt connected with the birds and other animals. This childhood interest became transformed into an enduring spiritual quest in adulthood. Eddie had found peace in spiritual retreats throughout his adult life; he had developed a keen eye for beauty and felt he was able to "commune with nature"—which, he acknowledged, had felt safer than intimate human relationships. He also put great stock in his relationship with his spiritual guide, whose equanimity and benevolence offered a dramatic contrast to his stepfather.

Eddie's spirituality was derailed by his symptoms; he couldn't sleep and couldn't concentrate, so he was unable to rely on meditation. He was so ashamed of his violent thoughts and images that he told no one about them. He felt utterly alienated from others and from himself. Driven by desperation and buoyed by courage, Eddie gradually talked in psychotherapy about what was going on in his mind. Despite his upbringing, it was evident to me that Eddie was tenderhearted, and his violent images were at great variance with the character he had cultivated. Of course, his worst fear was that he would become like his stepfather, despite lifelong efforts to be the opposite. In treatment, he was able to appreciate how the assault had rekindled long-buried violent fantasies toward his stepfather. As his anxiety abated and he regained his capacity to concentrate, he resumed his meditation and was able to take a mindful stance toward his intrusive images: striving to be compassionate toward himself, he was able to detach from them rather than identify with them; accordingly, he could allow them to come and go in his mind without being so disruptive. Importantly, he became able to talk with his spiritual advisor about all this experience, thus opening the door to further healing.

I like Thomas Plante's (2009) broad definition of *spirituality* as "being attentive to what is sacred and is connected to a concept, belief, or power greater than oneself" (p. 4). I include consideration of spirituality in this chapter because, like religion, spirituality can be a resource for finding meaning and healing in conjunction with trauma—a potential pathway for feeling less alone and alienated and more at home in the world. For those who are disinclined to believe in God for reasons of temperament, upbringing, education, or disillusionment, spirituality provides another pathway to a *feeling of connection*. In my view, spirituality has two opposites—if that's possible (see Figure 6–1). First, spirituality is opposite to self-absorption. In his evocatively titled *The Little Book of Atheist Spirituality*, André Comte-Sponville (2007) wrote, "The self is a prison. To be aware of our own puniness…is to break free of that prison. This is why sensing nature in all its immensity is a spiritual experience" (pp. 147–148). Second, spirituality is opposite to what Pruyser (1987a) dubbed "flat-footed realism" (p. 197). In this vein, Nagel (2010) refers to a popular secular stance of "hardheaded atheism" as follows: "The universe exists and meets a certain [scientific] description; one of the things it has generated is us; end of story" (p. 8). Fair enough, with the full backing of the Enlightenment.

Yet, to use a vulgarism, flat-footed realism leaves the trauma survivor with a barren theodicy: *shit happens*. Hardly satisfying, this view leaves us needing more, as Charles Taylor (2002) made plain: "People go on feeling

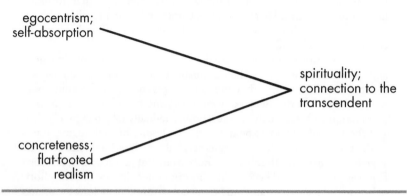

egocentrism;
self-absorption

spirituality;
connection to the
transcendent

concreteness;
flat-footed
realism

FIGURE 6–1.   Spirituality and its opposites.

a sense of unease at the world of unbelief: some sense that something big, something important has been left out, some level of profound desire has been ignored, some greater reality outside us has been closed off" (p. 56). As I see it, spirituality provides a middle ground for persons who are not disposed to belief in the God of theism but who feel a need for more— something sacred and transcendent. But there are degrees of transcendence within spirituality (Pargament 2007). In his engaging book *Spirituality for the Skeptic*, Robert Solomon (2002) advocates a naturalized spirituality encapsulated as the thoughtful love of life and embedded in relatedness: "Whatever else it may be, spirit is social. It represents our sense of participation and membership in a humanity and a world much larger than our individual selves" (p. 9).

From Nagel's (2010) perspective, such humanistic spirituality is a *partial* solution to the absence of God inasmuch as "the universe does not offer any sense to our lives, but we are not alone in it" (p. 10). Nagel seeks something broader, asking, "Is there a way to live in harmony with the universe, and not just in it?" (p. 5). He points to a harmony that I find immensely appealing in its reverence and spiritual connotations. Linking the desire for harmony with a religious temperament, he puts it thus:

> Having, amazingly, burst into existence, one is a representative of existence itself—of the whole of it—not just because one is part of it but because it's present to one's consciousness. In each of us, *the universe has come to consciousness*, and therefore our existence is not merely our own. (p. 6, emphasis added)

Thus, Nagel proposes, "Each of us, on this view, is a part of the lengthy process of the universe gradually waking up" (p. 17).

In whatever way we might choose to construe it, at the highest level of spirituality, we must accept our dependence on the universe, and we also must find a way of feeling *at home in the universe*. This metaphor captures a sense of connection or belonging that constitutes the antithesis of trauma as I've construed it—namely, feeling alone and alienated in emotional pain. Pruyser (1974) pointed to the possibility of the universe appearing as a "friendly abode," and he captured this spirit beautifully in the following comment, referring to existential philosopher and psychiatrist Karl Jaspers: "Jaspers once called the world as a whole 'the encompassing'…which I find a nice term. I would be inclined to be slightly more metaphorical and *warm* about it, by calling it 'the *embracing*'" (p. 224, emphasis added).

I emphasize connection and highlight Pruyser's warm term *embracing* to link spirituality to secure attachment. Yet I don't want to stretch the concept of attachment too far. As described in the previous section, God can be an attachment figure par excellence in meeting all the key criteria for an attachment relationship. Embracing as it might be, the "universe" cannot serve the attachment functions of either persons or a personified God. But, as Eddie's experience exemplifies, there's no question that spirituality is an existential resource that can be crucial in conjunction with trauma—not only a resource for meaning and acceptance but also for a feeling of emotional security. This takes me back to my central interest, psychotherapy.

Integrating Religion and Spirituality into Psychotherapy

For many patients, religion and spirituality aren't prominent concerns, and we therapists certainly shouldn't impose them in our practice. Yet we must be able to address them with ease when they arise. Pargament (2007) presents a strong case for the relevance of spiritually integrated psychotherapy to patients with a history of trauma. He observes that traumatic experiences may lead persons to become either more or less religious; consistent with attachment research, childhood abuse is associated with less likelihood of maintaining religious beliefs taught in the family and with more negative characterizations of God. He points out that spirituality is a "double-edged sword" (p. 276) and is "linked to life at its best and life at its worst" (p. 128).

Pargament (2011) distinguishes among three types of religious struggle: 1) internal—for example, doubts about faith and conflicts between higher and lower aspects of the self; 2) interpersonal—for example, conflicts with friends, family members, and congregations about spiritual beliefs; and 3) divine—for example, negative feelings toward God. He also distinguishes between positive religious coping (e.g., feeling connected with God and supported by God in active problem solving) and negative religious coping (e.g., being bogged down in religious struggles). Struggles associated with trauma can lead to spiritual growth and transformation (e.g., a greater capacity for acceptance and letting go), but these struggles are by no means invariably successful and also can lead to disengagement. On balance, however, he proposes that "spirituality does more good than harm" and is "more often involved in resolving psychological problems than promoting them" (Pargament 2007, p. 182).

Accordingly, we therapists have ample reason to address our patients' religious concerns and struggles. Attachment conflicts with God merit therapeutic exploration for the same reason that their human counterparts do: recognizing the influence of the past on the present can pave the way for greater security in both domains. Extensive evidence shows a relation between religious commitment and a feeling of positive connection with God, on the one hand, and good mental and physical health, on the other hand (Plante 2009). Of course, these health benefits as well as positive religious experiences are embedded in secure attachment.

Pargament (2007) proposes an eminently straightforward approach to broaching spiritual concerns:

> When spirituality seems to be salient in treatment, I will say to the client something like "It seems as though there may be a spiritual dimension to your problems" or "It sounds like spirituality may be a potential resource for you in dealing with your problems." Then, I would ask, "How would you feel about exploring the spiritual side of your situation?" These kinds of statements and questions are merely starting points. (pp. 208–209)

My favorite example of an openhearted exploration of spirituality comes from the practice of my colleague Jim Lomax (Lomax et al. 2011). His patient had been unable to talk about a profoundly significant and highly personal spiritual experience, which she revealed only months after the fact. Little wonder: her parents consistently had responded to her thoughts and feelings in an oddly accusatory, punishing, or dismissive fashion. Understandably, she was reluctant to disclose what she labeled "weird" and "paranormal" experiences. Eventually, she developed enough trust to broach the subject, starting with what seemed to be a supernatural childhood experience. Having put her toe into the water without drowning, she went on to reveal the particularly poignant adulthood experience that she'd been holding back. This experience related to a loving attachment she'd developed to her mentor, who became terminally ill. She was far away on vacation when he died, and she learned of his death a day later. Yet, right around the actual time of his death, she heard his voice, letting her know that he had died and expressing his love for her. Far from replicating her parents' attitudes, when she sought his reaction, Jim remarked that she'd told him "a beautiful love story." She then revealed a subsequent supernatural experience that cemented her feeling of connection to her deceased mentor, and she asked if other people had similar experiences. Jim responded, "Only if they are extremely lucky." Jim's responses illustrate the ideal I have in mind when I claim that effective mentalizing in therapy comes down to skill in being human.

As we therapists explore spirituality and religion, we also must be mindful of practicing within the limits of our competence. We have no religious authority and cannot provide answers to religious questions; rather, as Pargament (2007) proposes, we must aspire to help our patients "discover and live out the truths of *their* own lives as *they* perceive and experience these truths" (p. 19, emphasis in original). We can encourage patients to make use of spiritual and religious resources, but we cannot teach them how to do so. Thus, we can help our patients by referring them to members of the clergy and religious experts, and we mental health professionals can benefit from consulting and collaborating with members of the clergy, just as they can benefit from working with us (Plante 2009).

Spiritually integrated psychotherapy covers an extremely wide range. At one end of the continuum, therapists can make use of interventions derived from spiritual practices in the conduct of secular psychotherapy; mindfulness practice is a common example. In the mid-range of this continuum, therapists can encourage participation in a wide array of spiritual and religious activities (Plante 2009). On the other end of the continuum, therapists should be aware that there is an emerging field of spiritually focused psychotherapy (Pargament 2007). Although research is in its early stages, Everett Worthington Jr. and colleagues (2011) concluded that these specialized treatments are equal in effectiveness to their secular counterparts in relation to psychological outcomes, and they have greater benefit in relation to enhancing spirituality. Given the benefits of honoring patients' preferences, specialized interventions merit consideration, particularly for persons who are highly religious or spiritual.

Cultivating Hope

In conducting educational groups on trauma and depression, my favorite topic has been hope. I start with Aristotle's point that we're more likely to achieve our aim if we have a target (Bartlett and Collins 2011). Thus, we must strive to think clearly about hope. Then I invite each patient in the group to answer the question, "What gives you hope?" Plainly, "Nothing!"

is a fair answer for patients who feel utterly hopeless. But even in our in-patient setting, where patients often are at their most desperate, "Nothing!" is a rare response.

Sometimes I am asked what gives me hope. The multitude of positive answers to this question that I've heard over the years gives me hope. But my most profound basis for hope stems from having worked with patients who felt utterly hopeless and were utterly determined for prolonged periods of time to die by suicide; they didn't want to use psychotherapy as an opportunity for change but rather sought companionship in what they wished to be their last days. I've been privileged to hear from such patients many years later and to know that they are glad to be alive. Indeed, only one such patient would be reason for me to maintain hope in the face of suicidal despair.

We have reason to think clearly about hope; yet, as Karl Menninger (1959/1987) pointed out a half century ago, hope has been sadly neglected in the psychiatric literature, a fact that remains largely true:

> Our shelves hold many books now on the place of *faith* in science and psychiatry, and on the vicissitudes of man's efforts to *love* and to be loved. But when it comes to hope, our shelves are bare. The journals are silent. The *Encyclopedia Britannica* devotes many columns to the topic of love, and many more to faith. But hope, poor little hope! She is not even listed. (pp. 447–448, emphasis in original)

In what follows, I address two prominent themes in the literature: linking hope to sound expectations for the future and viewing hope as an existential stance. I conclude by placing hope in the cradle of attachment. Table 6–2 provides an overview of contributors to hope as I view them.

Sound Expectations

When I ask patients in educational groups about their understanding of hope, the first responses invariably point to positive expectations for the future. In being future oriented, hope overlaps with wishing and optimism. Following Pruyser (1987b), I start defining *hope* by distinguishing it from these two companions. Wishing focuses on desirable objects or events—wishing for a winning lottery ticket, a new home, or an ideal mate. Often, the preface "I hope…" is followed by a wish. There's nothing inherently wrong with wishing; we all do it. But I steer the group discussion toward several key distinctions. Wishing is easy; maintaining hope is hard. Wishing can be unrealistic; hope must not be. Wishing is passive; hope is active. Wishing can be a means of escaping reality; hope entails facing reality.

TABLE 6–2. Contributors to hope

- Ability to keep going in the face of uncertainty
- Tolerance for doubt, fear, and despair as they alternate with hope
- Capacity to face reality with realistic expectations
- Ability to imagine alternative futures
- Combining agency (active engagement) and pathways (sense of direction)
- Capacity to borrow hope from others who see hope for you
- Capacity to derive personal growth from trauma
- Connection to benevolence; secure attachment

We have reason to praise optimism. Extensive research associates optimism with good mood, good health, popularity, perseverance, and success (Peterson and Chang 2003). Conversely, often embedded in depression, pessimism is associated with alienation, passivity, failure, and ill health. For better or for worse, optimism and pessimism are associated with self-fulfilling prophecies: optimists strive for goals and thus are more likely to succeed; pessimists don't try or give up easily and thus fail. Valuable though it may be, optimism isn't equivalent to hope. In my view, optimism is too lighthearted a word to capture what is needed in the oftentimes-grueling process of healing from trauma.

Our traumatized patients come to the hospital in profoundly difficult—if not downright dire—circumstances. Optimism seems almost out of place, although some are sufficiently buoyed by finding their way to potentially helpful treatment that they express optimism. Most, however, are not so straightforwardly confident and are much less cheerfully optimistic; they need hope. But we walk a fine line in promoting hope, as Menninger (1959/1987) cautioned: "It is a responsibility of the teacher to the student, just as it is of the young doctor to his patient to inspire the right amount of hope—some, but not too much. Excess of hope is presumption and leads to disaster. Deficiency of hope is despair and leads to decay" (p. 449). Menninger went on to propose that our professional knowledge enables us therapists

> to replace therapeutic nihilism with constructive effort, to replace unsound expectations—first with hope, and then with *sound expectations*…for our patients—miserable, apprehensive, discouraged, and often desperate— what can we do better than that? What can we do better than to dispel their false expectations—good and bad—and then light for them a candle of hope to show them possibilities that may become sound expectations? (p. 461, emphasis added)

One of the greatest professional challenges I face is developing sound expectations, patient by patient. After I started to write books on trauma, I realized belatedly that one of the main driving forces behind my effort was my desire to learn as much as possible, so that I could develop realistic expectations. The present book is no exception. Knowledge helps, as does clinical experience. But knowing how much to expect is never easy. Cultivating hope is most difficult when patients express suicidal despair as they continue to founder in the face of trauma-related problems discussed throughout this book—*despite having worked hard for years in sound treatment*. How often I hear, "I'm exhausted." "I feel like giving up." "I can't keep fighting." "I want it to end." I bring to mind patients who have felt this way, continued the struggle, and been glad they did. This experience prevents me from joining patients in their wish to give up.

Hope enables us to keep going in the face of uncertainty; in this respect, hope overlaps faith—confidence without a basis in tangible evidence. In turn, faith overlaps trust—the link to attachment. Often enough, I begin psychotherapy with a patient who enters the hospital in a state of deep depression in conjunction with extremely stressful circumstances that present seemingly insurmountable obstacles. I cannot imagine a way out—just as the patient cannot do. When all else fails, I keep in mind the response of a young woman to my question, "What gives you hope?" With uncommon wisdom, she replied, "I can be surprised!" So I persist, as any patient who remains alive is doing. I take comfort in a passage from John Dewey (1922/1988):

> Man continues to live because he is a living creature not because reason convinces him of the certainty or probability of future satisfactions and achievements. He is instinct with activities that carry him on. Individuals here and there cave in, and most individuals sag, withdraw and seek refuge at this and that point. But man as man still has the *dumb pluck* of the animal. He has endurance, hope, curiosity, eagerness, love of action. These traits belong to him by structure, not by taking thought. (pp. 199–200; emphasis added)

"Dumb pluck" captures the one-foot-in-front-of-the-other mentality that therapists and patients must embrace in the face of despair and uncertainty. I often make the provocative point to patients that hopelessness is a form of arrogance in implying a sense of certainty about the future. Hope requires tolerance for uncertainty as well as a sense of humility in not knowing, a cardinal feature of the mentalizing stance.

For several years, I've been leading a weekly peer-supervision group at The Menninger Clinic in which we clinicians gather and discuss patients and families who have us most frustrated, anxious, flummoxed, and discouraged. Often in this group, as I experience at the beginning with despairing patients in individual psychotherapy, I cannot imagine how the treatment can progress to a satisfactory outcome. Practicing what we preach, we in the group find that talking helps—plain old therapy for us therapists. In this group, we reliably find understanding, sympathy, support, and encouragement—and occasionally some good advice. But we often end the group session in a muddle, just as we began. Yet the clinicians don't quit easily—dumb pluck indeed. Amazingly, in ways unforeseen, the patient and the clinicians get unstuck. Not always, by any means; sometimes patients bolt out of treatment, and sometimes clinicians conclude that the patients are not using treatment and must seek help elsewhere. But, often enough to keep hope alive, the situation improves, sometimes dramatically so. If I've learned anything from this process, it is our inability to predict how things will go and how important it is for us to maintain confidence in the unforeseeable—the territory of faith.

While proceeding with dumb pluck, we do so without blind optimism. In a fine paper that echoes Karl Menninger's advocacy of sound expectations, Kaethe Weingarten (2010) proposed that we therapists cultivate *reasonable hope,* hope that is realistic as well as "sensible and moderate" (p. 7).

An Existential Stance

Following Pruyser (1987b), I've come to see hope as an existential stance:

> To hope…one must have a tragic sense of life, an undistorted view of reality, a degree of modesty vis-à-vis the power and workings of nature or the cosmos, some feeling of commonality, if not communion, with other people, and some capacity to abstain from impulsive, unrealistic wishing. (p. 465)

I believe that hope invariably is accompanied by doubt; Weingarten (2010) adds despair: "Doubt and despair are not antithetical to reasonable hope but rather can run in parallel" (p. 10). Similarly, fear is hope's companion. This emotional complexity fits the tragic circumstances that call for hope: without fear, doubt, and despair, we would have no need for hope. As Weingarten states, "reasonable hope accepts that life can be messy. It embraces contradiction" (p. 10).

Hope is embodied in an existential *stance* inasmuch as hope is an active process, as contrasted with passive wishing. In Weingarten's (2010) words, "With reasonable hope, the present is filled with working not waiting; we scaffold ourselves to prepare for the future" (p. 7). She goes on to

propose, "Reasonable hope is a practice; it is something we do with others" (p. 8). Her view is consistent with Menninger's (1959/1987) point
that "hope implies a process; it is an adventure, a going forward, a confident search" (p. 452). As he elaborated,

> In a way it seems curious that the psychoanalytic process, which is so ob-
> viously diagnostic, has generally come to be called treatment. Diagnosis is
> the hopeful search for a way out; but the setting forth on the way which
> one discovers and the unflinching persistence in making the effort—*that* is
> the treatment; that is the self-directed, self-administered change. (p. 460,
> emphasis in original)

Continuing in this vein, Menninger proposed that hope is a motive
force for a plan of action. Similarly, Rick Snyder (1994) construed hope as
requiring a combination of agency and pathways. Agency entails initiative
and taking responsibility—at bottom, doing something. But Snyder argued that agency isn't enough: hope requires pathways, some sense of direction. It's not enough to have the energy and the will; you also need a
plan. In this sense, I view hope as an *outcome* of treatment: hope sustains
the capacity to keep moving forward. I keenly remember making a point
about the need for a pathway in an educational group, wherein a therapy
patient of mine queried, "What do you think about blind faith?" I responded, "Blind faith is not enough"—one of innumerable stupid statements I've made in my professional lifetime. It was in the aftermath of
this naïve response that I came to prize Dewey's (1922/1988) point
about dumb pluck. Weingarten (2010) puts it more eloquently: "reasonable hope thrives in advance of a coherent image of the future" (p. 9). You
must keep going without a plan until you can develop one.

Hope also is an active process in requiring imagination. Here we face
a paradox: hopelessness typically is embedded in depression, and the depressed person is liable to feel the heavy weight of innumerable burdens
with a mind that is sluggish and mired down in concrete ruminations.
Cultivating hope in the face of hopelessness requires a challenging mental
feat. Mentalizing is included in the feat: the patient must appreciate the
crucial distinction between *feeling* hopeless and *being* hopeless. When patients come to feel less hopeless, they're able to use imagination to see
that they're not hopeless. Their outward situation is unlikely to change,
but they're able to see possibilities that had been obscured by their depressive hopelessness.

I remember making the statement in an educational group on depression that hopelessness is not justified because recovery from depression is
difficult but not impossible: the vast majority of depressed persons recover. A wise young man piped up with a protest: "I can tell you doc, it

was impossible for me to recover *on my own!*" I couldn't agree more. I reiterate Weingarten's (2010) point that hope is something we do with others. With less fettered imaginations, others can see possibilities that the patient who feels hopeless cannot. Others can help with problem solving. And others can provide what we've come to call *borrowed hope:* many patients who feel hopeless can be sustained by the hope that others—family, friends, and us therapists—have for them. Others can see what the patient cannot see, and the patient may be able to take it on faith that others may be right.

Quite often when I ask patients, "What gives you hope?" they respond by stating something they *hope for:* "to be reunited with my family," "to be a better mother to my daughter," "to get my old self back," "to be able to return to work," and so forth. In this vein, I remember a traumatized patient stating that it was not enough for her to survive; she wanted to *thrive.* Here we have grounds for hope in the common observation that trauma leads not only to impairment but also to growth, which we should not overlook (Ryff and Singer 2003). Janoff-Bulman and Yopyk (2004) summarize research indicating that 75%–90% of survivors report benefits from their traumatic experiences. As Armstrong (2010) documented, compassion is borne of suffering. I've worked with patients who credit the trauma they've survived with their capacity for concern for others, caring, empathy, and intimacy. They take pride in their resilience—what I like to call pluck, dumb or not.

I'm loath to push the idea of posttraumatic growth when I work with patients who are in the midst of suffering the damage wrought by traumatic experience. But there is something to be said for the process of paying attention to benefits gleaned from challenging or painful experience. As this chapter attests, trauma can be a pathway to spirituality in the sense of developing a greater sense of meaning, a clearer philosophy of life, and renewed appreciation for life, perhaps coupled with a keener appreciation for mortality. In the context of thinking about shattered assumptions, Janoff-Bulman and Yopyk (2004) comment,

> Survivors' greater strength may also reflect the psychological advantages of a more flexible, less rigid, assumptive world; that is, in rebuilding their fundamental assumptions, survivors recognize the limits and naïvete of their earlier assumptions and reconstruct fundamental schemas that can now account for their traumatic experience, without being wholly negative. (pp. 128–129)

Janoff-Bulman and Yopyk (2004) also note that trauma can have the effect of prompting "appreciation through existential reevaluation," a process "that is related to questions of meaning, and particularly meaning in the sense of significance" (p. 128). This reevaluation can lead to greater appreciation of life, which can encompass close relationships as well as connections with nature and spirituality. Greater appreciation for life is a positive outcome indeed. Remarking on the perennial complaint that life is too short, Stoic philosopher Seneca countered that human life is plenty long, but "slight is the portion of life we live" (Hadas 1958, p. 49).

Attachment

By this point, it shouldn't seem surprising that I find hope in attachment theory and research. Secure attachment is conducive to hope. Although it's true that attachment trauma is the greatest threat to secure attachment, we also know that attachment security can change, given the opportunity for a trustworthy relationship. I take heart in a study we conducted in our specialized trauma program at The Menninger Clinic in which we asked female patients simply to list the number of persons with whom they felt they had a relatively secure attachment relationship (Allen et al. 2001). Responses covered the full range of possible attachment relationships: partners (spouses and romantic partners); members of their extended family of marriage; mothers, fathers, and siblings; members of their extended family of origin; friends; and professionals (e.g., clergy and clinicians). Some respondents also listed children; many listed pets with whom they had close emotional bonds. Some listed God. The average number of relatively secure human attachments reported by these women was four—not greatly different from the average number (six) reported by a community control group. I'm keenly aware that many traumatized persons go for extended periods of time with no secure attachments, but I conclude that most persons don't give up on attachment, despite their history of abuse, neglect, and betrayal. I recognize, however, that we therapists are working with a biased group of patients; seeking our help attests to the fact that they've not given up on attachment. For many, this persistence is an act of faith.

Having inundated you with quotations throughout this chapter, I've saved my favorite for last. Pruyser (1987b) concluded, "hoping is based on a belief that there is *some benevolent disposition toward oneself somewhere in the universe, conveyed by a caring person*" (p. 467, emphasis in original). I love the way Pruyser placed an attachment perspective—a benevolent disposition exemplified by a caring person—within such an open-ended frame: somewhere in the universe. This existential view of hope encompasses human relationships, spirituality, and religion: "From the experience of the self as a caring and cared-for object, as well as the other as a caring and cared-for object, stem our cognitive gropings about the rest of reality, our metaphysical speculations, our creative imaginations, our leading thoughts, and our religious ideas" (Pruyser 1974, p. 180).

The wellsprings of hope, as Pruyser construed it, run deep. In grounding attachment in evolutionary biology, John Bowlby (1982) was clear that we're wired for it by nature (i.e., natural selection). We are in the company of innumerable mammalian species in this regard, although we're unique in being self-conscious in the connections we make. In focusing on traumatic attachment relationships, I've concentrated on the ways in which attachment can go wrong. But secure attachment is the norm. Accordingly, benevolence is the norm, as evidenced in children's natural proclivity to be caring and empathic from the earliest years (Tomasello 2009). Without benevolence from a community, our humanity would not have gotten off the ground: our capacity for empathic connection evolved in the context of psychological attunement by mothers and others, to co-opt Sara Hrdy's (2009) felicitous title. To drive home my overarching thesis: our very existence as a species is founded in mentalizing in the context of attachment relationships.

These reflections bring me back to Mikulincer's conviction, mentioned in Chapter 5 (see Cultivation of Internal Secure Base), that all of us have islands of security (Shaver and Mikulincer 2011). Perhaps such islands are what led the women in our trauma treatment program to develop a handful of relatively secure attachments despite their history (Allen et al. 2001). And these islands also can be a foundation for a secure relationship with oneself, as I've construed the internal secure base. To this extent, hope can come from within as well as from without. Adopting Pruyser's (1987b) view that sources of hope abound, I've endeavored in this chapter to take the widest purview on resources for grappling with trauma. But I intend also to have conveyed that from the beginning of life until the end, there's no substitute for a *caring person*.

Key Points

◆ Trauma extends beyond psychiatric disorders, confronting patients and therapists with existential-spiritual concerns that require a search for meaning and connection. Therapists typically aren't equipped by professional training to grapple with these concerns, and they may be less inclined than their patients to address them.

◆ The problem of evil pertains to the most grievous forms of trauma, including trauma in attachment relationships. Thus, therapists potentially have much to learn from the literature on evil, not least from philosophical and scientific literature implicating mentalizing failures in actions that result in intolerable harm.

♦ For patients who are religious, attachment trauma can contribute to insecurity in their relationship with God. Psychotherapy can be beneficial in exploring these problematic attachments, and pastoral counseling can be a crucial adjunct in fostering positive religious coping. A mentalizing stance is optimal for therapists to relate to diversity in patients' religious beliefs.

♦ Cultivating hope is a mainstay of trauma treatment, and hope is a crucial treatment outcome. Hope must be grounded in realistic expectations, and such expectations are not easily achieved in working with complex psychiatric and existential consequences of trauma. Ultimately, hope rests on conviction in benevolence, with secure attachment as the model.

References

Adams R: Watership Down. New York, Scribner, 1972

Ainsworth MDS: Attachments beyond infancy. Am Psychol 44:709–716, 1989

Ainsworth MDS, Blehar MC, Waters E, et al: Patterns of Attachment: A Psychological Study of the Strange Situation. Hillsdale, NJ, Erlbaum, 1978

Allen JG: The spectrum of accuracy in memories of childhood trauma. Harv Rev Psychiatry 3:84–95, 1995

Allen JG: Traumatic Relationships and Serious Mental Disorders. Chichester, UK, Wiley, 2001

Allen JG: What stabilizes stable instability? Commentary on "Plausibility and possible determinants of sudden 'remissions' in borderline patients." Psychiatry 66:120–123, 2003

Allen JG: Coping With Trauma: Hope Through Understanding, 2nd Edition. Washington, DC, American Psychiatric Publishing, 2005

Allen JG: Coping With Depression: From Catch-22 to Hope. Washington, DC, American Psychiatric Publishing, 2006

Allen JG: Evil, mindblindness, and trauma: challenges to hope. Smith Coll Stud Soc Work 77:9–31, 2007

Allen JG: Psychotherapy: the artful use of science. Smith Coll Stud Soc Work 78:159–187, 2008

Allen JG: Mentalizing suicidal states, in Building a Therapeutic Alliance With the Suicidal Patient. Edited by Michel K, Jobes DA. Washington, DC, American Psychological Association, 2011, pp 81–91

Allen JG, Fonagy P: Preface, in Handbook of Mentalization-Based Treatment. Edited by Allen JG, Fonagy P. Chichester, UK, Wiley, 2006, pp ix–xxi

Allen JG, Fonagy P: Constructing an evidence base for a psychodynamic approach to treating trauma, in Handbook of Contemporary Psychodynamic Approaches to Psychopathology. Edited by Luyten P, Mayes LC, Fonagy P, et al. New York, Guilford (in press)

Allen JG, Newsom GE, Gabbard GO, et al: Scales to assess the therapeutic alliance from a psychoanalytic perspective. Bull Menninger Clin 48:383–400, 1984

Allen JG, Huntoon J, Evans RB: Complexities in complex posttraumatic stress disorder in inpatient women: evidence from cluster analysis of MCMI-III personality disorder scales. J Pers Assess 73:449–471, 1999

Allen JG, Coyne L, Console DA: Course of illness following specialized inpatient treatment for women with trauma-related psychopathology. Bull Menninger Clin 64:235–256, 2000

Allen JG, Huntoon J, Fultz J, et al: A model for brief assessment of attachment and its application to women in inpatient treatment for trauma-related psychiatric disorders. J Pers Assess 76:420–446, 2001

Allen JG, Fonagy P, Bateman AW (eds): Mentalizing in Clinical Practice. Washington, DC, American Psychiatric Publishing, 2008

Allen JG, O'Malley F, Freeman C, et al: Brief treatment, in Handbook of Mentalizing in Mental Health Practice. Edited by Bateman AW, Fonagy P. Washington, DC, American Psychiatric Publishing, 2012, pp 159–196

American Psychiatric Association: Diagnostic and Statistical Manual of Mental Disorders, 3rd Edition. Washington, DC, American Psychiatric Association, 1980

American Psychiatric Association: Diagnostic and Statistical Manual of Mental Disorders, 4th Edition. Washington, DC, American Psychiatric Association, 1994

American Psychiatric Association: Diagnostic and Statistical Manual of Mental Disorders, 4th Edition, Text Revision. Washington, DC, American Psychiatric Association, 2000

Andreski P, Chilcoat H, Breslau N: Post-traumatic stress disorder and somatization symptoms: a prospective study. Psychiatry Res 79:131–138, 1998

Andrews B, Brewin CR, Philpott R, et al: Delayed-onset posttraumatic stress disorder: a systematic review of the evidence. Am J Psychiatry 164:1319–1326, 2007

Andrews B, Brewin CR, Stewart L, et al: Comparison of immediate-onset and delayed-onset posttraumatic stress disorder in military veterans. J Abnorm Psychol 118:767–777, 2009

Andrews G, Charney DS, Sirovatka PJ, et al (eds): Stress-Induced and Fear Circuitry Disorders: Refining the Research Agenda for DSM-V. Washington, DC, American Psychiatric Publishing, 2009

Arendt H: The Life of the Mind: I. Thinking. New York, Harcourt, 1971

Arendt H: Eichmann in Jerusalem: A Report on the Banality of Evil (1963). New York, Penguin, 1994

Arendt H: Responsibility and Judgment. New York, Schocken, 2003

Armstrong K: A History of God: The 4,000-Year Quest of Judaism, Christianity, and Islam. New York, Knopf, 1993

Armstrong K: The Case for God. New York, Knopf, 2009

Armstrong K: Twelves Steps to a Compassionate Life. New York, Knopf, 2010

Arnsten AF: The biology of being frazzled. Science 280:1711–1712, 1998

Asen E, Fonagy P: Mentalization-based family therapy, in Handbook of Mentalizing in Mental Health Practice. Edited by Bateman AW, Fonagy P. Washington, DC, American Psychiatric Publishing, 2012, pp 107–128

Asmundson GJ, Stapleton JA, Taylor S: Are avoidance and numbing distinct PTSD symptom clusters? J Trauma Stress 17:467–475, 2004

Ball JS, Links PS: Borderline personality disorder and childhood trauma: evidence for a causal relationship. Curr Psychiatry Rep 11:63–68, 2009

Barlow MR, Freyd JJ: Adaptive dissociation: information processing and response to betrayal, in Dissociation and the Dissociative Disorders: DSM-V and Beyond. Edited by Dell PF, O'Neil JA. New York, Routledge, 2009, pp 93–105

Baron-Cohen S: Mindblindness: An Essay on Autism and Theory of Mind. Cambridge, MA, MIT Press, 1995

Baron-Cohen S: The Science of Evil: On Empathy and the Origins of Cruelty. New York, Basic Books, 2011

Bartlett RC, Collins SD: Aristotle's Nicomachean Ethics. Chicago, IL, University of Chicago Press, 2011

Bateman A, Fonagy P: Effectiveness of partial hospitalization in the treatment of borderline personality disorder: a randomized controlled trial. Am J Psychiatry 156:1563–1569, 1999

Bateman A, Fonagy P: Treatment of borderline personality disorder with psychoanalytically oriented partial hospitalization: an 18-month follow-up. Am J Psychiatry 158:36–42, 2001

Bateman A, Fonagy P: Mentalization-Based Treatment for Borderline Personality Disorder: A Practical Guide. New York, Oxford University Press, 2006a

Bateman A, Fonagy P: Mentalizing and borderline personality disorder, in Handbook of Mentalization-Based Treatment. Edited by Allen JG, Fonagy P. Chichester, UK, Wiley, 2006b, pp 185–200

Bateman A, Fonagy P: 8-year follow-up of patients treated for borderline personality disorder: mentalization-based treatment versus treatment as usual. Am J Psychiatry 165:631–638, 2008

Bateman A, Fonagy P: Randomized controlled trial of outpatient mentalization-based treatment versus structured clinical management for borderline personality disorder. Am J Psychiatry 166:1355–1364, 2009

Bateman A, Fonagy P (eds): Handbook of Mentalizing in Mental Health Practice. Washington, DC, American Psychiatric Publishing, 2012a

Bateman A, Fonagy P: Individual techniques of the basic model, in Handbook of Mentalizing in Mental Health Practice. Edited by Bateman AW, Fonagy P. Washington, DC, American Psychiatric Publishing, 2012b, pp 67–80

Baumeister RF: Evil: Inside Human Violence and Cruelty. New York, Freeman, 1997

Beck AT, Rush AJ, Shaw BF, et al: Cognitive Therapy of Depression. New York, Guilford, 1979

Becker CB, Zayfert C: Eating disorders, in The Encyclopedia of Psychological Trauma. Edited by Reyes G, Elhai JD, Ford JD. New York, Wiley, 2008, pp 240–241

Bedics JD, Atkins DC, Comtois KA, et al: Treatment differences in the therapeutic relationship and introject during a 2-year randomized controlled trial of dialectical behavior therapy versus nonbehavioral psychotherapy experts for borderline personality disorder. J Consult Clin Psychol November 7, 2011 [Epub ahead of print]

Beebe B, Jaffe J, Markese S, et al: The origins of 12-month attachment: a microanalysis of 4-month mother-infant interaction. Attach Hum Dev 12:3–141, 2010

Belsky J: Attachment theory and research in ecological perspective: insights from the Pennsylvania Infant and Family Development Project and the NICHD study of early child care, in Attachment From Infancy to Adulthood: The Major Longitudinal Studies. Edited by Grossman KE, Grossman K, Waters E. New York, Guilford, 2005, pp 71–97

Belsky J, Fearon RMP: Precursors of attachment security, in Handbook of Attachment: Theory, Research, and Clinical Applications, 2nd Edition. Edited by Cassidy J, Shaver PR. New York, Guilford, 2008, pp 295–316

Bender DS, Oldham JM: Psychotherapies for borderline personality disorder, in Understanding and Treating Borderline Personality Disorder. Edited by Gunderson J, Hoffman PD. Washington, DC, American Psychiatric Publishing, 2005, pp 21–41

Berant E, Obegi JH: Attachment-informed psychotherapy research with adults, in Attachment Theory and Research in Clinical Work With Adults. Edited by Obegi JH, Berant E. New York, Guilford, 2009, pp 461–489

Berlin LJ, Cassidy J, Appleyard K: The influence of early attachments on other relationships, in Handbook of Attachment: Theory, Research, and Clinical Applications, 2nd Edition. Edited by Cassidy J, Shaver PR. New York, Guilford, 2008, pp 333–347

Bernet CZ, Stein MB: Relationship of childhood maltreatment to the onset and course of major depression in adulthood. Depress Anxiety 9:169–174, 1999

Berntsen D, Rubin DC: When a trauma becomes a key to identity: enhanced integration of trauma memories predicts posttraumatic stress disorder symptoms. Appl Cogn Psychol 21:417–431, 2007

Berntsen D, Willert M, Rubin DC: Splintered memories or vivid landmarks? Qualities and organization of traumatic memories with and without PTSD. Appl Cogn Psychol 17:675–693, 2003

Beutler LE, Blatt SJ: Participant factors in treating dysphoric disorders, in Principles of Therapeutic Change That Work. Edited by Castonguay LG, Beutler LE. New York, Oxford University Press, 2006, pp 13–63

Beutler LE, Castonguay LG: The task force on empirically based principles of change, in Principles of Therapeutic Change That Work. Edited by Castonguay LG, Beutler LE. New York, Oxford University Press, 2006, pp 3–10

Bifulco A, Moran PM: Wednesday's Child: Research Into Women's Experience of Neglect and Abuse in Childhood, and Adult Depression. London, Routledge, 1998

Bifulco A, Harris T, Brown GW, et al: Mourning or early inadequate care? Reexamining the relationship of maternal loss in childhood with adult depression and anxiety. Dev Psychopathol 4:433–439, 1992

Bifulco A, Moran PM, Baines R, et al: Exploring psychological abuse in childhood II: association with other abuse and adult clinical depression. Bull Menninger Clin 66:241–258, 2002

Blatt SJ: Experiences of Depression: Theoretical, Clinical, and Research Perspectives. Washington, DC, American Psychological Association, 2004

Blatt SJ: Polarities of Experience: Relatedness and Self-Definition in Personality Development, Psychopathology, and the Therapeutic Process. Washington, DC, American Psychological Association, 2008

Blatt SJ, Luyten P: Reactivating the psychodynamic approach to the classification of psychopathology, in Contemporary Directions in Psychopathology: Scientific Foundations of the DSM-V and ICD-11. Edited by Millon T, Krueger RF, Simonson E. New York, Guilford, 2010, pp 483–514

Blumenthal SJ: An overview and synopsis of risk factors, assessment, and treatment of suicidal patients over the life cycle, in Suicide Over the Life Cycle: Risk Factors, Assessment, and Treatment of Suicidal Patients. Edited by Blumenthal SJ, Kupfer DJ. Washington, DC, American Psychiatric Press, 1990, pp 685–723

Bowlby J: The nature of the child's tie to his mother. Int J Psychoanal 39:350–373, 1958

Bowlby J: Attachment and Loss, Volume II: Separation. New York, Basic Books, 1973

Bowlby J: Attachment and Loss, Volume III: Loss, Sadness, and Depression. New York, Basic Books, 1980

Bowlby J: Attachment and Loss, Volume I: Attachment, 2nd Edition. New York, Basic Books, 1982

Bowlby J: A Secure Base: Parent-Child Attachment and Healthy Human Development. New York, Basic Books, 1988

Brady KT, Dansky BS, Sonne SC, et al: Posttraumatic stress disorder and cocaine dependence. Order of onset. Am J Addict 7:128–135, 1998

Bremner JD: Neurobiology of dissociation: a view from the trauma field, in Dissociation and the Dissociative Disorders: DSM-V and Beyond. Edited by Dell PF, O'Neil JA. New York, Routledge, 2009, pp 329–336

Bremner JD, Southwick SM, Johnson DR, et al: Childhood physical abuse and combat-related posttraumatic stress disorder in Vietnam veterans. Am J Psychiatry 150:235–239, 1993

Brennan KA, Clark CL, Shaver PR: Self-report measurement of adult attachment: an integrative overview, in Attachment Theory and Close Relationships. Edited by Simpson JA, Rholes WS. New York, Guilford, 1998, pp 46–75

Bretherton I, Munholland KA: Internal working models in attachment relationships: elaborating a central construct in attachment theory, in Handbook of Attachment: Theory, Research, and Clinical Applications, 2nd Edition. Edited by Cassidy J, Shaver PR. New York, Guilford, 2008, pp 102–127

Brewin CR: Posttraumatic Stress Disorder: Malady or Myth? New Haven, CT, Yale University Press, 2003

Brewin CR: Encoding and Retrieval of Traumatic Memories, in Neuropsychology of PTSD: Biological, Cognitive, and Clinical Perspectives. Edited by Vasterling JJ, Brewin CR. New York, Guilford, 2005, pp 131–150

Brewin CR: The nature and significance of memory disturbance in posttraumatic stress disorder. Annu Rev Clin Psychol 7:203–227, 2011

Brewin CR, Reynolds M, Tata P: Autobiographical memory processes and the course of depression. J Abnorm Psychol 108:511–517, 1999

Brewin CR, Lanius RA, Novac A, et al: Reformulating PTSD for DSM-V: life after Criterion A. J Trauma Stress 22:366–373, 2009

Brodsky BS, Oquendo M, Ellis SP, et al: The relationship of childhood abuse to impulsivity and suicidal behavior in adults with major depression. Am J Psychiatry 158:1871–1877, 2001

Broman-Fulks JJ, Ruggiero KJ, Green BA, et al: Taxometric investigation of PTSD: data from two nationally representative samples. Behav Ther 37:364–380, 2006

Brown D, Hammond DC, Scheflin AW: Memory, Trauma Treatment, and the Law. New York, WW Norton, 1998

Brown GW: Psychosocial origins of depressive and anxiety disorders, in Diagnostic Issues in Depression and Generalized Anxiety Disorder: Refining the Research Agenda for DSM-V. Edited by Goldberg D, Kendler KS, Sirovatka PJ, et al. Washington, DC, American Psychiatric Publishing, 2010, pp 303–331

Brown GW, Harris TO: Social Origins of Depression: A Study of Psychiatric Disorder in Women. New York, Free Press, 1978

Brown GW, Bifulco A, Veiel HO, et al: Self-esteem and depression. II. Social correlates of self-esteem. Soc Psychiatry Psychiatr Epidemiol 25:225–234, 1990

Brown GW, Harris TO, Hepworth C: Loss, humiliation and entrapment among women developing depression: a patient and non-patient comparison. Psychol Med 25:7–21, 1995

Bryant RA: Treating the full range of posttraumatic reactions, in Clinician's Guide to Posttraumatic Stress Disorder. Edited by Rosen GM, Frueh BC. New York, Wiley, 2010, pp 205–234

Burgess AW, Holmstrom LL: Rape trauma syndrome. Am J Psychiatry 131:981–986, 1974

Cahill SP, Foa EB: Psychological theories of PTSD, in Handbook of PTSD: Science and Practice. Edited by Friedman MJ, Keane TM, Resick PA. New York, Guilford, 2007, pp 55–77

Cahill SP, Rothbaum BO, Resick PA, et al: Cognitive-behavioral therapy for adults, in Effective Treatments for PTSD: Practice Guidelines From the International Society for Traumatic Stress Studies. Edited by Foa EB, Keane TM, Friedman MJ, et al. New York, Guilford, 2009, pp 139–222

Card C: The Atrocity Paradigm: A Theory of Evil. New York, Oxford University Press, 2002

Carlson EA: A prospective longitudinal study of attachment disorganization/disorientation. Child Dev 69:1107–1128, 1998

Carlson EA, Egeland B, Sroufe LA: A prospective investigation of the development of borderline personality symptoms. Dev Psychopathol 21:1311–1334, 2009a

Carlson EA, Yates TM, Sroufe LA: Dissociation and the development of the self, in Dissociation and the Dissociative Disorders: DSM-V and Beyond. Edited by Dell PF, O'Neil JA. New York, Routledge, 2009b, pp 39–52

Carnes P: The Betrayal Bond. Deerfield Beach, FL, Health Communications, 1997

Cassidy J: The nature of the child's ties, in Handbook of Attachment: Theory, Research, and Clinical Applications, 2nd Edition. Edited by Cassidy J, Shaver PR. New York, Guilford, 2008, pp 3–22

Cassidy J, Shaver PR, Mikulincer M, et al: Experimentally induced security influences responses to psychological pain. J Soc Clin Psychol 28:463–478, 2009

Castonguay LG, Beutler LE (eds): Principles of Therapeutic Change That Work. New York, Oxford University Press, 2006

Castonguay LG, Holtforth MG, Coombs MM, et al: Relationship factors in treating dysphoric disorders, in Principles of Therapeutic Change That Work. Edited by Castonguay LG, Beutler LE. New York, Oxford University Press, 2006, pp 65–81

Chambless DL, Ollendick TH: Empirically supported psychological interventions: controversies and evidence. Annu Rev Psychol 52:685–716, 2001

Chekhov A: The Cherry Orchard (1904). London, Nick Hern, 1998

Clarkin JF, Yeomans FE, Kernberg OF: Psychotherapy for Borderline Personality. New York, Wiley, 1999

Clarkin JF, Levy KN, Lenzenweger MF, et al: Evaluating three treatments for borderline personality disorder: a multiwave study. Am J Psychiatry 164:922–928, 2007

Coan JA: Toward a neuroscience of attachment, in Handbook of Attachment: Theory, Research, and Clinical Applications, 2nd Edition. Edited by Cassidy J, Shaver PR. New York, Guilford, 2008, pp 241–265

Coan JA, Schaefer HS, Davidson RJ: Lending a hand: social regulation of the neural response to threat. Psychol Sci 17:1032–1039, 2006

Comte-Sponville A: The Little Book of Atheist Spirituality. London, Penguin, 2007

Connor KM, Davidson JR, Lee LC: Spirituality, resilience, and anger in survivors of violent trauma: a community survey. J Trauma Stress 16:487–494, 2003

Connors R: Self-injury in trauma survivors: 1. Functions and meanings. Am J Orthopsychiatry 66:197–206, 1996

Coons PM: Depersonalization and derealization, in Handbook of Dissociation: Theoretical, Empirical, and Clinical Perspectives. Edited by Michelson LK. Ray WJ. New York, Plenum, 1996, pp 291–305

Cormier JF, Thelen MH: Professional skepticism of multiple personality disorder. Professional Psychology: Research and Practice 29:163–167, 1998

Courtois CA, Ford JD (eds): Treating Complex Traumatic Stress Disorders: An Evidence-Based Guide. New York, Guilford, 2009

Courtois CA, Ford JD, Cloitre M: Best practices in psychotherapy for adults, in Treating Complex Traumatic Stress Disorders: An Evidence-Based Guide. Edited by Courtois CA, Ford JD. New York, Guilford, 2009, pp 82–103

Craske MG, Kircanski K, Zelikowsky M, et al: Optimizing inhibitory learning during exposure therapy. Behav Res Ther 46:5–27, 2008

Critchfield KL, Benjamin LS: Integration of therapeutic factors in treating personality disorders, in Principles of Therapeutic Change That Work. Edited by Castonguay LG, Beutler LE. New York, Oxford University Press, 2006, pp 253–271

Crowell JA, Waters E: Attachment representations, secure-base behavior, and the evolution of adult relationships: The Stony Brook Adult Relationship Project, in Attachment From Infancy to Adulthood: The Major Longitudinal Studies. Edited by Grossman KE, Grossman K, Waters E. New York, Guilford, 2005, pp 223–244

Crowell JA, Fraley RC, Shaver PR: Measurement of individual differences in adolescent and adult attachment, in Handbook of Attachment: Theory, Research, and Clinical Applications, 2nd Edition. Edited by Cassidy J, Shaver PR. New York, Guilford, 2008, pp 599–634

Dalenberg C, Paulson K: The case for the study of "normal" dissociation processes, in Dissociation and the Dissociative Disorders: DSM-V and Beyond. Edited by Dell PF, O'Neil JA. New York, Routledge, 2009, pp 145–154

Davidson J, Allen JG, Smith WH: Complexities in the hospital treatment of a patient with multiple personality disorder. Bull Menninger Clin 51:561–568, 1987

Deklyen M, Greenberg MT: Attachment and psychopathology in childhood, in Handbook of Attachment: Theory, Research, and Clinical Applications, 2nd Edition. Edited by Cassidy J, Shaver PR. New York, Guilford, 2008, pp 637–665

Dell PF: The long struggle to diagnose multiple personality disorder (MPD): MPD, in Dissociation and the Dissociative Disorders: DSM-V and Beyond. Edited by Dell PF, O'Neil JA. New York, Routledge, 2009a, pp 383–402

Dell PF: The phenomena of pathological dissociation, in Dissociation and the Dissociative Disorders: DSM-V and Beyond. Edited by Dell PF, O'Neil JA. New York, Routledge, 2009b, pp 225–237

Dell PF: Understanding dissociation, in Dissociation and the Dissociative Disorders: DSM-V and Beyond. Edited by Dell PF, O'Neil JA. New York, Routledge, 2009c, pp 709–825

Dewey J: Human Nature and Conduct (1922). Carbondale, Southern Illinois University Press, 1988

Diamond D, Stovall-McClough C, Clarkin JF, et al: Patient-therapist attachment in the treatment of borderline personality disorder. Bull Menninger Clin 67:227–259, 2003

Doering S, Hörz S, Rentrop M, et al: Transference-focused psychotherapy v. treatment by community psychotherapists for borderline personality disorder: randomised controlled trial. Br J Psychiatry 196:389–395, 2010

Dohrenwend BP: Toward a typology of high-risk major stressful events and situations in posttraumatic stress disorder and related psychopathology. Psychol Inj Law 3:89–99, 2010

Dohrenwend BP, Turner JB, Turse NA, et al: The psychological risks of Vietnam for U.S. veterans: a revisit with new data and methods. Science 313:979–982, 2006

Dostoevsky F: The Brothers Karamazov (1912). New York, Barnes & Noble Classics, 2005

Doyle TP: Roman Catholic clericalism, religious duress, and clergy sexual abuse. Pastoral Psychol 51:189–231, 2003

Dozier M, Stovall-McClough KC, Albus KE: Attachment and psychopathology in adulthood, in Handbook of Attachment: Theory, Research, and Clinical Applications, 2nd Edition. Edited by Cassidy J, Shaver PR. New York, Guilford, 2008, pp 718–744

Dubo ED, Zanarini MC, Lewis RE, et al: Childhood antecedents of self-destructiveness in borderline personality disorder. Can J Psychiatry 42:63–69, 1997

Dutra L, Bianchi I, Siegel DJ, et al: The relational context of dissociative phenomena, in Dissociation and the Dissociative Disorders: DSM-V and Beyond. Edited by Dell PF, O'Neil JA. New York, Routledge, 2009, pp 83–92

Eagle MN, Wolitzky DL: Adult psychotherapy from the perspectives of attachment theory and psychoanalysis, in Attachment Theory and Research in Clinical Work With Adults. Edited by Obegi JH, Berant E. New York, Guilford, 2009, pp 351–378

Ehlers A, Clark DM, Hackmann A, et al: Cognitive therapy for post-traumatic stress disorder: development and evaluation. Behav Res Ther 43:413–431, 2005

Elhai JD, Biehn TL, Armour C, et al: Evidence for a unique PTSD construct represented by PTSD's D1-D3 symptoms. J Anxiety Disord 25:340–345, 2011a

Elhai JD, Carvalho LF, Miguel FK, et al: Testing whether posttraumatic stress disorder and major depressive disorder are similar or unique constructs. J Anxiety Disord 24:404–410, 2011b

Ellenberger HF: The Discovery of the Unconscious: The History and Evolution of Dynamic Psychiatry. New York, Basic Books, 1970

Elliott R, Bohart AC, Watson JC, et al: Empathy, in Psychotherapy Relationships That Work: Evidence-Based Responsiveness. Edited by Norcross JC. New York, Oxford University Press, 2011, pp 132–152

Epstein JN, Saunders BE, Kilpatrick DG, et al: PTSD as a mediator between childhood rape and alcohol use in adult women. Child Abuse Negl 22:223–234, 1998

Erickson MF, Egeland B: Child neglect, in The APSAC Handbook on Child Maltreatment. Edited by Briere J, Berliner L, Bulkley JA, et al. Thousand Oaks, CA, Sage, 1996, pp 4–20

Fanselow MS, Lester LS: A functional behavioristic approach to aversively motivated behavior: predatory imminence as a determinant of the topography of defensive behavior, in Evolution and Learning. Edited by Bolles RC, Beecher MD. Hillsdale, NJ, Erlbaum, 1988, pp 185–212

Farber BA, Doolin EM: Positive regard and affirmation, in Psychotherapy Relationships That Work: Evidence-Based Responsiveness. Edited by Norcross JC. New York, Oxford University Press, 2011, pp 168–186

Favazza AR: Bodies Under Siege: Self-Mutilation in Culture and Psychiatry. Baltimore, MD, Johns Hopkins University Press, 1987

Favazza AR: A cultural understanding of nonsuicidal self-injury, in Understanding Nonsuicidal Self-Injury: Origins, Assessment, and Treatment. Edited by Nock MK. Washington, DC, American Psychological Association, 2009, pp 19–35

Feeney JA: Adult romantic attachment: developments in the study of couple relationships, in Handbook of Attachment: Theory, Research, and Clinical Applications, 2nd Edition. Edited by Cassidy J, Shaver PR. New York, Guilford, 2008, pp 456–481

Felitti VJ, Anda RF: The relationship of adverse childhood experiences to adult medical disease, psychiatric disorders and sexual behavior: implications for healthcare, in The Impact of Early Life Trauma on Health and Disease: The Hidden Epidemic. Edited by Lanius RA, Vermetten E, Pain C. New York, Cambridge University Press, 2010, pp 77–87

Fergusson DM, Horwood LJ: Generalized anxiety disorder and major depression: common and reciprocal causes, in Diagnostic Issues in Depression and Generalized Anxiety Disorder: Refining the Research Agenda for DSM-V. Edited by Goldberg D, Kendler KS, Sirovatka PJ, et al. Washington, DC, American Psychiatric Publishing, 2010, pp 179–189

Feuerbach L: The Essence of Religion (1873). Amherst, NY, Prometheus, 2004

First MB, Spitzer RL, Gibbon ML, et al: User's Guide for the Structured Clinical Interview for DSM-IV Axis I Disorders: Clinician Version, SCID-I. Washington, DC, American Psychiatric Press, 1997

Fischer S, Stojek M, Hartzell E: Effects of multiple forms of child abuse and sexual assault on current eating disorder symptoms. Eat Behav 11:190–192, 2010

Florsheim P, McArthur L: An interpersonal approach to attachment and change, in Attachment Theory and Research in Clinical Work With Adults. Edited by Obegi JH, Berant E. New York, Guilford, 2009, pp 379–409

Foa EB, Kozak MJ: Emotional processing: theory, research, and clinical implications for anxiety disorders. Emotion, Psychotherapy, and Change. Edited by Safran JD, Greenberg LS. New York, Guilford, 1991, pp 21–49

Foa EB, Rothbaum BO: Treating the Trauma of Rape: Cognitive-Behavioral Therapy for PTSD. New York, Guilford, 1998

Foa EB, Ehlers A, Clark DN, et al: The posttraumatic cognitions inventory (PTCI): Development and validation. Psychol Assess 11:303–314, 1999

Foa EB, Huppert JD, Cahill SP: Emotional processing theory: an update, in Pathological Anxiety: Emotional Processing in Etiology and Treatment. Edited by Rothbaum BO. New York, Guilford, 2006, pp 3–24

Foa EB, Hembree EA, Rothbaum BO: Prolonged Exposure Therapy for PTSD: Emotional Processing of Traumatic Experiences. New York, Oxford University Press, 2007

Foa EB, Keane TM, Friedman MJ, et al (eds): Effective Treatments for PTSD: Practice Guidelines From the International Society for Traumatic Stress Studies. New York, Guilford, 2009a

Foa EB, Keane TM, Friedman MJ, et al: Introduction, in Effective Treatments for PTSD: Practice Guidelines from the International Society for Traumatic Stress Studies. Edited by Foa EB, Keane TM, Friedman MJ, et al. New York, Guilford, 2009b, pp 1–20

Follette VM, Iverson KM, Ford JD: Contextual behavior trauma therapy, in Treating Complex Traumatic Stress Disorders: An Evidence-Based Guide. Edited by Courtois CA, Ford JD. New York, Guilford, 2009, pp 264–285

Fonagy P: Early life trauma and the psychogenesis and prevention of violence. Ann N Y Acad Sci 1036:181–200, 2004

Fonagy P, Bateman A: The development of borderline personality disorder: a mentalizing model. J Pers Disord 22:4–21, 2008

Fonagy P, Luyten P: A developmental, mentalization-based approach to the understanding and treatment of borderline personality disorder. Dev Psychopathol 21:1355–1381, 2009

Fonagy P, Target M: Attachment and reflective function: their role in self-organization. Dev Psychopathol 9:679–700, 1997

Fonagy P, Target M: Bridging the transmission gap: an end to an important mystery of attachment research? Attach Hum Dev 7:333–343, 2005

Fonagy P, Steele H, Steele M: Maternal representations of attachment during pregnancy predict the organization of infant-mother attachment at one year of age. Child Dev 62:891–905, 1991a

Fonagy P, Steele M, Steele H: The capacity for understanding mental states: the reflective self in parent and child and its significance for security of attachment. Infant Ment Health J 12:201–218, 1991b

Fonagy P, Steele M, Steele H, et al: Attachment, the reflective self, and borderline states: the predictive specificity of the Adult Attachment Interview and pathological emotional development, in Attachment Theory: Social, Developmental, and Clinical Perspectives. Edited by Goldberg S, Muir R, Kerr J. New York, Analytic Press, 1995, pp 233–278

Fonagy P, Leigh T, Steele M, et al: The relation of attachment status, psychiatric classification, and response to psychotherapy. J Consult Clin Psychol 64:22–31, 1996

Fonagy P, Gergely G, Jurist EL: Affect Regulation, Mentalization, and the Development of the Self. New York, Other Press, 2002

Fonagy P, Gergely G, Target M: The parent-infant dyad and the construction of the subjective self. J Child Psychol Psychiatry 48:288–328, 2007

Fonagy P, Gergely G, Target M: Psychoanalytic constructs and attachment theory and research, in Handbook of Attachment: Theory, Research, and Clinical Applications, 2nd Edition. Edited by Cassidy J, Shaver PR. New York, Guilford, 2008, pp 783–810

Fonagy P, Bateman A, Luyten P: Introduction and overview, in Handbook of Mentalizing in Mental Health Practice. Edited by Bateman AW, Fonagy P. Washington, DC, American Psychiatric Publishing, 2012, pp 3–42

Ford JD: Dissociation in complex posttraumatic stress disorder or disorders of extreme stress not otherwise specified (DESNOS), in Dissociation and the Dissociative Disorders: DSM-V and Beyond. Edited by Dell PF, O'Neil JA. New York, Routledge, 2009, pp 471–483

Ford JD, Courtois CA: Defining and understanding complex trauma and complex traumatic stress disorders, in Treating Complex Traumatic Stress Disorders: An Evidence-Based Guide. Edited by Courtois CA, Ford JD. New York, Guilford, 2009, pp 13–30

Ford JD, Fallot RD, Harris M: Group therapy, in Treating Complex Traumatic Stress Disorders: An Evidence-Based Guide. Edited by Courtois CA, Ford JD. New York, Guilford, 2009, pp 415–440

Frank JD: Persuasion and Healing. New York, Schocken Books, 1961

Freud S: The Future of an Illusion (1927). Translated by Robson-Scott WD. Revised and edited by Strachey J. Garden City, NY, Doubleday Anchor, 1964

Freyd JJ: Betrayal Trauma: The Logic of Forgetting Childhood Abuse. Cambridge, MA, Harvard University Press, 1996

Friedman MJ: Interrelationships between biological mechanisms and pharmacotherapy of posttraumatic stress disorder, in Posttraumatic Stress Disorder: Etiology, Phenomenology, and Treatment. Edited by Wolf ME, Mosnaim AD. Washington, DC, American Psychiatric Press, 1990, pp 204–225

Friedman MJ, Karam EG: Posttraumatic stress disorder, in Stress-Induced and Fear Circuitry Disorders: Refining the Research Agenda for DSM-V. Edited by Andrews G, Charney DS, Sirovatka PJ, et al. Washington, DC, American Psychiatric Publishing, 2009, pp 3–29

Friedman MJ, Resick PA, Keane TM: Key questions and an agenda for future research, in Handbook of PTSD: Science and Practice. Edited by Friedman MJ, Keane TM, Resick PA. New York, Guilford, 2007, pp 540–561

Friedman MJ, Cohen JA, Foa EB, et al: Integration and summary, in Effective Treatments for PTSD: Practice Guidelines From the International Society for Traumatic Stress Studies. Edited by Foa EB, Keane TM, Friedman MJ, et al. New York, Guilford, 2009, pp 617–642

Fromm E: The Anatomy of Human Destructiveness. New York, Holt, Rinehart, & Winston, 1973

Frueh BC, Grubaugh AL, Cusack KJ, et al: Exposure-based cognitive-behavioral treatment of PTSD in adults with schizophrenia or schizoaffective disorder: a pilot study. J Anxiety Disord 23:665–675, 2009

Frueh BC, Elhai JD, Gold PB, et al: The future of posttraumatic stress disorder in the DSM. Psychol Inj Law 3:260–270, 2010

Gabbard GO: Psychodynamic Psychiatry in Clinical Practice. Washington, DC, American Psychiatric Press, 2000

George C, Solomon J: The caregiving system: a behavioral systems approach to parenting, in Handbook of Attachment: Theory, Research, and Clinical Applications, 2nd Edition. Edited by Cassidy J, Shaver PR. New York, Guilford, 2008, pp 833–856

Geraerts E: Posttraumatic memory, in Clinician's Guide to Posttraumatic Stress Disorder. Edited by Rosen GM, Frueh BC. New York, Wiley, 2010, pp 77–95

Ginzburg K, Butler LD, Saltzman K, et al: Dissociative reactions in PTSD, in Dissociation and the Dissociative Disorders: DSM-V and Beyond. Edited by Dell PF, O'Neil JA. New York, Routledge, 2009, pp 457–469

Glodich A, Allen JG, Fultz J, et al: School-based psychoeducational groups on trauma designed to decrease reenactment, in Handbook of Community-Based Clinical Practice. Edited by Lightburn A, Sessions P. New York, Oxford University Press, 2006, pp 349–363

Gold SD, Marx BP, Soler-Baillo JM, et al: Is life stress more traumatic than traumatic stress? J Anxiety Disord 19:687–698, 2005

Goldberg D: The relationship between generalized anxiety disorder and major depressive episode, in Diagnostic Issues in Depression and Generalized Anxiety Disorder: Refining the Research Agenda for DSM-V. Edited by Goldberg D, Kendler KS, Sirovatka PJ, et al. Washington, DC, American Psychiatric Publishing, 2010, pp 355–361

Granqvist P, Kirkpatrick LA: Attachment and religious representations and behavior, in Handbook of Attachment: Theory, Research, and Clinical Applications, 2nd Edition. Edited by Cassidy J, Shaver PR. New York, Guilford, 2008, pp 906–933

Grey N, Holmes EA: "Hotspots" in trauma memories in the treatment of post-traumatic stress disorder: a replication. Memory 16:788–796, 2008

Grienenberger J, Kelly K, Slade A: Maternal reflective functioning, mother-infant affective communication, and infant attachment: exploring the link between mental states and observed caregiving behaviour in the intergenerational transmission of attachment. Attach Hum Dev 7:299–311, 2005

Griffin MG: A prospective assessment of auditory startle alterations in rape and physical assault survivors. J Trauma Stress 21:91–99, 2008

Groat M, Allen JG: Promoting mentalizing in experiential psychoeducational groups: from agency and authority to authorship. Bull Menninger Clin 75:315–343, 2011

Grossman K, Grossman KE, Kindler H, et al: A wider view of attachment and exploration: the influence of mothers and fathers on the development of psychological security from infancy to young adulthood, in Handbook of Attachment: Theory, Research, and Clinical Applications, 2nd Edition. Edited by Cassidy J, Shaver PR. New York, Guilford, 2008, pp 857–879

Grossman KE, Grossman K, Waters E (eds): Attachment From Infancy to Adulthood: The Major Longitudinal Studies. New York, Guilford, 2005

Grubaugh AL, Magruder KM, Waldrop AE, et al: Subthreshold PTSD in primary care: prevalence, psychiatric disorders, healthcare use, and functional status. J Nerv Ment Dis 193:658–664, 2005

Hadas M: The Stoic Philosophy of Seneca: Essays and Letters. New York, WW Norton, 1958

Hammen C: Stress and depression. Annu Rev Clin Psychol 1:293–319, 2005

Harkness KL, Monroe SM: Childhood adversity and the endogenous versus non-endogenous distinction in women with major depression. Am J Psychiatry 159:387–393, 2002

Harris EC, Barraclough B: Suicide as an outcome for mental disorders: a meta-analysis. Br J Psychiatry 170:205–228, 1997

Hayes SC, Strosahl KD, Wilson KG: Acceptance and Commitment Therapy: An Experiential Approach to Behavior Change. New York, Guilford, 1999

Hazan C, Shaver P: Romantic love conceptualized as an attachment processes. J Pers Soc Psychol 52:511–524, 1987

Hembree EA, Foa EB: Cognitive behavioral treatments for PTSD, in Clinician's Guide to Posttraumatic Stress Disorder. Edited by Rosen GM, Frueh BC. New York, Wiley, 2010, pp 177–203

Herink R (ed): The Psychotherapy Handbook. New York, New American Library, 1980

Herman JL: Father-Daughter Incest. Cambridge, MA, Harvard University Press, 1981

Herman JL: Complex PTSD: a syndrome in survivors of prolonged and repeated trauma. J Trauma Stress 5:377–391, 1992a

Herman JL: Trauma and Recovery. New York, Basic Books, 1992b

Herman JL: Sequelae of prolonged and repeated trauma: evidence for a complex posttraumatic syndrome (DESNOS), in Posttraumatic Stress Disorder: DSM-IV and Beyond. Edited by Davidson JRT, Foa EB. Washington, DC, American Psychiatric Press, 1993, pp 213–228

Herman JL: Foreword, in Treating Complex Traumatic Stress Disorders: An Evidence-Based Guide. Edited by Courtois CA, Ford JD. New York, Guilford, 2009, pp xiii–xvii

Hesse E: The Adult Attachment Interview: protocol, method of analysis, and empirical studies, in Handbook of Attachment: Theory, Research, and Clinical Applications, 2nd Edition. Edited by Cassidy J, Shaver PR. New York, Guilford, 2008, pp 552–598

Hoffmann SG, Sawyer AT, Witt AA, et al: The effect of mindfulness-based therapy on anxiety and depression: a meta-analytic review. J Consult Clin Psychol 78:169–183, 2010

Holmes EA, Brown RJ, Mansell W, et al: Are there two qualitatively distinct forms of dissociation? A review and some clinical implications. Clin Psychol Rev 25:1–23, 2005a

Holmes EA, Grey N, Young KA: Intrusive images and "hotspots" of trauma memories in posttraumatic stress disorder: an exploratory investigation of emotions and cognitive themes. J Behav Ther Exp Psychiatry 36:3–17, 2005b

Holmes J: The Search for the Secure Base: Attachment Theory and Psychotherapy. London, Routledge, 2001

Holmes J: From attachment research to clinical practice: getting it together, in Attachment Theory and Research in Clinical Work With Adults. Edited by Obegi JH, Berant E. New York, Guilford, 2009, pp 490–514

Holmes J: Exploring in Security: Towards an Attachment-Informed Psychoanalytic Psychotherapy. New York, Routledge, 2010

Holmes J: Attachment theory and the suicidal patient, in Building a Therapeutic Alliance With the Suicidal Patient. Edited by Michel K, Jobes DA. Washington, DC, American Psychological Association, 2011, pp 149–167

Horvath AO, Del Re AC, Flükiger C, et al: Alliance in individual psychotherapy, in Psychotherapy Relationships That Work: Evidence-Based Responsiveness. Edited by Norcross JC. New York, Oxford University Press, 2011, pp 25–69

Horwitz L: The capacity to forgive: intrapsychic and developmental perspectives. JAMA 53:485–511, 2005

Horwitz L, Gabbard GO, Allen JG, et al: Borderline Personality Disorder: Tailoring the Therapy to the Patient. Washington, DC, American Psychiatric Press, 1996

Hrdy SB: Mothers and Others: The Evolutionary Origins of Mutual Understanding. Cambridge, MA, Harvard University Press, 2009

Insel TR: Is social attachment an addictive disorder? Physiol Behav 79:351–357, 2003

Insel TR, Cuthbert B, Garvey M, et al: Research Domain Criteria (RDoC): toward a new classification framework for research on mental disorders. Am J Psychiatry 167:748–751, 2010

Jackson C, Nissenson K, Cloitre M: Cognitive-behavioral therapy, in Treating Complex Traumatic Stress Disorders: An Evidence-Based Guide. Edited by Courtois CA, Ford JD. New York, Guilford, 2009, pp 243–263

Jacques-Tiura AJ, Tkatch AJ, Abbey A, et al: Disclosure of sexual assault: characteristics and implications for posttraumatic stress symptoms among African American and Caucasian survivors. J Trauma Dissociation 11:174–192, 2010

James W: The Varieties of Religious Experience (1902). New York, Modern Library, 1994

Jamison KR: Night Falls Fast: Understanding Suicide. New York, Random House, 1999

Janoff-Bulman R: Shattered Assumptions: Towards a New Psychology of Trauma. New York, The Free Press, 1992

Janoff-Bulman R, Yopyk DJ: Random outcomes and valued commitments: existential dilemmas and the paradox of meaning, in Handbook of Experimental Existential Psychology. Edited by Greenberg J, Koole SL, Pyszczynski T. New York, Guilford, 2004, pp 122–138

Jelinek L, Randjbar S, Seifert D, et al: The organization of autobiographical and nonautobiographical memory in posttraumatic stress disorder (PTSD). J Abnorm Psychol 118:288–298, 2009

Jobes DA: Managing Suicidal Risk: A Collaborative Approach. New York, Guilford, 2006

Jobes DA, Nelson KN: Shneidman's contributions to the understanding of suicidal thinking, in Cognition and Suicide: Theory, Research, and Therapy. Edited by Ellis TE. Washington, DC, American Psychological Association, 2006, pp 29–49

Johnson JG, Cohen P, Brown J, et al: Childhood maltreatment increases risk for personality disorders during early adulthood. Arch Gen Psychiatry 56:600–606, 1999

Johnson JG, Cohen P, Chen H, et al: Parenting behaviors associated with risk for offspring personality disorder during adulthood. Arch Gen Psychiatry 63:579–587, 2006

Johnson SM: Couple and family therapy: an attachment perspective, in Handbook of Attachment: Theory, Research, and Clinical Applications, 2nd Edition. Edited by Cassidy J, Shaver PR. New York, Guilford, 2008, pp 811–829

Johnson SM: Attachment theory and emotionally focused therapy for individuals and couples, in Attachment Theory and Research in Clinical Work With Adults. Edited by Obegi JH, Berant E. New York, Guilford, 2009, pp 410–433

Johnson SM, Courtois CA: Couple therapy, in Treating Complex Traumatic Stress Disorders: An Evidence-Based Guide. Edited by Courtois CA, Ford JD. New York, Guilford, 2009, pp 371–390

Joiner TE: Depression in its interpersonal context, in Handbook of Depression. Edited by Gotlib IH, Hammen C. New York, Guilford, 2002, pp 295–313

Joiner TE: Why People Die by Suicide. Cambridge, MA, Harvard University Press, 2005

Joiner TE, Sachs-Ericsson NJ, Wingate LR, et al: Childhood physical and sexual abuse and lifetime number of suicide attempts: a persistent and theoretically important relationship. Behav Res Ther 45:539–547, 2007

Kabat-Zinn J: Full Catastrophe Living: Using the Wisdom of Your Body and Mind to Face Stress, Pain, and Illness. New York, Delta, 1990

Kaplan LJ: Female Perversions: The Temptations of Emma Bovary. New York, Doubleday, 1991

Karen R: Becoming Attached: First Relationships and How They Shape Our Capacity to Love. New York, Oxford University Press, 1998

Kazdin AE: Mediators and mechanisms of change in psychotherapy research. Annu Rev Clin Psychol 3:1–27, 2007

Kazdin AE, Blasé SL: Rebooting psychotherapy research and practice to reduce the burden of mental illness. Perspect Psychol Sci 6:21–37, 2011

Keane TM, Brief DJ, Pratt EM, et al: Assessment of PTSD and its comorbidities in adults, in Handbook of PTSD: Science and Practice. Edited by Friedman MJ, Keane TM, Resick PA. New York, Guilford, 2007, pp 279–305

Kekes J: The Roots of Evil. Ithaca, NY, Cornell University Press, 2005

Kempe CH, Silverman FN, Steele BF, et al: The battered-child syndrome. JAMA 181:105–112, 1962

Kendler KS, Kessler RC, Walters EE, et al: Stressful life events, genetic liability, and onset of an episode of major depression in women. Am J Psychiatry 152:833–842, 1995

Kendler KS, Gardner CO, Prescott CA: Toward a comprehensive developmental model of major depression in women. Am J Psychiatry 159:1133–1145, 2002

Kernberg OF, Diamond D, Yeomans F, et al: Mentalization and attachment in borderline patients in transference focused psychotherapy, in Mind to Mind: Infant Research, Neuroscience, and Psychoanalysis. Edited by Jurist EL, Slade A, Bergner A. New York, Other Press, 2008, pp 167–198

Kessler RC, Sonnega A, Bromet E, et al: Posttraumatic stress disorder in the National Comorbidity Survey. Arch Gen Psychiatry 52:1048–1060, 1995

Kessler RC, Gruber M, Hettema JM, et al: Major depression and generalized anxiety disorder in the National Comorbidity Survey follow-up survey, in Diagnostic Issues in Depression and Generalized Anxiety Disorder: Refining the Research Agenda for DSM-V. Edited by Goldberg D, Kendler KS, Sirovatka PJ, et al. Washington, DC, American Psychiatric Publishing, 2010, pp 139–170

Kimerling R, Ouimette P, Weitlauf JC: Gender issues in PTSD, in Handbook of PTSD: Science and Practice. Edited by Friedman MJ, Keane TM, Resick PA. New York, Guilford, 2007, pp 207–228

Kirkpatrick LA: Attachment, Evolution, and the Psychology of Religion. New York, Guilford, 2005

Kleim S, Kroger C, Kosfelder J: Dialectical behavior therapy for borderline personality disorder: a meta-analysis using mixed-effects modeling. J Consult Clin Psychol 78:936–951, 2010

Kluft RP: Basic principles in conducting the psychotherapy of multiple personality disorder, in Current Perspectives on Multiple Personality Disorder. Edited by Kluft RP, Fine CG. Washington, DC, American Psychiatric Press, 1993, pp 19–50

Koenen KC, Moffitt TE, Poulton R, et al: Early childhood factors associated with the development of post-traumatic stress disorder: results from a longitudinal birth cohort. Psychol Med 37:181–192, 2007

Kolden GG, Klein MH, Wang CC: Congruence/genuineness, in Psychotherapy Relationships That Work: Evidence-Based Responsiveness. Edited by Norcross JC. New York, Oxford University Press, 2011, pp 187–202

Lanius RA, Vermetten E, Loewenstein RJ, et al: Emotion modulation and PTSD: clinical and neurobiological evidence for a dissociative subtype. Am J Psychiatry 167:640–647, 2010

Lebell S: Epictetus: The Art of Living. New York, HarperCollins, 1995

Lee CW, Taylor G, Drummond PD: The active ingredient in EMDR: is it traditional exposure or dual focus of attention? Clin Psychol Psychother 13:97–107, 2006

Leibenluft E, Gardner DL, Cowdry RW: The inner experience of the borderline self-mutilator. J Pers Disord 1:317–324, 1987

Leichsenring F: Applications of psychodynamic psychotherapy to specific disorders: efficacy and indications, in Textbook of Psychotherapeutic Treatments. Edited by Gabbard GO. Washington, DC, American Psychiatric Publishing, 2009, pp 97–132

Levy KN: Psychotherapies and lasting change. Am J Psychiatry 165:556–559, 2008

Levy KN, Meehan KB, Kelly KM, et al: Change in attachment patterns and reflective function in a randomized control trial of transference-focused psychotherapy for borderline personality disorder. J Consult Clin Psychol 74:1027–1040, 2006

Levy KN, Ellison WD, Scott LN, et al: Attachment style, in Psychotherapy Relationships That Work: Evidence-Based Responsiveness. Edited by Norcross JC. New York, Oxford University Press, 2011, pp 377–401

Lewis L, Kelly KA, Allen JG: Restoring Hope and Trust: An Illustrated Guide to Mastering Trauma. Baltimore, MD, Sidran Press, 2004

Linehan MM: Cognitive-Behavioral Treatment of Borderline Personality Disorder. New York, Guilford, 1993a

Linehan MM: Skills Training Manual for Treating Borderline Personality Disorder. New York, Guilford, 1993b

Linehan MM, Armstrong HE, Suarez A, et al: Cognitive-behavioral treatment of chronically parasuicidal borderline patients. Arch Gen Psychiatry 48:1060–1064, 1991

Linehan MM, Comtois KS, Murray AM, et al: Two-year randomized controlled trial and follow-up of dialectical behavior therapy vs therapy by experts for suicidal behaviors and borderline personality disorder. Arch Gen Psychiatry 63:757–766, 2006

Liotti G: Attachment and dissociation, in Dissociation and the Dissociative Disorders: DSM-V and Beyond. Edited by Dell PF, O'Neil JA. New York, Routledge, 2009, pp 53–65

Liotti G: Attachment disorganization and the clinical dialogue: theme and variations, in Disorganized Attachment and Caregiving. Edited by Solomon J, George C. New York, Guilford, 2011, pp 383–413

Littleton HL: The impact of social support and negative disclosure reactions on sexual assault victims: a cross-sectional and longitudinal investigation. J Trauma Dissociation 11:210–227, 2010

Livesley WJ: Confusion and incoherence in the classification of personality disorder: commentary on the preliminary proposals for DSM-5. Psychol Inj Law 3:304–313, 2010

Loftus EF: The reality of repressed memories. Am Psychol 48:518–537, 1993

Lomax JW, Kripal JJ, Pargament KI: Perspectives on "sacred moments" in psychotherapy. Am J Psychiatry 168:1–7, 2011

Long ME, Elhai JD, Schweinle A, et al: Differences in posttraumatic stress disorder diagnostic rates and symptom severity between Criterion A1 and non-Criterion A1 stressors. J Anxiety Disord 22:1255–1263, 2008

Luyten P, van Houdenhove B: Common versus specific factors in the psychotherapeutic treatment of patients suffering from chronic fatigue and pain. J Psychother Integr (in press)

Luyten P, Vliegen N, Blatt SJ: Equifinality, multifinality, and the rediscovery of the importance of early experiences: pathways from early adversity to psychiatric and (functional) somatic disorders. Psychoanal Study Child 63:27–60, 2008

Luyten P, Fonagy P, Lemma A, et al: Depression, in Handbook of Mentalizing in Mental Health Practice. Edited by Bateman AW, Fonagy P. Washington, DC, American Psychiatric Publishing, 2012, pp 385–417

Lynn SJ, Rhue JW: Fantasy proneness: hypnosis, developmental antecedents, and psychopathology. Am Psychol 43:35–44, 1988

Lyons-Ruth K, Jacobvitz D: Attachment disorganization: genetic factors, parenting contexts, and developmental transformation from infancy to adulthood, in Handbook of Attachment: Theory, Research, and Clinical Applications, 2nd Edition. Edited by Cassidy J, Shaver PR. New York, Guilford, 2008, pp 666–697

Lyons-Ruth K, Yellin C, Melnick S, et al: Expanding the concept of unresolved mental states: hostile/helpless states of mind on the Adult Attachment Interview are associated with disrupted mother-infant communication and infant disorganization. Dev Psychopathol 17:1–23, 2005

MacDonald HZ, Beeghly M, Grant-Knight W, et al: Longitudinal association between infant disorganized attachment and childhood posttraumatic stress symptoms. Dev Psychopathol 20:493–508, 2008

Main M, Hesse E: Parents' unresolved traumatic experiences are related to infant disorganized attachment status: is frightened and/or frightening parental behavior the linking mechanism? In Attachment in the Preschool Years: Theory, Research, and Intervention. Edited by Greenberg MT, Cicchetti D, Cummings EM. Chicago, IL, University of Chicago Press, 1990, pp 161–182

Main M, Morgan H: Disorganization and disorientation in infant Strange Situation behavior: phenotypic resemblance to dissociative states, in Handbook of Dissociation: Theoretical, Empirical, and Clinical Perspectives. Edited by Michelson LK. Ray WJ. New York, Plenum, 1996, pp 107–138

Main M, Solomon J: Procedures for identifying infants as disorganized/disoriented during the Ainsworth Strange Situation, in Attachment in the Preschool Years: Theory, Research, and Intervention. Edited by Greenberg MT, Cicchetti D, Cummings EM. Chicago, IL, University of Chicago Press, 1990, pp 121–160

Main M, Kaplan N, Cassidy J: Security in infancy, childhood, and adulthood: a move to the level of representation, in Growing Points of Attachment Theory and Research. Edited by Bretherton I, Waters E. Monographs of the Society for Research in Child Development 50:66–104, 1985

Main M, Hesse E, Kaplan N, et al: Predictability of attachment behavior and representational processes at 1, 6, and 19 years of age, in Attachment From Infancy to Adulthood: The Major Longitudinal Studies. Edited by Grossman KE, Grossman K, Waters E. New York, Guilford, 2005, pp 245–304

Main M, Hesse E, Goldwyn R: Studying differences in language usage in recounting attachment history: an introduction to the AAI, in Clinical Applications of the Adult Attachment Interview. Edited by Steele H, Steele M. New York, Guilford, 2008, pp 31–68

Malik ML, Beutler KE, Alimohamed S, et al: Are all cognitive therapies alike? A comparison of cognitive and noncognitive therapy process and implications for the application of empirically supported treatments. J Consult Clin Psychol 71:150–158, 2003

Mallinckrodt B, McCreary BA, Robertson AK: Co-occurrence of eating disorders and incest: the role of attachment, family environment, and social competencies. J Counsel Psychol 42:178–186, 1995

Mallinckrodt B, Daly K, Wang CDC: An attachment approach to adult psychotherapy, in Attachment Theory and Research in Clinical Work With Adults. Edited by Obegi JH, Berant E. New York, Guilford, 2009, pp 234–268

Marvin R, Cooper G, Hoffman K, et al: The Circle of Security project: attachment-based intervention with caregiver-pre-school child dyads. Attach Hum Dev 4:107–124, 2002

McBride C, Atkinson L: Attachment theory and cognitive-behavioral therapy, in Attachment Theory and Research in Clinical Work With Adults. Edited by Obegi JH, Berant E. New York, Guilford, 2009, pp 434–458

McCauley J, Kern DE, Kolodner K, et al: Clinical characteristics of women with a history of childhood abuse. JAMA 277:1362–1368, 1997

McFarlane AC: Epidemiological evidence about the relationship between PTSD and alcohol abuse: the nature of the association. Addict Behav 23:813–825, 1998

McNally RJ: On eye movements and animal magnetism: a reply to Greenwald's defense of EMDR. J Anxiety Disord 13:617–620, 1999

Meins E, Fernyhough C, Johnson F, et al: Mind-mindedness in children: individual differences in internal-state talk in middle childhood. Br J Dev Psychol 24:181–196, 2006

Melnick S, Finger B, Hans S, et al: Hostile-helpless states of mind in the AAI: a proposed additional AAI category with implications for identifying disorganized infant attachment in high-risk samples, in Clinical Applications of the Adult Attachment Interview. Edited by Steele H, Steele M. New York, Guilford, 2008, pp 399–423

Menninger KA: Man Against Himself. New York, Harcourt, Brace, 1938

Menninger KA: Hope (1959). Bull Menninger Clin 51:447–462, 1987

Michel K, Valach L: The narrative interview with the suicidal patient, in Building a Therapeutic Alliance With the Suicidal Patient. Edited by Michel K, Jobes DA. Washington, DC, American Psychological Association, 2011, pp 63–80

Michelson LK, Ray WJ (eds): Handbook of Dissociation: Theoretical, Empirical, and Clinical Perspectives. New York, Plenum, 1996

Mikulincer M, Shaver PR: Security-based self-representations in adulthood: contents and processes, in Adult Attachment: Theory, Research, and Clinical Implications. Edited by Rholes WS, Simpson JA. New York, Guilford, 2004, pp 159–195

Mikulincer M, Shaver PR: Attachment in Adulthood: Structure, Dynamics, and Change. New York, Guilford, 2007a

Mikulincer M, Shaver PR: Reflections on security dynamics: core constructs, psychological mechanisms, relational contexts, and the need for an integrative theory. Psychol Inq 18:197–209, 2007b

Mikulincer M, Florian V, Hirschberger G: Terror of death and the quest for love: an existential perspective on close relationships, in Handbook of Experimental Existential Psychology. Edited by Greenberg J, Koole SL, Pyszczynski T. New York, Guilford, 2004, pp 287–304

Moffitt TE, Caspi A, Harrington H, et al: Generalized anxiety disorder and depression: childhood risk factors in a birth cohort followed to age 32 years, in Diagnostic Issues in Depression and Generalized Anxiety Disorder: Refining the Research Agenda for DSM-V. Edited by Goldberg D, Kendler KS, Sirovatka PJ, et al. Washington, DC, American Psychiatric Publishing, 2010, pp 217–239

Mohr JJ: Same-sex romantic attachment, in Handbook of Attachment: Theory, Research, and Clinical Applications, 2nd Edition. Edited by Cassidy J, Shaver PR. New York, Guilford, 2008, pp 482–502

Morgan HG, Burns-Cox CJ, Pocock H, et al: Deliberate self-harm: clinical and socioeconomic characteristics of 368 patients. Br J Psychiatry 127:564–574, 1975

Morrison JA: The therapeutic relationship in prolonged exposure therapy for posttraumatic stress disorder: the role of cross-theoretical dialogue in dissemination. Behavior Therapist 34:20–26, 2011

Moss E, Bureau J-F, St-Laurent D, et al: Understanding disorganized attachment at preschool and school age: examining divergent pathways of disorgnaized and controlling children, in Disorganized Attachment and Caregiving. Edited by Solomon J, George C. New York, Guilford, 2011, pp 52–79

Murphy JG: Getting Even: Forgiveness and Its Limits. New York, Oxford University Press, 2003

Nagel T: The View From Nowhere. New York, Oxford University Press, 1985

Nagel T: Secular Philosophy and the Religious Temperament. New York, Oxford University Press, 2010

Najavits LM, Ryngala, Back SE, et al: Treatment of PTSD and comorbid disorders, in Effective Treatments for PTSD: Practice Guidelines From the International Society for Traumatic Stress Studies. Edited by Foa EB, Keane TM, Friedman MJ, et al. New York, Guilford, 2009, pp 508–535

Neff KD: Self-Compassion. New York, HarperCollins, 2011

Neiman S: Evil in Modern Thought: An Alternative History of Philosophy. Princeton, NJ, Princeton University Press, 2002

Newman MG, Stiles WB, Janeck A, et al: Integration of therapeutic factors in anxiety disorders, in Principles of Therapeutic Change That Work. Edited by Castonguay LG, Beutler LE. New York, Oxford University Press, 2006, pp 187–200

Nijenhuis ER, Vanderlinden J, Spinhoven P: Animal defensive reactions as a model for trauma-induced dissociative reactions. J Trauma Stress 11:243–260, 1998

Nock MK (ed): Understanding Nonsuicidal Self-Injury: Origins, Assessment, and Treatment. Washington, DC, American Psychological Association, 2009

Nock MK, Cha CB: Psychological models of nonsuicidal self-injury, in Understanding Nonsuicidal Self-Injury: Origins, Assessment, and Treatment. Edited by Nock MK. Washington, DC, American Psychological Association, 2009, pp 65–77

Nock MK, Favazza AR: Nonsuicidal self-injury: definition and classification, in Understanding Nonsuicidal Self-Injury: Origins, Assessment, and Treatment. Edited by Nock MK. Washington, DC, American Psychological Association, 2009, pp 9–18

Nolen-Hoeksema S: The role of rumination in depressive disorders and mixed anxiety/depressive symptoms. J Abnorm Psychol 109:504–511, 2000

Norcross JC (ed): Psychotherapy Relationships That Work: Evidence-Based Responsiveness. New York, Oxford University Press, 2011

Norcross JC, Lambert MJ: Evidence-based therapy relationships, in Psychotherapy Relationships That Work: Evidence-Based Responsiveness. Edited by Norcross JC. New York, Oxford University Press, 2011, pp 3–21

Norcross JC, Wampold BE: Conclusions and guidelines, in Psychotherapy Relationships That Work: Evidence-Based Responsiveness. Edited by Norcross JC. New York, Oxford University Press, 2011, pp 423–430

Norris F: Epidemiology of trauma: frequency and impact of different potentially traumatic events on different demographic groups. J Consult Clin Psychol 60:409–418, 1992

Nussbaum MC: Upheavals of Thought: The Intelligence of the Emotions. Cambridge, UK, Cambridge University Press, 2001

O'Donnell ML, Creamer M, Cooper J: Criterion A: controversies and clinical implications, in Clinician's Guide to Posttraumatic Stress Disorder. Edited by Rosen GM, Frueh BC. New York, Wiley, 2010, pp 51–75

Obegi JH, Berant E (eds): Attachment Theory and Research in Clinical Work With Adults. New York, Guilford, 2009a

Obegi JH, Berant E: Introduction, in Attachment Theory and Research in Clinical Work With Adults. Edited by Obegi JH, Berant E. New York, Guilford, 2009b, pp 1–14

Oldham JM: Psychodynamic psychotherapy for personality disorders. Am J Psychiatry 164:1465–1467, 2007

Oldham JM: Epilogue, in Mentalizing in Clinical Practice. Edited by Allen JG, Fonagy P, Bateman AW. Washington, DC, American Psychiatric Publishing, 2008, pp 341–346

Oldham JM, Skodol AE, Kellman HD, et al: Diagnosis of DSM-III-R personality disorders by two structured interviews: patterns of comorbidity. Am J Psychiatry 149:213–220, 1992

Orbach I: Therapeutic empathy with the suicidal wish: principles of therapy with suicidal individuals. Am J Psychother 55:166–184, 2001

Orbach I: Taking an inside view: stories of pain, in Building a Therapeutic Alliance With the Suicidal Patient. Edited by Michel K, Jobes DA. Washington, DC, American Psychological Association, 2011, pp 111–128

Ozer EJ, Best SR, Lipsey TL, et al: Predictors of posttraumatic stress disorder and symptoms in adults: a meta-analysis. Psychol Bull 129:52–73, 2003

Pargament KI: Spiritually Integrated Psychotherapy: Understanding and Addressing the Sacred. New York, Guilford, 2007

Pargament KI: Religion and coping: the current state of knowledge, in Oxford Handbook of Stress, Health, and Coping. Edited by Folkman S. New York, Oxford University Press, 2011, pp 269–288

Pennebaker JW: Writing to Heal: A Guided Journal for Recovering From Trauma and Emotional Upheaval. Oakland, CA, New Harbinger, 2004

Peterson C, Chang EC: Optimism and flourishing, in Flourishing: Positive Psychology and the Life Well-Lived. Edited by Keyes CL, Haidt J. Washington, DC, American Psychiatric Publishing, 2003, pp 55–79

Peterson M: The problem of evil, in A Companion to Philosophy of Religion. Edited by Quinn PL, Taliaferro C. Malden, MA, Blackwell, 1997, pp 393–401

Philips B, Kahn U, Bateman AW: Drug addiction, in Handbook of Mentalizing in Mental Health Practice. Edited by Bateman AW, Fonagy P. Washington, DC, American Psychiatric Publishing, 2012, pp 445–461

Pillemer DB: Momentous Events, Vivid Memories. Cambridge, MA, Harvard University Press, 1998

Plante TG: Spiritual Practices in Psychotherapy. Washington, DC, American Psychological Association, 2009

Pope HG Jr, Oliva PS, Hudson JI, et al: Attitudes toward DSM-IV dissociative disorder diagnoses among board-certified American psychiatrists. Am J Psychiatry 156:321–323, 1999

Porges SW: Reciprocal influences between body and brain in the perception and expression of affect, in The Healing Power of Emotion: Affective Neuroscience, Development, and Clinical Practice. Edited by Fosha D, Siegal DJ, Solomon MF. New York, WW Norton, 2009, pp 27–54

Porges SW: The Polyvagal Theory: Neurophysiological Foundations of Emotions, Attachment, Communication, and Self-Regulation. New York, WW Norton, 2011

Powers MB, Halpern JM, Ferenschak MP, et al: A meta-analytic review of prolonged exposure for posttraumatic stress disorder. Clin Psychol Rev 30:635–641, 2010

Prinstein MJ, Guerry JD, Browne CB, et al: Interpersonal models of nonsuicidal self-injury, in Understanding Nonsuicidal Self-Injury: Origins, Assessment, and Treatment. Edited by Nock MK. Washington, DC, American Psychological Association, 2009, pp 79–98

Pruyser PW: Between Belief and Unbelief. New York, Harper & Row, 1974

Pruyser PW: Epilogue, in Changing Views of the Human Condition. Edited by Pruyser PW. Macon, GA, Mercer University Press, 1987a, pp 196–200

Pruyser PW: Maintaining hope in adversity. Bull Menninger Clin 51:463–474, 1987b

Pruyser PW: A transformational understanding of humanity, in Changing Views of the Human Condition. Edited by Pruyser PW. Macon, GA, Mercer University Press, 1987c, pp 1–10

Resick PA, Schnicke MK: Cognitive processing therapy for sexual assault victims. J Consult Clin Psychol 60:748–756, 1992

Resick PA, Monson CM, Rizvi SL: Posttraumatic stress disorder, in Clinical Handbook of Psychological Disorders: A Step-by-Step Treatment Manual, 4th Edition. Edited by Barlow DH. New York, Guilford, 2008, pp 65–122

Resnick HS, Yehuda R, Acierno R: Acute post-rape plasma cortisol, alcohol use, and PTSD symptom profile among recent rape victims. Ann N Y Acad Sci 821:433–436, 1997

Riggs DS, Monson CM, Glynn SM, et al: Couple and family therapy for adults, in Effective Treatments for PTSD: Practice Guidelines From the International Society for Traumatic Stress Studies. Edited by Foa EB, Keane TM, Friedman MJ, et al. New York, Guilford, 2009, pp 458–478

Rizzuto A-M: The Birth of the Living God: A Psychoanalytic Study. Chicago, IL, University of Chicago Press, 1979

Robins CJ, Ivanoff AM, Linehan MM, et al: Dialectical behavior therapy, in Handbook of Personality Disorders: Theory Research, and Treatment. Edited by Livesley WJ. New York, Guilford, 2001, pp 437–459

Rodham K, Hawton K: Epidemiology and phenomenology of nonsuicidal self-injury, in Understanding Nonsuicidal Self-Injury: Origins, Assessment, and Treatment. Edited by Nock MK. Washington, DC, American Psychological Association, 2009, pp 37–62

Roemer L, Orsillo SM: Mindfulness- and Acceptance-Based Behavioral Therapies in Practice. New York, Guilford, 2009

Rogers CR: Client-Centered Therapy: Its Current Practice, Implications, and Theory. Boston, MA, Houghton Mifflin, 1951

Rogers CR: The necessary and sufficient conditions of therapeutic personality change (1957). J Consult Clin Psychol 60:827–832, 1992

Rosen GM, Frueh BC, Lilienfeld SO, et al: Afterword: PTSD's future in the DSM: implications for clinical practice, in Clinician's Guide to Posttraumatic Stress Disorder. Edited by Rosen GM, Frueh BC. New York, Wiley, 2010, pp 263–276

Ross C: Dissociative amnesia and dissociative fugue, in Dissociation and the Dissociative Disorders: DSM-V and Beyond. Edited by Dell PF, O'Neil JA. New York, Routledge, 2009, pp 429–434

Roth A, Fonagy P: What Works for Whom? A Critical Review of Psychotherapy Research, 2nd Edition. New York, Guilford, 2005

Rudd MD: Fluid vulnerability theory: a cognitive approach to understanding the process of acute and chronic suicide risk, in Cognition and Suicide: Theory, Research, and Therapy. Edited by Ellis TE. Washington, DC, American Psychological Association, 2006, pp 355–368

Rudd MD, Brown GK: A cognitive theory of suicide: building hope in treatment and strengthening the therapeutic relationship, in Building a Therapeutic Alliance With the Suicidal Patient. Edited by Michel K, Jobes DA. Washington, DC, American Psychological Association, 2011, pp 169–181

Ruzek JI, Polusny MA, Abeug FR: Assessment and treatment of concurrent post-traumatic stress disorder and substance abuse, in Cognitive-Behavioral Therapies for Trauma. Edited by Follette VM, Ruzek JI, Abueg FR. New York, Guilford, 1998, pp 226–255

Ryff CD, Singer V: Flourishing under fire: resilience as a prototype of challenged thriving, in Flourishing: Positive Psychology and the Life Well-Lived. Edited by Keyes CL, Haidt J. Washington, DC, American Psychiatric Publishing, 2003, pp 15–36

Sadler LS, Slade A, Mayes LC: Minding the Baby: a mentalization-based parenting program, in Handbook of Mentalization-Based Treatment. Edited by Allen JG, Fonagy P. Chichester, UK, Wiley, 2006, pp 271–288

Safran J, Segal ZV: Interpersonal Processes in Cognitive Therapy. New York, Basic Books, 1990

Safran JD, Muran JC, Eubanks-Carte C: Repairing alliance ruptures, in Psychotherapy Relationships That Work: Evidence-Based Responsiveness. Edited by Norcross JC. New York, Oxford University Press, 2011, pp 224–238

Sahdra BK, Shaver PR, Brown KW: A scale to measure nonattachment: a Buddhist complement to Western research on attachment and adaptive functioning. J Pers Assess 92:116–127, 2010

Schjoedt U, Stodkilde-Jorgenson H, Geertz AW, et al: Highly religious participants recruit areas of social cognition in personal prayer. Soc Cogn Affect Neurosci 4:199–207, 2009

Schore AN: Attachment trauma and the developing right brain: origins of pathological dissociation, in Dissociation and the Dissociative Disorders: DSM-V and Beyond. Edited by Dell PF, O'Neil JA. New York, Routledge, 2009, pp 107–141

Segal ZV, Bieling P, Young T, et al: Antidepressant monotherapy vs sequential pharmacotherapy and mindfulness-based cognitive therapy, or placebo, for relapse prophylaxis in recurrent depression. Arch Gen Psychiatry 67:1256–1264, 2010

Segman R, Shalev AY, Gelernter J: Gene-environment interactions: twin studies and gene research in the context of PTSD, in Handbook of PTSD: Science and Practice. Edited by Friedman MJ, Keane TM, Resick PA. New York, Guilford, 2007, pp 190–206

Seidler GH, Wagner FE: Comparing the efficacy of EMDR and trauma-focused cognitive-behavioral therapy in the treatment of PTSD: a meta-analytic study. Psychol Med 36:1515–1522, 2006

Shapiro F: Eye Movement Desensitization and Reprocessing (EMDR): evaluation of controlled PTSD research. J Behav Ther Exp Psychiatry 27:209–218, 1996

Shaver PR, Mikulincer M: Clinical implications of attachment theory. Lecture presented at Creating Connections: International Conference on Attachment, Neuroscience, Mentalization Based Treatment, and Emotionally Focused Therapy, Kaatsheuvel, The Netherlands, April 19–20, 2011

Shaver PR, Lavy S, Saron C, et al: Social foundations of the capacity for mindfulness: an attachment perspective. Psychol Inq 18:264–271, 2007

Shea MT, Stout R, Gunderson J, et al: Short-term diagnostic stability of schizotypal, borderline, avoidant, and obsessive-compulsive personality disorders.
Am J Psychiatry 159:2036–2041, 2002

Shea MT, McDevitt-Murphy M, Ready DJ, et al: Group therapy, in Effective
Treatments for PTSD: Practice Guidelines From the International Society for
Traumatic Stress Studies. Edited by Foa EB, Keane TM, Friedman MJ, et al.
New York, Guilford, 2009, pp 306–326

Sher G: In Praise of Blame. New York, Oxford University Press, 2006

Sher L, Stanley B: Biological models of nonsuicidal self-injury, in Understanding
Nonsuicidal Self-Injury: Origins, Assessment, and Treatment. Edited by
Nock MK. Washington, DC, American Psychological Association, 2009, pp
99–116

Siegel DJ: The Developing Mind: Toward a Neurobiology of Interpersonal Experience. New York, Guilford, 1999

Simeon D: Depersonalization disorder, in Dissociation and the Dissociative Disorders: DSM-V and Beyond. Edited by Dell PF, O'Neil JA. New York, Routledge, 2009, pp 435–444

Skårderud F, Fonagy P: Eating disorders, in Handbook of Mentalizing in Mental
Health Practice. Edited by Bateman AW, Fonagy P. Washington, DC, American Psychiatric Publishing, 2012, pp 347–383

Slade A: Reflective parenting program: theory and development. Psychoanal Inq
26:640–657, 2006

Slade A: The implications of attachment theory and research for adult psycho-
therapy: research and clinical perspectives, in Handbook of Attachment:
Theory, Research, and Clinical Applications, 2nd Edition. Edited by Cassidy
J, Shaver PR. New York, Guilford, 2008a, pp 762–782

Slade A: Mentalization as a frame for working with parents in child psychotherapy, in Mind to Mind: Infant Research, Neuroscience, and Psychoanalysis.
Edited by Jurist EL, Slade A, Bergner A. New York, Other Press, 2008b, pp
307–334

Slade A, Sadler LS, de Dios-Kenn C, et al: Minding the Baby: A Manual. New Haven, CT, Yale Child Study Center, 2004

Slade A, Grienenberger J, Bernbach E, et al: Maternal reflective functioning, attachment, and the transmission gap: a preliminary study. Attach Hum Dev
7:283–298, 2005

Smith TL, Barrett MS, Benjamin LS, et al: Relationship factors in treating personality disorders, in Principles of Therapeutic Change That Work. Edited by
Castonguay LG, Beutler LE. New York, Oxford University Press, 2006, pp
219–238

Snyder CR: The Psychology of Hope. New York, Free Press, 1994

Solomon J, George C: Disorganization of maternal caregiving across two generations:
the origins of caregiving helplessness, in Disorganized Attachment and Caregiving. Edited by Solomon J, George C. New York, Guilford, 2011, pp 25–51

Solomon RC: Spirituality for the Skeptic: The Thoughtful Love of Life. New
York, Oxford University Press, 2002

Somer E: Opioid use disorder and dissociation, in Dissociation and the Dissociative Disorders: DSM-V and Beyond. Edited by Dell PF, O'Neil JA. New York, Routledge, 2009, pp 511–518

Spangler G: Genetic and environmental determinants of attachment disorganization, in Disorganized Attachment and Caregiving. Edited by Solomon J, George C. New York, Guilford, 2011, pp 110–130

Spates CR, Koch E, Pagoto S, et al: Eye movement desensitization and reprocessing, in Effective Treatments for PTSD: Practice Guidelines From the International Society for Traumatic Stress Studies. Edited by Foa EB, Keane TM, Friedman MJ, et al. New York, Guilford, 2009, pp 279–305

Spitzer RL, First MB, Wakefield JC: Saving PTSD from itself in DSM-V. J Anxiety Disord 21:233–241, 2007

Sroufe LA, Waters E: Attachment as an organizational construct. Child Dev 48:1184–1199, 1977

Sroufe LA, Egeland B, Carlson EA, et al: The Development of the Person: The Minnesota Study of Risk and Adaptation From Birth to Adulthood. New York, Guilford, 2005

Steele H, Steele M, Fonagy P: Associations among attachment classifications of mothers, fathers, and their infants. Child Dev 67:541–555, 1996

Steele K, Dorahy MJ, van der Hart O, et al: Dissociation versus alterations in consciousness: related but different concepts, in Dissociation and the Dissociative Disorders: DSM-V and Beyond. Edited by Dell PF, O'Neil JA. New York, Routledge, 2009a, pp 155–169

Steele K, van der Hart O, Nijenhuis ERS: The theory of trauma-related structural dissociation of the personality, in Dissociation and the Dissociative Disorders: DSM-V and Beyond. Edited by Dell PF, O'Neil JA. New York, Routledge, 2009b, pp 239–258

Steinberg M: Interviewer's Guide to the Structured Clinical Interview for DSM-IV Dissociative Disorders (SCID-D). Washington, DC, American Psychiatric Press, 1993

Stewart SH, Pihl RO, Conrod PJ, et al: Functional associations among trauma, PTSD, and substance-related disorders. Addict Behav 23:797–812, 1998

Stiles WB, Wolfe BE: Relationship factors in treating anxiety disorders, in Principles of Therapeutic Change That Work. Edited by Castonguay LG, Beutler LE. New York, Oxford University Press, 2006, pp 155–165

Stovall-McClough KC, Cloitre M, McClough JL: Adult attachment and posttraumatic stress disorder in women with histories of childhood abuse, in Clinical Applications of the Adult Attachment Interview. Edited by Steele H, Steele M. New York, Guilford, 2008, pp 320–340

Strathearn L: Maternal neglect: oxytocin, dopamine and the neurobiology of attachment. J Neuroendocrinol 23:1054–1065, 2011

Swanton C: Virtue Ethics: A Pluralistic View. New York, Oxford, 2003

Swift JK, Callahan JL, Vollmer BM: Preferences, in Psychotherapy Relationships That Work: Evidence-Based Responsiveness. Edited by Norcross JC. New York, Oxford University Press, 2011, pp 301–315

Swirsky D, Mitchell V: The binge-purge cycle as a means of dissociation: somatic trauma and somatic defense in sexual abuse and bulimia. Dissociation 9:18–27, 1996

Taliaferro C: Contemporary Philosophy of Religion. Malden, MA, Blackwell, 1998

Tangney JP, Mashek DJ: In search of the moral person: do you have to feel really bad to be good? In Handbook of Experimental Existential Psychology. Edited by Greenberg J, Koole SL, Pyszczynski T. New York, Guilford, 2004, pp 156–166

Taylor C: Varieties of Religion Today: William James Revisited. Cambridge, MA, Harvard University Press, 2002

Taylor C: A Secular Age. Cambridge, MA, Harvard University Press, 2007

Tellegen A, Atkinson G: Openness to absorbing and self-altering experiences ("absorption"), a trait related to hypnotic susceptibility. J Abnorm Psychol 83:268–277, 1974

Terr L: Unchained Memories: True Stories of Traumatic Memories, Lost and Found. New York, Basic Books, 1994

Thompson R: Early attachment and later relationships: familiar questions, new answers, in Handbook of Attachment: Theory, Research, and Clinical Applications, 2nd Edition. Edited by Cassidy J, Shaver PR. New York, Guilford, 2008, pp 348–365

Tomasello M: Why We Cooperate. Cambridge, MA, MIT Press, 2009

Toth SL, Rogosch FA, Cicchetti D: Attachment-theory-informed intervention and reflective functioning in depressed mothers, in Clinical Applications of the Adult Attachment Interview. Edited by Steele H, Steele M. New York, Guilford, 2008, pp 154–172

Ullman SE, Foynes MM, Tang SS: Benefits and barriers to disclosing sexual trauma: a contextual approach. J Trauma Dissociation 11:127–133, 2010

van der Hart O, Dorahy M: History of the concept of dissociation, in Dissociation and the Dissociative Disorders: DSM-V and Beyond. Edited by Dell PF, O'Neil JA. New York, Routledge, 2009, pp 3–26

van der Kolk BA: The separation cry and the trauma response: developmental issues in the psychobiology of attachment and separation, in Psychological Trauma. Edited by van der Kolk BA. Washington, DC, American Psychiatric Press, 1986, pp 31–62

van der Kolk BA: The body keeps the score: memory and the evolving psychobiology of posttraumatic stress. Harv Rev Psychiatry 1:253–265, 1994

van der Kolk BA, d'Andrea W: Towards a developmental trauma disorder diagnosis for childhood interpersonal trauma, in The Impact of Early Life Trauma on Health and Disease: The Hidden Epidemic. Edited by Lanius RA, Vermetten E, Pain C. New York, Cambridge University Press, 2010, pp 57–68

van IJzendoorn MH, Bakermans-Kranenburg MJ: The distribution of adult attachment representations in clinical groups: a meta-analytic search for patterns of attachment in 105 AAI studies, in Clinical Applications of the Adult Attachment Interview. Edited by Steele H, Steele M. New York, Guilford, 2008, pp 69–96 van IJzendoorn MH, Schuengel C, Bakermans-Kranenburg MJ: Disorganized attachment in early childhood: meta-analysis of precursors, concomitants, and sequelae. Dev Psychopathol 11:225–249, 1999

Vaughn BE, Bost KK, van IJzendoom MH: Attachment and temperament: additive and interactive influences on behavior, affect, and cognition during infancy and childhood, in Handbook of Attachment: Theory, Research, and Clinical Applications, 2nd Edition. Edited by Cassidy J, Shaver PR. New York, Guilford, 2008, pp 192–216

Vermote R, Lowyck B, Luyten P, et al: Process and outcome in psychodynamic hospitalization-based treatment for patients with a personality disorder. J Nerv Ment Dis 198:110–115, 2010

Vermote R, Lowyck B, Luyten P, et al: Patterns of inner change and their relation with patient characteristics and outcome in a psychoanalytic hospitalization-based treatment for personality disordered patients. Clin Psychol Psychother 18:303–313, 2011

Vermote R, Lowyck B, Vandeneede B, et al: Psychodynamically oriented therapeutic settings, in Handbook of Mentalizing in Mental Health Practice. Edited by Bateman AW, Fonagy P. Washington, DC, American Psychiatric Publishing, 2012, pp 247–269

Vogt DS, King DW, King LA: Risk pathways for PTSD: making sense of the literature, in Handbook of PTSD: Science and Practice. Edited by Friedman MJ, Keane TM, Resick PA. New York, Guilford, 2007, pp 99–115

Wachtel PL: Relational Theory and the Practice of Psychotherapy. New York, Guilford, 2008

Waelde LC, Silvern L, Carlson E, et al: Dissociation in PTSD, in Dissociation and the Dissociative Disorders: DSM-V and Beyond. Edited by Dell PF, O'Neil JA. New York, Routledge, 2009, pp 447–456

Walker LE: The Battered Woman. New York, Harper & Row, 1979

Watson D: Differentiating the mood and anxiety disorders: a quadripartite model. Annu Rev Clin Psychol 5:221–247, 2009

Weiner H: Perturbing the Organism: The Biology of Stressful Experience. Chicago, IL, University of Chicago Press, 1992

Weinfield NS, Sroufe LA, Egeland B, et al: Individual differences in infant-caregiver attachment: conceptual and empirical aspects of security, in Handbook of Attachment: Theory, Research, and Clinical Applications, 2nd Edition. Edited by Cassidy J, Shaver PR. New York, Guilford, 2008, pp 78–101

Weingarten K: Reasonable hope: construct, clinical applications, and supports. Fam Process 49:5–25, 2010

Welch SS, Rothbaum BO: Emerging treatments for PTSD, in Handbook of PTSD: Science and Practice. Edited by Friedman MJ, Keane TM, Resick PA. New York, Guilford, 2007, pp 469–496

Wenzel A, Beck AT: A cognitive model of suicidal behavior: theory and treatment. Appl Prev Psychol 12:189–201, 2008

Wenzel A, Brown GK, Beck AT: Cognitive Therapy for Suicidal Patients: Scientific and Clinical Applications. Washington, DC, American Psychological Association, 2009

Whitlock J, Purington A, Gershkovich M: Media, the Internet, and nonsuicidal self-injury, in Understanding Nonsuicidal Self-Injury: Origins, Assessment, and Treatment. Edited by Nock MK. Washington, DC, American Psychological Association, 2009, pp 139–155

Wilson SA, Becker LA, Tinker RH: Eye Movement Desensitization and Reprocessing (EMDR) treatment for psychologically traumatized individuals. J Consult Clin Psychol 63:928–937, 1995

Wilson SA, Becker LA, Tinker RH: Fifteen-month follow-up of Eye Movement Desensitization and Reprocessing (EMDR) treatment for posttraumatic stress disorder and psychological trauma. J Consult Clin Psychol 65:1047–1056, 1997

Wilson SC, Barber TX: The fantasy-prone personality: implications for understanding imagery, hypnosis, and parapsychological phenomena, in Imagery: Current Theory, Research, and Application. Edited by Sheikh AA. New York, Wiley, 1983, pp 340–387

Worthington EL Jr, Hook JN, Davis DE, et al: Religion and spirituality, in Psychotherapy Relationships That Work: Evidence-Based Responsiveness. Edited by Norcross JC. New York, Oxford University Press, 2011, pp 402–419

Yalom ID: The Theory and Practice of Group Psychotherapy. New York, Basic Books, 1970

Yates TM: Developmental pathways from child maltreatment to nonsuicidal self-injury, in Understanding Nonsuicidal Self-Injury: Origins, Assessment, and Treatment. Edited by Nock MK. Washington, DC, American Psychological Association, 2009, pp 117–137

Yudofsky SC: Fatal Flaws: Navigating Destructive Relationships With People With Disorders of Personality and Character. Washington, DC, American Psychiatric Publishing, 2005

Zanarini MC, Williams AA, Lewis RE, et al: Reported pathological childhood experiences associated with the development of borderline personality disorder. Am J Psychiatry 154:1101–1106, 1997

Zanetti CA, Powell B, Cooper G, et al: The Circle of Security intervention: using the therapeutic relationship to ameliorate attachment security in disorganized dyads, in Disorganized Attachment and Caregiving. Edited by Solomon J, George C. New York, Guilford, 2011, pp 318–342

Zeifman D, Hazan C: Pair bonds as attachments: reevaluating the evidence, in Handbook of Attachment: Theory, Research, and Clinical Applications, 2nd Edition. Edited by Cassidy J, Shaver PR. New York, Guilford, 2008, pp 436–455

Index

Page numbers printed in **boldface** *type refer to tables or figures.*